Endocrine Physiology II

Publisher's Note

The *International Review of Physiology* remains a major force in the education of established scientists and advanced students of physiology throughout the world. It continues to present accurate, timely, and thorough reviews of key topics by distinguished authors charged with the responsibility of selecting and critically analyzing new facts and concepts important to the progress of physiology from the mass of information in their respective fields.

Following the successful format established by the earlier volumes in this series, new volumes of the *International Review of Physiology* will concentrate on current developments in neurophysiology and cardiovascular, respiratory, gastrointestinal, liver, endocrine, kidney and urinary tract, environmental, and reproductive physiology. New volumes on a given subject generally appear at two-year intervals, or according to the demand created by new developments in the field. The scope of the series is flexible, however, so that future volumes may cover areas not included earlier.

University Park Press is honored to continue publication of the *International Review of Physiology* under its sole sponsorship beginning with Volume 9. The following is a list of volumes published and currently in preparation for the series:

Volume 1: **CARDIOVASCULAR PHYSIOLOGY**
(A. C. Guyton and C. E. Jones)
Volume 2: **RESPIRATORY PHYSIOLOGY** (J. G. Widdicombe)
Volume 3: **NEUROPHYSIOLOGY** (C. C. Hunt)
Volume 4: **GASTROINTESTINAL PHYSIOLOGY**
(E. D. Jacobson and L. L. Shanbour)
Volume 5: **ENDOCRINE PHYSIOLOGY** (S. M. McCann)
Volume 6: **KIDNEY AND URINARY TRACT PHYSIOLOGY** (K. Thurau)
Volume 7: **ENVIRONMENTAL PHYSIOLOGY** (D. Robertshaw)
Volume 8: **REPRODUCTIVE PHYSIOLOGY** (R. O. Greep)
Volume 9: **CARDIOVASCULAR PHYSIOLOGY II**
(A. C. Guyton and A. W. Cowley, Jr.)
Volume 10: **NEUROPHYSIOLOGY II** (R. Porter)
Volume 11: **KIDNEY AND URINARY TRACT PHYSIOLOGY II** (K. Thurau)
Volume 12: **GASTROINTESTINAL PHYSIOLOGY II** (R. K. Crane)
Volume 13: **REPRODUCTIVE PHYSIOLOGY II** (R. O. Greep)
Volume 14: **RESPIRATORY PHYSIOLOGY II** (J. G. Widdicombe)
Volume 15: **ENVIRONMENTAL PHYSIOLOGY II** (D. Robertshaw)
Volume 16: **ENDOCRINE PHYSIOLOGY II** (S. M. McCann)

Consultant Editor: Arthur C. Guyton, M.D., Department of Physiology and Biophysics, University of Mississippi Medical Center

INTERNATIONAL
REVIEW OF PHYSIOLOGY

Volume 16

Endocrine
Physiology II

Edited by

S. M. McCann, M.D.

Professor and Chairman
Department of Physiology
The University of Texas
Health Science Center at Dallas

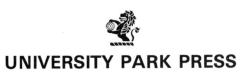

UNIVERSITY PARK PRESS
Baltimore · London · Tokyo

UNIVERSITY PARK PRESS
International Publishers in Science and Medicine
233 East Redwood Street
Baltimore, Maryland 21202

Typeset by The Composing Room of Michigan, Inc.
Manufactured in the United States of America by Universal Lithographers, Inc.,
and The Optic Bindery Incorporated

Library of Congress Cataloging in Publication Data

Main entry under title:

Endocrine physiology II.

   (International review of physiology ; v. 16)
   Edition for 1974 by S. M. McCann and published
   under title: Endocrine physiology.
   Includes index.
   1. Endocrinology. I. McCann, Samuel McDonald,
1925—   II. McCann, Samuel McDonald, 1925—
Endocrine physiology. III. Series. [DNLM:
1. Endocrine glands—Physiology. 2. Hormones—
Physiology. W1 IN834F v. 16 / WK102 E553]
QP1.P62 vol. 16 [QP187]   599'.01'08s
ISBN 0-8391-1064-2 [599'.01'42]   77-11727

Consultant Editor's Note

In 1974 the first series of the *International Review of Physiology* appeared. This new review was launched in response to unfulfilled needs in the field of physiological science, most importantly the need for an in-depth review written especially for teachers and students of physiology throughout the world. It was not without trepidation that this publishing venture was begun, but its early success seems to ensure its future. Therefore, we need to repeat here the philosophy, the goals, and the concept of the *International Review of Physiology.*

The *International Review of Physiology* has the same goals as all other reviews for accuracy, timeliness, and completeness, but it also has policies that we hope and believe engender still other important qualities often missing in reviews, the qualities of critical evaluation, integration, and instructiveness. To achieve these goals, the format allows publication of approximately 2,500 pages per series, divided into eight subspecialty volumes, each organized by experts in their respective fields. This extensiveness of coverage allows consideration of each subject in great depth. And, to make the review as timely as possible, a new series of all eight volumes is published approximately every two years, giving a cycle time that will keep the articles current.

Yet, perhaps the greatest hope that this new review will achieve its goals lies in its editorial policies. A simple but firm request is made to each author that he utilize his expertise and his judgment to sift from the mass of biennial publications those new facts and concepts that are important to the progress of physiology; that he make a conscious effort not to write a review consisting of an annotated list of references; and that the important material that he does choose be presented in thoughtful and logical exposition, complete enough to convey full understanding, as well as woven into context with previously established physiological principles. Hopefully, these processes will continue to bring to the reader each two years a treatise that he will use not merely as a reference in his own personal field but also as an exercise in refreshing and modernizing his whole store of physiological knowledge.

A. C. Guyton

Contents

Preface

In *Endocrine Physiology I*, published in 1974, we presented comprehensive reviews of nearly all aspects of endocrine physiology, together with sufficient background information to make the review understandable to readers new to the subject. Latest research was also discussed, so that the reviews would be useful to the specialist in the field as well. In this second volume we have continued along the same line, and have covered those areas of endocrinology that have made the most rapid advances in the time since the publication of the initial review. For example, the hypothalamic releasing and inhibiting hormones have continued to be one of the most active areas in endocrinology; consequently, a chapter on this topic is included. Important new information has come to light in the area of neurohypophysis and this subject has also been reviewed. The pituitary–target gland interrelationships are considered in a chapter on the pituitary adrenal system. The role of hormones in the control of electrolyte metabolism is considered by evaluating their place in control of sodium excretion. The advances in our understanding of hormone control of mineral metabolism are also discussed. An extensive review of the role of glucagon in the control of carbohydrate metabolism is presented because of the dramatic advances that have been made in this area. Finally, the mechanism of hormone action through the cyclic nucleotides is considered. (Because of a lack of space, certain areas, such as the pineal, growth hormone, and pituitary thyroid interrelationships, have not been covered in this volume, but they will be reviewed in *Endocrine Physiology III*.) We wish to thank the authors for presenting up-to-date and critical reviews of the subjects considered.

S. M. McCann

Endocrine Physiology II

International Review of Physiology
Endocrine Physiology II, Volume 16
Edited by S. M. McCann
Copyright 1977   University Park Press   Baltimore

1
The Neurohypophysis

B. A. CROSS and J. B. WAKERLEY

A. R. C. Institute of Animal Physiology, Babraham, Cambridge, England

The foundations for current investigations of the neurohypophysis and its neural control were laid near the start of this century when the vasopressor, oxytocic, milk-ejecting, and antidiuretic properties of neurohypophysial extracts were discovered (1–4) and subsequently shown to be caused by just two active principles (5). The true morphological relationship between the neurohypophysis and the neurons of the paraventricular (PV) and supraoptic (SO) nuclei

1

emerged when histological methods were developed for visualizing neurosecretory material in the hypothalamo-neurohypophysial system (6). The PV and SO cells were then recognized as neurons with a neurosecretory function (7). Later, their secretory products, vasopressin and oxytocin, were characterized and synthesized (8, 9).

Two factors have contributed to the rapid advances achieved over the last few years: 1) the anatomically and functionally well defined nature of the hypothalamo-neurohypophysial system and 2) the development of powerful new investigative techniques. Every stage of the neurosecretory process has been the subject of careful scrutiny by these new methods. Quantitative electron microscopic techniques (10, 11) yield detailed information about the subcellular organization of neurosecretory cells. In vivo application of radioactive precursors, with subsequent extraction and measurement of labeled products (12, 13) or their localization by autoradiography (14, 15), throws light on the elaboration, intracellular movement, and storage of neurosecretory granules; similar methods can be used to study the secretory activity of neurosecretory cells cultured in vitro (16). Intracellular (17) and extracellular (18–22) recording techniques, combined with microiontophoresis (23, 24), reveal the neuronal properties of PV and SO cells. Studies with isolated neurohypophyses in solutions containing radioactive tracers (25) or membrane-active substances (26, 27), for example, elucidate the events leading to the exocytotic discharge of neurosecretory granules. Exocytosis may be viewed by electron microscopy of normal (28) and freeze-etched material (29, 30). Antibodies to the oxytocin or the vasopressin carrier proteins (neurophysins), combined with immunofluorescent (31–33) or immunoperoxidase (34) histochemistry, permit the identification of neurosecretory products in tissue sections. Quantitative determinations of the hormones in blood (35–37) and cerebrospinal fluid (CSF) (38) can be made by radioimmunoassay. Finally, the discovery of a strain of rats with an inherited inability to secrete vasopressin (Brattleboro strain) is being extensively exploited (39).

In the review which follows, the recent work on the physiology of the neurohypophysis is described from a particular standpoint. Our working hypothesis is that the hypothalamo-neurohypophysial system consists of two distinct populations of oxytocin- and vasopressin-releasing cells. Other postulated neurohypophysial hormones, e.g., coherin (40), for which no convincing evidence exists, are not discussed. Nor is much attention paid to the mode of action and metabolism of neurohypophysial hormones. To fill in these and other gaps, the reader is referred to previous reviews (41–43).

SUBCELLULAR ORGANIZATION AND NEUROSECRETORY MECHANISMS

Ultrastructure of Neurosecretory Cells

The structure of PV and SO neurons reflects their secretory function. The perikarya of the cells are larger (30–40 μm) than surrounding nonsecretory neurons of the hypothalamus (>10 μm) but have fewer dendrites (44). The cells contain an extensive endoplasmic reticulum (with varying degrees of dilatation), a distinctive perinuclear Golgi region, a large nucleus, dense lysosomal bodies, and, most significantly, membrane-bound neurosecretory granules (0.1–0.3 μm in diameter) (45–47). Under the usual conditions of fixation, the latter have a dense cored appearance (48) and contain neurosecretory material (49–51). The unmyelinated axon of the neurosecretory cells which usually emerges from the dorsal pole of the perikaryon has the appearance of a thick dendrite, rather than of a typical axon hillock, and is unbranched (44). At intervals there are dilatations in which neurosecretory granules, mitochondria, and microtubules are common (52, 53). On entering the neurohypophysis, the axons make numerous expanded contacts with the basement membrane of fenestrated capillaries. These terminal dilatations, which number 2,000–6,000 per cell (54), contain many neurosecretory granules, mitochondria, and microvesicles. There are also nonterminal dilatations (600–4,000 per cell) containing large numbers of granules, but no microvesicles (54).

The subcellular organelles in neurosecretory cells undergo pronounced morphological changes in response to an increased demand for hormone secretion. Stimulating secretion of vasopressin in rats by osmotic stress results in a 25% increase in cytoplasmic area (11, 55), with widening of the endoplasmic reticulum and extension of the perinuclear Golgi apparatus (19, 11). Ultrastructural changes induced by dehydration may commence very early; Hatton and Walters (56) observed an increase in the number of rat SO cells containing multiple nucleoli after only 2 hr of water deprivation. Regression of the ultrastructural response which is associated with increased lysosomal activity occurs within about 2 days (11). The regulatory mechanisms governing the subcellular changes during hypersecretion are unknown, although it has been suggested (56) that SO cells may release a tropic substance from their endings which acts as a feedback signal to the cell body.

Because of their obvious relation to neurosecretion, much attention has been paid to changes in the number, size, and appearance of neurosecretory granules in the hypothalamo-neurohypophysial system. These have been studied during water deprivation (10, 52), hemorrhage (57), saline treatment (11, 53), gestation (10), suckling (58), and in hereditary diabetes insipidus (59). The most consistent feature is a loss of granules, and this has been shown to correlate with a fall in the hormone content of the hypothalamo-neurohypophysial system (48). Conversely, an experimentally induced increase of granule numbers is associated with an elevated hormone content (60).

It has been thought that depletion of neurohypophysial hormone causes an abundance of "empty" granules (electron translucent) in the neurosecretory terminals (57, 61). Recent work by Morris and Cannata (48), however, showed that "filled" or "empty" vesicles can be produced at will by controlling pH of the fixation medium, and their appearance has nothing to do with physiological release of hormone.

Neurosecretory granules grow larger as they descend the hypothalamo-neurohypophysial system (46). An accelerated turnover of material might, therefore, be expected to reduce the size of the neurosecretory granules within the neurohypophysis. Krisch (10) recently observed that dehydration for 10 days reduced the mean diameter of neurosecretory granules within the terminals from 140 to 110 mm. Under these conditions, presumably, the period from the manufacture to the release of the granule is shortened.

Although no special function has yet been demonstrated for them, it should be mentioned that pituicytes may undergo marked ultrastructural changes with increased demand for neurohypophysial hormone secretion (62).

Mechanisms for Hormone Synthesis

It is now well established that oxytocin and vasopressin are synthesized in the perikarya of the PV and SO cells and transported down their axons to the neurohypophysis for storage and release. The hormones are stored in granules in association with carrier proteins—neurophysin I for oxytocin and neurophysin II for vasopressin (12, 50, 54).

Initial hormone synthesis probably involves a ribosomal step because vaso-pressin production can be inhibited by puromycin, both in vivo (63) and in vitro (64). Also, in organ-cultured hypothalamo-neurohypophysial systems, the ability to synthesize vasopressin develops in parallel with a rise in RNA levels (16) and may be inhibited by bromotubercidin, an inhibitor of RNA synthesis (64). It has been suggested that although hormone synthesis starts on ribosomes attached to the rough endoplasmic reticulum, active hormone is not formed until a later stage, perhaps at the site of the Golgi region where packaging into granules occurs (63, 64). The final synthetic step may involve cleavage of a large precursor molecule (54).

Present evidence suggests that the neurophysins I and II are synthesized in parallel with oxytocin and vasopressin. Incorporation of labeled substrate into neurophysin follows the same time course as incorporation into vasopressin and labeled vasopressin, and neurophysin appears simultaneously in the various subcellular fractions (65). The arrival of labeled oxytocin and vasopressin in the neurohypophysis exactly parallels that of labeled neurophysin, and a 1:1 molar ratio of neurophysin to hormone is always maintained (12). The condition of hereditary diabetes insipidus is associated with the absence of both vasopressin and its specific neurophysin (39).

Final completion of hormone synthesis probably occurs as the neurosecre-tory granule is transported toward the neurohypophysis. After maturation the neurosecretory granules change their fixation properties; at a pH of 8.0, many more granules preserve their dense core in the perikarya of SO cells than in their neurosecretory terminals (66). Oxytocin to vasopressin ratio is lower in the hypothalamus than in the neurohypophysis (67). After damming back of neuro-secretory granules by hypophysectomy, the oxytocin to vasopressin ratio in the hypothalamus increases (68).

Transport of neurosecretory granules down the hypothalamo-neurohypo-physial stalk is extraordinarily fast (1–4 mm/hr) compared to the rate of axoplasmic flow (1 mm/day) (12). There may also be a slow (0.5 mm/day) transport mechanism (13). Transport rates go up with a greater demand for hormone secretion (69). Two mechanisms of transport may be considered. One is that the neurosecretory axon displays peristaltic movements so that axonal swellings, containing large numbers of granules, move toward the neurohypo-physis. Convincing morphological evidence for such a dynamic mechanism may prove difficult to obtain. A more plausible hypothesis is that microtubules are involved. The main evidence for this comprises observations that colchicine treatment (which causes disruption of microtubules) leads to a damming up of neurosecretory granules (64). Also, there is a correlation between microtubular number and transport activity (70).

In common with most peptide-secreting endocrine cells, the neurosecretory cells of the PV and SO nuclei store vast quantities of hormone in relation to the daily requirements for release. The neurohypophysis of the rat may contain some 500–600 mU of oxytocin and vasopressin, whereas less than 50 mU are released daily (12). The structural basis for this prodigious store is the terminal and preterminal dilatations of the neurosecretory axons, which contain large numbers of granules (53, 54, 57, 58). Recent autoradiographic work (15) has emphasized the dynamic nature of the storage mechanisms. Granules first appear at the terminal dilatations, but if they are not released they later move in an antidromic direction to preterminal dilatations. A maximal demand for hormone may then cause the old granules to be transported to the terminals again. The newest granules, within terminal dilatations, might constitute the so-called "readily releasable pool" of hormone (63). However, the whole concept of a readily releasable pool has been recently questioned by Nordmann (71), who suggests that the fall-off in hormone output during severe stimulation may have little to do with the nonavailability of hormone, but rather with an inactivation of calcium channels within the terminal membrane.

What happens to old granules which are not released? Their most likely fate is to be broken down by lysosomal activity (54); we may suppose the products are transported in a retrograde direction to the perikaryon for reincorporation into new hormone.

Mechanisms for Hormone Release

In order to reach the blood, the oxytocin or vasopressin within the neurosecre-tory granule has to overcome several barriers: 1) the membrane of the granule, 2) the membrane of the nerve terminal, and 3) the basement membrane of the fenestrated endothelium of the neurohypophysial capillaries. The latter is thought to be by simple diffusion. Only the first two barriers are traversed by an active process.

One hypothesis on the mechanism of hormone discharge, reviewed by Douglas (72), was that molecular dispersion occurs within the granule, followed by release of the hormone into the cytoplasm and diffusion out of the terminal. The appearance of empty granules in the neurohypophysis was adduced as supporting evidence, but, as has been seen, this is now known to be an artifact of fixation (48). Furthermore, the release of neurophysin in association with hormone (35, 36) argues against the diffusion theory, because neurophysin is a very large molecule to move through the terminal membrane. Cytoplasmic enzymes, for example, do not traverse it (73). According to another hypothesis, the microvesicles of the neurosecretory terminals were supposed to contain acetylcholine, which was somehow involved in release. However, Lederis and Livingstone (74) showed that the microvesicle fraction of neurohypophysial homogenates contained little acetylcholine activity.

Undoubtedly the most convincing hypothesis is that hormone release occurs by simple fusion of the neurosecretory granule membrane with the axon membrane—a process of exocytosis (72, 75). The sequence of events involved may now be described in detail. The first event is depolarization of the axon terminal membrane. Hormone release from neurohypophyses in vitro may be triggered by electrical stimulation (76, 77), even after action potential activity is blocked by tetrodotoxin (TDX) or a reduced extracellular sodium concentration (78). Depolarization of the terminal by increasing extracellular potassium is a powerful procedure for releasing hormone (79). The next important event is the movement of calcium into the neurosecretory terminal. Neurohypophyses in a calcium-free medium show diminished hormone release (79, 80), and the application of ionophores (which form membrane channels for calcium movement) greatly increases hormone output (26, 81). Pharmacological blockade of calcium uptake prevents hormone release (27). The action of calcium once inside the neurosecretory terminal is unknown. Calcium might form ionic bridges between the negatively charged granule membrane and the negatively charged intracellular side of the axon membrane (82). Fusion of these membranes is facilitated by their similarity of structure (75). Fusion results in the discharge of all the granular contents, which explains the release of neurophysin as well as hormone (35, 36).

All the above events are accomplished extremely rapidly, and it is not surprising that good ultrastructural evidence for exocytosis has only recently been obtained (28–30, 83).

A problem which had to be overcome before the exocytosis theory could be finally accepted was the fate of the neurosecretory granule membrane, for without some means of recapture there would be an unacceptable expansion of the neurosecretory cell. Elegant studies with horseradish peroxidase (84) or tritiated water (25) have demonstrated the occurrence of pinocytosis, whereby membrane is recaptured as small vesicles. The proliferation of microvesicles in terminal neurosecretory endings has been recognized for many years (61).

Under physiological conditions, exocytosis is triggered by action potentials arriving at the neurosecretory terminal. Electrical stimulation of the neurohypophysial stalk in vivo releases hormone (85, 86), but not if impulse traffic is blocked below the site of stimulation by reversible heat blockade (87). For both oxytocin (86, 88) and vasopressin (21, 22) cells, there is good evidence that hormone discharge is correlated with an increased frequency of firing. Lincoln (89), using information on the activity of oxytocin cells during milk ejection in the lactating rat (86, 88), has calculated that during activation of the neurosecretory cell each spike releases some 50 granules of oxytocin. Under resting conditions, the amount of hormone released per action potential is 100-fold less, suggesting a phenomenon of facilitation, as in nonendocrine neurons. This explains the need for a high stimulation frequency for oxytocin release (85, 86). A complicating factor, at least under experimental conditions, is that anesthetics can also influence the rate of hormone release from the neurohypophysis (90).

CHARACTERIZATION OF
SEPARATE OXYTOCIN AND VASOPRESSIN CELLS

Evidence for Two Cell Types

Suckling or milking causes a preferential release of oxytocin, as shown by direct measurement of plasma hormones (91), by radioimmunoassay of the plasma concentrations of neurophysin I and II (92), and by simultaneous monitoring of milk ejection and urine flow rates (93). Conversely, hemorrhage (94) or carotid occlusion (21, 95) may favor the release of vasopressin, and hemorrhage results in a specific release of neurophysin II (97). The only explanation for these findings, at least with our existing information about neuronal function, is that the neurohypophysis is innervated by separate populations of oxytocin and vasopressin cells. The preparation of purified oxytocin- and vasopressin-containing neurosecretosomes (pinched-off nerve terminals) from the neurohypophysis (96) supports this view. Neurosecretory granules themselves may be partitioned in a similar fashion (49, 50). The hypothalamo-neurohypophysial system of rats with inherited diabetes insipidus (Brattleboro strain), which are unable to synthesize vasopressin or its carrier protein (39), has a morphological appearance entirely consistent with the one-hormone—one-cell hypothesis. There is an absence of neurosecretory granules in a discrete population of SO and PV cells (97), and in the neurohypophysis there are bundles of empty nerve terminals scattered among more heavily staining (oxytocin?) endings (98). The above circumstantial evidence for the existence of two neuronal populations has been largely superseded by the development of means of identifying individual oxytocin and vasopressin cells. The most spectacular advances have been made in the field of immunohistochemistry with the use of antibodies raised against neurophysin I or II to discriminate the cell types in histological sections. Livett et al. (31), studying the pig, were the first to label cells with antibodies specific to neurophysin II. A discrete population of hypothalamic vasopressin cells was revealed, with the remainder of cells in the PV and SO nuclei showing no fluorescence. Subsequent workers have employed specific antibodies to neuro-

physin I and II to detect oxytocin or vasopressin cells in the bovine hypothalamo-neurohypophysial system (33). Studies with antibodies which are not
specific for one or the other of the neurophysins are, in this context, only of
interest when performed in the Brattleboro rat. Here, as might be expected,
there is an absence of neurophysin in a selected proportion of cells projecting to
the neurohypophysis (99). Very recently, labeling of cells with specific antibodies to oxytocin or vasopressin has been achieved. Vandesande and Dierickx
(100) employed an immunoenzyme histochemical double staining method to
identify simultaneously the two kinds of neuronal perikarya in the PV and SO
nuclei of the rat. No cells were found to contain both hormones. Swaab et al.
(101) obtained a similar separation of oxytocin and vasopressin cells, also in the
rat. These findings cast doubt on an earlier report by Le Clerc and Pelletier (102)
that all the cells projecting to the neurohypophysis of the rat had an affinity for
vasopressin antibodies.

Oxytocin and vasopressin cells may now be separated by electrophysiological
means, according to their patterns of spike discharge during conditions favoring
the release of one or the other of the neurohypophysial hormones (see also
under "Physiological Roles of Oxytocin Cells," and "Physiological Roles of
Vasopressin Cells"). During the selective relase of oxytocin evoked by suckling
in the lactating rat, a proportion of SO and PV cells displays an explosive burst
of firing (86, 88). Other cells react in a highly characteristic fashion when release
of vasopressin is induced by hemorrhage (22) or carotid occlusion (21).

Are there differences in ultrastructural characteristics of oxytocin and vasopressin cells? Morris and Cannata (48) found that at a critical pH of 7.0 some
axons in the supraopticohypophysial tract contained either exclusively pale
(oxytocin?) granules or dark (vasopressin?) granules. Rodriguez (103) claimed
that granules within vasopressin cells were generally smaller than those in
oxytocin cells. However, the differences in fixation properties or granule size
tend to be of a statistical nature and, as yet, there is no certain way of deciding
the precise secretory function of any given cell on the basis of ultrastructural
appearance.

Distribution of Cell Types

Perhaps because of their distinct functions (see under "Physiological Roles of
Oxytocin Cells" and "Physiological Roles of Vasopressin Cells"), it has been
tempting to suggest that the two cell types of the hypothalamo-neurohypophysial system have become anatomically separated, such that oxytocin cells lie
in the PV nucleus and vasopressin cells in the SO nucleus. Determination of the
oxytocin and vasopressin content of the two nuclei (104), the effects of
electrical stimulation of discrete hypothalamic regions on blood hormone levels
(105), and the effects of hypothalamic lesions on neurohypophysial function
(106) all produced results to support this view. More recent work suggests that a
functional dichotomy does not exist in all species. In the rat, which has been
more investigated, there is little difference in function between the two magnocellular cell groups. Burford and co-workers (107) studied the incorporation of

radioactivity into neurophysin I and II after intranuclear injections of labeled substrate ([^{35}S]cysteine) and showed that both nuclei synthesized both hormones. This accords with earlier findings that Brattleboro rats were able to synthesize oxytocin even after destruction of their PV nuclei (108) and that the oxytocin to vasopressin ratio in the PV nucleus in rats does not differ substantially from that of the SO nucleus (60, 68).

The availability of methods for identifying oxytocin and vasopressin cells in the rat has provided a means of accurately determining quantitatively the proportion of each cell type in the two nuclei. Swaab et al. (101), using immunofluorescent labeling, showed that oxytocin cells comprised 31% of the SO and 40% of the PV nuclei, whereas vasopressin cells comprised 53% of the SO and 50% of the PV nuclei, with 10–20% of cells showing no staining reaction. Dierickx and Vandesande (100) also found roughly equal numbers of immunoreactive cell types in each nuclei. In electrophysiological studies, in which oxytocin neurons were identified by their characteristic discharge preceding milk ejection, there was no substantial difference in the proportion of PV and SO cells activated by suckling (86, 88). Since the SO nucleus of the rat contains about 3 times more neurosecretory cells than the PV nucleus (109), it would appear that the former may be quantitatively more important for release of both vasopressin and oxytocin. Certainly, elimination of the input to the PV nucleus does not seriously affect reflex release of oxytocin during suckling (110).

In certain other species, an unequal distribution of oxytocin and vasopressin cells between the PV and SO nuclei has been confirmed. In the guinea pig, the SO nucleus contains relatively little oxytocin (111) and does not appear to be involved in the milk-ejection reflex (112). In the ox, Zimmerman et al. (113) found equal amounts of oxytocin and vasopressin, together with their carrier proteins, in the PV nucleus, but vasopressin and neurophysin II were 4 times greater in the SO nucleus. This difference is also reflected in the immunofluorescent reaction of the cells in the bovine hypothalamus (33).

For many years, it has been known that some neurosecretory cells lie outside of the main body of the SO and PV nuclei in what have been termed the accessory neurosecretory nuclei (109). Recent immunofluorescent work has shown that a number of neurophysin-containing cells are also to be found in the suprachiasmatic nucleus (33, 99). Moreover, this nucleus contains a significant amount of radioimmunoassayable vasopressin (114). No one knows where these suprachiasmatic cells project to, but the median eminence contains neurophysin (99), and there are significant amounts of both neurophysin and vasopressin in hypophysial portal blood (38).

PHYSIOLOGICAL ROLES OF OXYTOCIN CELLS

Milk Ejection

Without question, the best established role of mammalian oxytocin cells is in initiating contraction of the myoepithelial cells of the lactating mammary gland to cause the ejection of milk. Evidence implicating neurohypophysial oxytocin in reflex milk ejection has been obtained in the cat (115), dog (116), rabbit (117), and rat (118). In certain ruminants, however, milk can be removed from the mammary gland without the involvement of oxytocin (119, 120).

A striking feature of oxytocin release during suckling or milking is that the hormone appears in the blood only transiently. Blood samples taken serially show wide fluctuations in oxytocin content, suggesting a pulsatile or spurt-like oxytocin release. This pattern appears to be common to all the species so far investigated (cow (119, 121), goat (120), pig (119), and woman (122)). Intra-mammary pressure records taken during suckling reflect the intermittent nature of oxytocin release. In the woman, for example, 15 min of suckling evoked three consecutive pressure curves which were best mimicked by giving separate injections of 30, 20, and 20 mU of oxytocin, rather than by slowly infusing the same amount of hormone (123). Between species there may be considerable differences in the size and frequency of the oxytocin pulses. During the nursing period of the rabbit, which lasts 4 min, there occurs a single oxytocin pulse (124). The lactating rat, on the other hand, nurses its young for 30–40 min at a time, and from the behavioral reaction of the pups it may be deduced that 6–8 oxytocin pulses are discharged (125, 126).

Within the last few years, electrophysiological recording in the PV (96) and SO nuclei (88) of anesthetized lactating rats has provided a detailed description of the way in which oxytocin cells react during suckling to initiate a series of oxytocin pulses. No change in spike activity occurs until some 10–15 min after attachment of the pups when brief (2–4) periods of activation are observed at intervals of 5–10 min (see Figure 1). Each burst is characterized by a 30–60-fold acceleration of firing to a peak of 20–80 spikes/s. The activity then subsides into 10–15 s of quiescence, followed by recovery to the initial rate of firing. Each burst is associated with a pulsatile release of 0.5–1.0 mU of oxytocin, and an abrupt rise in intramammary pressure follows at a latency of about 15 s. A similar latency to milk ejection is observed after electrical stimulation of the supraopticohypophysial system (86), and there can be little doubt that the burst of firing represents the neural trigger for release of oxytocin.

How is the afferent limb of the milk ejection reflex organized to provide the intermittent response in oxytocin neurons? In the rat, the periodicity in the suckling-induced response does not depend upon a negative feedback from the final common path because it remains undisturbed by electrical stimulation of the supraopticohypophysial tract (127) or by oxytocin injections (128). Another possibility, that the rhythmicity of neurosecretory activation stems from subtle alterations in the sucking stimulus, has also recently been excluded. Individually, rat pups do display short-term fluctuations in their sucking efforts and tend to suck in short episodes (1–2 s) about once every 20 s. However, these episodes seem to occur randomly between pups so that, collectively, the litter provides a constant sucking stimulus, and there is no observable trigger for each oxytocin pulse (129). This perplexing lack of correlation between the timing of

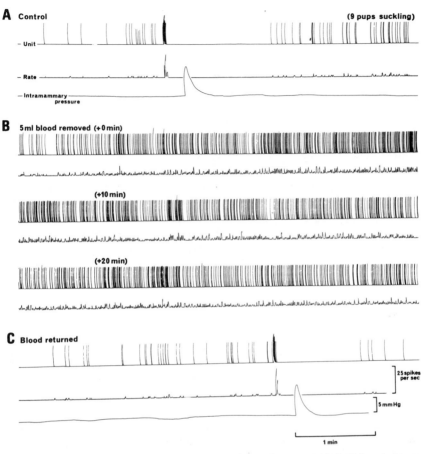

Figure 1. Polygraph records showing the unit activity of an oxytocin cell in relation to suckling and hemorrhage. The cell was antidromically identified from the neurohypophysis and histologically localized to the SO nucleus. *A,* 5 min of recording during suckling, spanning the occurrence of a reflex milk ejection (signaled by the abrupt rise in intramammary pressure); *B,* periods of activity at different times after removal of 5 ml of blood (pups still on the nipples); and *C,* after return of the blood, showing another reflex milk ejection. Note the dramatic increase in firing rate in this unit at the time of oxytocin release before milk ejection and the steady increase in background firing induced by hemorrhage. Compare these responses with those of the vasopressin cell shown in Figure 2.

oxytocin spurts and changes in stimulus intensity is not a peculiar feature of the rat; the timing of oxytocin release during milking in farm animals seems equally unpredictable (120, 121).

Certain observations in the rat (130) suggest the existence of a neural gating mechanism in the afferent limb of the milk-ejection reflex. Thus, 1) there is no excitation in PV and SO units during the intense sucking when the pups are first applied to the nipples; 2) following a period of neurosecretory activation the reflex becomes refractory, with no further bursts being initiated for at least 2–3 min; and 3) procedures which may trigger a burst during suckling (e.g., intra-mammary injection of saline solution) are ineffective if applied too soon after a preceding burst. The timing of the opening of the hypothetical neural gate might depend upon a pacemaker function inherent to the afferent path of the reflex. Factors which affect the frequency of milk ejection, such as the degree of mammary distension (126), electroencephalogram (EEG) state (131), or anes-thesia (126), might act by influencing the periodicity of the pacemaker. Once the neural gate opens, the magnitude of neurosecretory activation and of the oxytocin pulse which follows is, as a rule, proportional to the intensity of the afferent stimulus. Over the range of 6–10 pups, the relationship between pup number and the size of the burst of firing in individual neurons is linear (130, 131), suggesting a summation of input from each nipple. This explains why litter size influences the amount of oxytocin released during suckling (124, 132). It is noteworthy that the actual number of oxytocin cells which are activated at each milk ejection seems to remain constant because increasing the stimulus does not cause the recruitment of previously nonactivated neurons (130).

At present it is impossible to provide a complete account, in neurophysio-logical or neuroanatomical terms, of how suckling activates oxytocin cells. The majority of fiber connections of the PV or SO nuclei appear to arise from within the hypothalamus (133). However, some direct connections from extrahypo-thalamic sources have been shown by morphological methods; these originate from the brain stem (via the medial forebrain bundle), amygdala, septum, hippocampus, and olfactory tubercle (134). The convergence of input to these nuclei has been confirmed electrophysiologically by recording inhibition or excitation of antidromically identified neurosecretory cells after stimulation of a variety of different brain structures (17, 135–137). Microiontophoretic studies suggest that the final synapse mediating an inhibitory input is noradrenergic (23, 24, 138), and for an excitatory input is cholinergic (23, 24, 138, 139). Both monoaminergic (140, 141) and cholinergic (142) terminals have been demon-strated in the PV or SO nuclei.

According to the classic view of the milk-ejection reflex, the afferent barrage activating oxytocin cells arises from nerve endings within the nipple which respond to pressure and temperature stimulation (143). The afferents from the mammary gland enter the spinal cord segmentally and relay with secondary sensory neurons projecting ipsilaterally in the lateral funiculi (144, 145). There may also be a role for spinocervicothalamic and spinoreticular systems (146). In the brain stem, transmission of the suckling stimulus involves the reticular formation (133, 146, 147). At the level of the midbrain, a "milk ejection pathway" has been differentiated (148). This runs along the lateral tegmentum close to the medial leminiscus and later bifurcates into a dorsal component, perhaps associated with the medial longitudinal fasciculus and a ventral com-ponent associated with the medial forebrain bundle. However, the milk ejection pathway may be more diffuse than this description suggests because stimulation of a wide area of the midbrain tegmentum may release oxytocin (147). In addition, there is evidence for descending inputs to oxytocin cells (147, 149, 150) which might mediate the higher control of oxytocin release.

At the level of the hypothalamus, one may speculate that mechanisms lying within the PV and SO nuclei have a hand in fashioning the explosive but transient response of oxytocin neurons during suckling. Electrophysiological studies point to the existence of recurrent inhibitory collaterals in the hypo-thalamo-neurohypophysial system. Single pulses applied to the neurohypophysis cause a brief (80 ms) inhibition of neurosecretory cells (17, 151); more pro-longed stimulation (5 s) is followed by a long quiescent period identical with that following neurosecretory activation at milk ejection (152). The potent effect of iontophoretically applied oxytocin in exciting PV neurosecretory cells (153) might suggest that a facilitatory feedback system also operates.

Parturition

Unlike its function in milk ejection, when oxytocin is essential for normal removal of milk, the release of oxytocin during parturition is a helpful but not indispensable aid to delivery of the young. Parturition is a multifactorially regulated process involving maternal and fetal components where oxytocin release occurs as a belated event to accelerate the final evacuation of the uterine contents, when the fetus is in a dangerous no-man's-land between a parasitic and free living state (154). So far, attempts to demonstrate changes in activity of oxytocin cells in the maternal hypothalamus at term have been unsuccessful (155). Nonetheless, a picture can be pieced together of the behavior of the cells from measurements of oxytocin in the circulation. In the goat, Folley and Knaggs (156) found that oxytocin appeared in the blood intermittently, suggest-ing a spurt-like release. Highest levels were attained as the kid passed through the vagina. In an impressive study, exploiting a sensitive radioimmunoassay, Gibbens and Chard (157) examined hormone levels in 97 parturient women; the pattern of oxytocin release was pulsatile and bore no relation to the uterine contrac-tions. The oxytocin spurts became more frequent during stage 2 (the expulsive stage) of labor, recurring every few minutes. Thus, there is good evidence in the goat and human that oxytocin cells are activated intermittently (cf. suckling) during the second stages of labor. Whether the same applies to the small laboratory animals is less certain. However, in rats (158) and rabbits (159) only brief periods of neurohypophysial stimulation were required to induce parturi-tion, perhaps suggesting that reflex oxytocin release might also follow a pulsatile pattern.

The stimulus for the activation of oxytocin cells during parturition is apparently distension of the cervix or vagina, as first shown in the classic experiments of Ferguson (160). Release of oxytocin in response to stimulation of the reproductive tract has now been demonstrated either directly or by measuring milk ejection in the goat (161), sheep (162, 163), rat (164), and woman (165). Interestingly, the reflex appears to be very susceptible to the effects of ovarian hormones because estrogen enhances and progesterone depresses release of oxytocin (163); seasonal effects may also be demonstrated (161). The mechanism of action of the steroids is unknown, but recent work has shown that PV units are more likely to be excited by stimulation of the reproductive tract after estrogen treatment (166).

The spurt-like pattern of oxytocin release during labor is similar to that which occurs in suckling and so presumably the neural mechanisms proposed in the previous section may apply here also.

Other Functions

In both male and female mammals, there are indications that oxytocin may be released during coitus.

McNeilly and Ducker (167) studied hormone levels during mating in the estrous female goat and found a spurt-like release of oxytocin in 28 of the 36 matings examined. Plasma concentrations ranged from $2-190$ μU/ml. However, oxytocin release most often occurred before or after mounting, suggesting that intromission was not the major stimulus for release. Also, in diestrous animals, oxytocin release occurred in the absence of coitus. Evidently, the stimuli for activating oxytocin cells during mating are complex, for release could be triggered by the smell, sight, or sound of the male and by the presence of another female goat. Such observations not only challenge the assumption that the release of oxytocin which follows vaginal distension $(161-165)$ represents a reflex active during coitus, but also emphasizes the importance of careful controls in this type of experiment.

Oxytocin released in the female during coitus may increase uterine motility and so aid the movement of spermatozoa. These are known to be actively transported up the female reproductive tract (168). In estrogen-primed rabbits, Morton and Fitzpatrick (169) discovered that injections of 80 mU of oxytocin greatly facilitated the entry of semen into the uterus. However, when the same dose was given to untreated rabbits, no significant effect on sperm transport was detected. A significant role for oxytocin in the mated female has yet to be established.

Oxytocin is released in the copulating ram (170). Massage of the seminal vesicles may also release oxytocin in this species, as demonstrated in cross-circulation experiments involving a lactating ewe from which intramammary pressure records were taken (162). However, the sensory specificity of this stimulus is questionable, for stimulation of several other pelvic organs (e.g., bladder or rectum) is equally effective. Various actions of oxytocin on the male reproductive tract have been reported. Oxytocin may induce contractions of the vas deferens or epididymis (171, 172) and may increase the volume of semen ejaculated (173). However, Agmo (174) failed to detect any change in sperm density in ejaculates from oxytocin-treated rabbits, and it has yet to be shown that any male function is significantly impaired in the absence of oxytocin.

Although oxytocin is generally considered to be involved only in reproductive and lactational processes, more general roles, such as the control of renal function, have been proposed. The attraction of a role in kidney control is that it would explain why oxytocin is present in large quantities in both male and female nonbreeding mammals (104) and why the hormone is released in significant amounts during changes in the osmotic pressure of the blood (18). It has been known for many years that oxytocin may have a diuretic action, at least in the rat (175). This effect was originally thought to involve a change in glomerular filtration rate (176), but more recent work suggests that the diuresis may be secondary to a rise in sodium excretion (177).

PHYSIOLOGICAL ROLES OF VASOPRESSIN CELLS

Osmoregulation

Verney's (178) classic ablation and replacement experiments in the dog were crucial in establishing the role of vasopressin in osmoregulation. A striking example of the importance of vasopressin is provided by the Brattleboro strain of rats, which are unable to synthesize the hormone. The animals show a chronic diabetes insipidus which can be corrected by injections of synthetic vasopressin tannate (39).

In contrast to oxytocin, which can be detected by monitoring intra-mammary pressure, there is no simple on-line means of monitoring release of vasopressin. The most reliable information on hormone output from vasopressin cells during osmotic stimulation comes from direct hormone assays of collected blood samples. In the nonstimulated animal, plasma vasopressin is only just detectable; levels in the range of $1-5$ $\mu U/ml$ have been reported in the rat (179), dog (180), and human (181). During dehydration, in which increases in plasma osmotic pressure and decreases in blood volume both act to stimulate vaso-pressin release (182), there is a progressive increase in plasma hormone levels. For example, in rats (179) and humans (183) deprived of water for 3 days, levels are in the range $15-20$ $\mu U/ml$. Urinary excretion of vasopressin also increases (184).

The increase in vasopressin secretion associated with dehydration may be reproduced over a shorter time scale by administering hypertonic saline solution by either an intravenous (185), intracarotid (18), intraperitoneal (186), or intraventricular (187) route. The relation between the intensity of osmotic stimulation and the rate of vasopressin secretion has been accurately quantitatively determined in the conscious rat by Dunn and co-workers (186). The osmotic threshold for vasopressin secretion ($290-293$ mOsm/kg) was just below the normal plasma osmotic pressure (mean 294 ± 1.4 mOsm/kg). Thus, during normal conditions of hydration, vasopressin cells appear to be minimally activated; similar principles apply in man (182). Dunn and co-workers also found that, as the plasma osmotic pressure was increased above the osmotic threshold by intraperitoneal injections of saline solution, an almost exactly proportional increase in vasopressin levels occurred; the correlation between these two variables was always above 0.9. Furthermore, the slope of the regression line was such that even a 1% increase above the normal osmotic pressure regularly produced a significant change in vasopressin levels. These findings fully validate the earlier claims concerning the extraordinary sensitivity and precision of the osmoreceptor mechanism for regulating vasopressin secretion (178).

There have been many studies of hypothalamic unit activity during osmotic stimulation, starting with the work of Cross and Green (188) in the PV and SO nucleus of the rabbit. But electrophysiological identification of vasopressin neurons has only become possible very recently (21, 22). In most of the work, selection of neurons has been on the basis of antidromic identification of neurosecretory cells projecting to the neurohypophysis, which may have included oxytocin as well as vasopressin cells. In conformity with what is known about stimulus-secretion coupling within the hypothalamo-neurohypophysial system (54), the predominant effect of intravenous or intracarotid injections of hypertonic saline solution is to cause an increase in the firing of PV or SO neurosecretory cells (17, 19, 139). However, not all cells are excited; Dyball (18) described a proportion (30–40%) of cells in the rat which displayed several seconds of inhibition after intracarotid saline solution injections. In the unanesthetized monkey, the same procedure evokes in many SO cells a biphasic (excitatory-inhibitory) pattern of firing (189), which appears to be exclusive to neurons projecting to the neurohypophysis (19).

Perhaps more physiologically relevant are the electrophysiological data from animals subjected to chronic osmotic stimulation by having saline solution to drink or by water deprivation. In the rat, 3 days of saline solution treatment caused a significant increase in unit activity within the PV and SO nucleus, which was not observed in other hypothalamic areas (190). In a study of histologically identified rat SO cells, Walters and Hatton (191) reported similar effects after 5 days of water deprivation. Interestingly, in rats with hereditary diabetes insipidus, SO and PV unit activity seems to be permanently elevated (192). The increase in firing of SO units during chronic dehydration appears to be linearly proportional to the increase in osmotic pressure (193), which correlates well with the characteristics of vasopressin secretion (see above). Another aspect is that SO neurosecretory cells change their pattern of firing during water deprivation. Under normal conditions, some 20–30% of neurosecretory cells projecting to the neurohypophysis show a "phasic" (18, 139, 194) or "low frequency burster" (19) pattern. As dehydration progresses, it seems that cells first switch from a slow, irregular discharge to phasic firing so that the proportion of phasic cells in the monkey SO nucleus is significantly elevated by the 2nd day (195). The duration of the intermittent bursts also increases. Later, phasic cells seem to give way to fast firing, continuously active cells. A switching of pattern, from a quiescent or slow discharge to a phasic activity, may also be induced in a proportion of SO cells by slow infusions (196) or intraperitoneal injections (197) of hypertonic saline solution. These observations are especially significant in view of recent evidence (21, 22) equating phasic firing with vasopressin release (also see below).

If the electrophysiological correlate of osmotically induced vasopressin release is an excitation, probably with a change in pattern, in PV and SO neurosecretory cells, where is the receptor mechanism for this neural response? One suggestion is that part of the osmoreceptor mechanism is located in the liver and is affected by the osmotic pressure of the portal blood (198). However, there is little change in the afferent impulses arising from a perfused liver when the ionic concentration is varied by ±5%; so that the argument for hepatic osmoreceptors of the classic type is unconvincing (199). Jewell and Verney's (200) view that the osmoreceptors are located in or near the SO nucleus is supported by the ability of animals with deafferented hypothalamus to maintain their water balance (201) and by the effectiveness of osmotic stimuli to release vasopressin from the hypothalamo-neurohypophysial system in vitro (202). Observations on the osmotic activation of SO cells, without concomitant changes in the activity of other hypothalamic areas (190, 193), might suggest that the neurosecretory cells themselves are osmosensitive. However, Bridges and Thorn (203) have reasoned that since the release of antidiuretic hormone (ADH) in response to osmotic stimulation is prevented by autonomic blocking agents, a synaptic input is required for the osmotic excitation of vasopressin neurons. The precise intrahypothalamic location of the osmoreceptors, therefore, remains doubtful.

Although it is uncertain whether vasopressin cells depend upon synaptic connections for their osmoregulatory role, it may be assumed that extrahypothalamic inputs influence their activity. For example, SO neurosecretory cells in the thirsting monkey show an immediate inhibition when the animal drinks (204). Central pathways for regulating vasopressin release have been reviewed recently by Cross and Dyball (133). Evidence from intrahypothalamic (205) or intraventricular (206, 207) injections of transmitters suggests the membranes of vasopressin neurons contain both acetylcholine and norepinephrine receptors.

Blood Volume Regulation

The effectiveness of hemorrhage in releasing vasopressin has been confirmed by numerous reports (94, 208—210). However, to establish a primary role for vasopressin in regulating blood volume, physiological changes of the latter should be shown to modify the rate of vasopressin secretion. This has turned out to be a serious stumbling block because relatively large amounts of blood have to be removed before a rise in vasopressin levels is detectable. Although Claybaugh and Share (211) found that the anesthetized dog may release vasopressin after loss of as little as 2.5% of blood volume, it has been objected (212) that the animals were already sensitized by the hemorrhagic trauma associated with surgical preparation. Rats only released vasopressin after 10—15% blood loss, usually when the first substantial fall in blood pressure occurred (213). In man

(212) and sheep (210), less than 10% depletion of blood volume had no effect on vasopressin release. These negative results might reflect the use of insensitive methods of vasopressin assay.

A better explanation of why large hemorrhages are required to release detectable vasopressin is the exponential (rather than linear) relationship between percentage of blood depletion and hormonal response (186, 214). Removal of successive aliquots of blood initially causes a scarcely perceptible trickle of vasopressin, but eventually this becomes a torrent, as evidenced by the very high plasma levels of hormone attained during severe hemorrhage (213). The exponential stimulus-response relationship for hemorrhage contrasts with the linear relationship for osmotic change (186). Whereas a 1–2% change in plasma osmotic pressure causes a significant release of vasopressin, blood volume may have to be reduced by 10% to elicit the same response. Thus, under normal conditions of hydration the secretion of vasopressin probably represents a homeostatic response initiated by an osmotic rather than a volumetric stimulus.

There may be complicated interactions between the effects of blood volume and osmotic pressure on vasopressin neurons. Synergistically, volume reductions during dehydration may significantly increase the vasopressin response to a given plasma osmotic pressure (186, 210). Antagonistically, a hypovolemia may inhibit the diuresis normally associated with water infusion (215).

Hypothalamic control of hemorrhage-induced vasopressin release has recently been investigated in urethanized lactating rats (216). Vasopressin neurons in the SO nucleus were identified by a combination of antidromic activation from the neurohypophysis and a lack of response at milk ejection. During the withdrawal of 5 ml (20%) of blood, which resulted in plasma vasopressin levels in the range of 100–500 μU/ml, the neurons displayed a dramatic change in spike activity. From very slow firing rates (0.1 spikes/s), the cells accelerated to some 5–10 spikes/s and then after a period of 10–15 min switched to a phasic firing pattern, characterized by periods of quiescence and fast discharge alternating with a periodicity of 30–60 s (Figure 2). The phasic activity was observed in all vasopressin neurons and was maintained until blood was replaced, at which time the cells reverted to their slow discharge rate. The initial response of vasopressin cells during hemorrhage is, therefore, a period of continuous spike activity which later evolves into a phasic pattern.

Phasic firing is rarely observed in oxytocin cells (86, 88) (see also Figure 1) and seems to be a characteristic of vasopressin neurons. There are three notable features of the phasic activity.

1. The bursts are normally randomized between cells (190), so that collectively they release hormone in a continuous trickle rather than intermittently.
2. The lengths of the bursts may be modulated to change the rate of hormone secretion (22, 217).
3. An intense stimulus for vasopressin release, such as carotid occlusion, may synchronize the onset of the bursts in the population of phasic cells (21, 218).

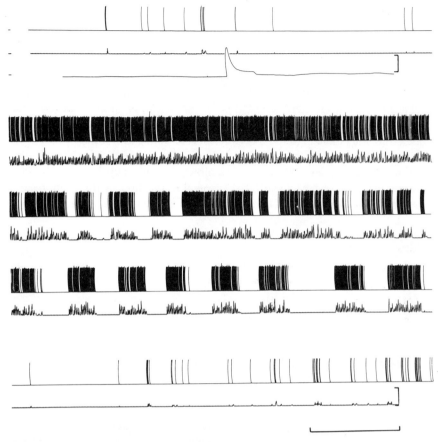

Figure 2. Effects of suckling and hemorrhage on the spike activity of a vasopressin cell. The cell was recorded in the SO nucleus after antidromic identification from the neurohypophysis. As in Figure 1, *A* shows the activity of the cell during oxytocin release at milk ejection; *B,* activity at different times after a 5-ml hemorrhage; and *C,* activity after return of the blood. Note that there was little change in the discharge of the cell during reflex milk ejection (cf. the cell in Figure 1), but hemorrhage induced a dramatic increase in firing rate which later evolved into a highly characteristic phasic pattern.

The receptors involved in the excitation of vasopressin neurons during blood volume reduction are probably carotid sinus baroreceptors and left atrial stretch receptors (219, 220). Baroreceptor involvement is indicated by the effectiveness of carotid occlusion in causing vasopressin release in cats (95) and dogs (221), provided the vagi are cut. In vagotomized dogs, perfusion of the carotid sinus at constant pressure during hemorrhage markedly attenuates the vasopressin response (222). In intact dogs, a drop in the perfusion pressure of the isolated carotid sinus, without hemorrhage, evokes a vasopressin response (223). Involvement of atrial stretch receptors in the vasopressin response to hemorrhage might be suggested by the finding that inflation of a balloon in the left atrium of the anesthetized dog inhibits vasopressin release (224). However, in the conscious dog, Goetz and colleagues (225) found no change in vasopressin secretion after reduction of atrial transmural pressure. Angiotensin II, which appears in the plasma during hemorrhage, may also participate in regulating vasopressin secretion (226, 227).

The afferent pathways from the pressure and stretch receptors have not been delineated. However, there seems to be no shortage of brain sites where stimulation elicits release of vasopressin (133). The neural organization involved in fashioning the phasic pattern of vasopressin cells during hemorrhage (216) is also unknown. There are three possibilities: 1) an intermittent excitatory input from outside the SO nucleus, 2) reciprocal inhibitory connections between the vasopressin neurons, and 3) an intrinsic pacemaker function in the membrane of vasopressin neurons, akin to that described for invertebrate neurosecretory cells (228).

Other Functions

A role for vasopressin cells in anterior pituitary regulation has been proposed. Interest in this area has been recently stimulated by reports that vasopressin is released into hypophysial portal blood (38), possibly from the median eminence (99, 229). Intravenous injections of vasopressin may stimulate the release of growth hormone (230) and ACTH (231). Vasopressin potentiates the actions of corticotropin-releasing factor (232).

Subcutaneous injections of vasopressin in microgram quantities significantly increase the preservation of a conditioned avoidance reaction (233). Local application of vasopressin in the posterior thalamic region is equally effective (234). Rats with hereditary diabetes insipidus display a deficiency in their ability to retain a conditioned avoidance reaction (235). However, the potency of vasopressin in influencing memory is not reduced by trypsin digestion (236), and at present the physiological significance of these findings is uncertain.

CONCLUSIONS

Despite their anatomical proximity, oxytocin and vasopressin cells show a clear dichotomy of function. Oxytocin cells regulate certain processes involved in reproduction in the female—the cells may have a role at the beginning (sperm transport) and end (parturition) of gestation. However, only during lactation are the cells essential, when elimination of oxytocin secretion abolishes milk ejection and death of the offspring ensues. Oxytocin release is usually evoked by exteroreceptive stimuli (e.g., suckling), and hormone release occurs in an intermittent fashion. The timing and amount of hormone release often bear little relation to the onset and intensity of the stimulus. Oxytocin cells have no established role outside reproduction, although they seem to be activated in combination with vasopressin cells during osmotic stimulation.

Vasopressin cells have an important homeostatic role, common to both males and females, in regulating the rate of water excretion by the kidney and so governing plasma osmotic pressure and blood volume. Elimination of vasopressin secretion produces a gross disturbance of water balance (diabetes insipidus). Vasopressin release is controlled by interoreceptive stimuli (e.g., elevated plasma osmotic pressure) and is probably continuous rather than episodic. Furthermore, the rate of hormone release is closely related to the intensity of the stimulus.

The research effort of the last few years has yielded considerable information about the day to day demands for oxytocin and vasopressin secretion and how the PV and SO cells which produce the hormones are organized to meet these secretory requirements. From a micromorphological, biochemical, and electrophysiological viewpoint, we can provide a fairly complete story of the cellular processes involved in the discharge of active neurohypophysial hormone into the circulation. However, when events preceding activation of the neurosecretory cells are considered, serious gaps in our understanding are revealed. What is the precise neural basis for the intermittent response of oxytocin cells during suckling? Where is the exact location of the osmoreceptor mechanism, and how does it provide for the graded output of hormone from vasopressin cells during a rise in plasma osmotic pressure? Only when answers to these and other such questions are found will we be able to write a full account of the physiology of the neurohypophysis.

REFERENCES

1. Oliver, G., and Schafer, E. A. (1895). On the physiological action of extracts of pituitary body and certain other glandular organs. J. Physiol. (London) 18:277.
2. Dale, H. H. (1909). The action of extracts of the pituitary body. Biochem. J. 4:427.
3. Ott, I., and Scott, J. C. (1910). The action of infundibulin upon the mammary secretion. Proc. Soc. Exp. Biol. Med. 8:48.
4. Von den Velden, R. (1913). Die Nierenwirkung von Hypophysenextrakten beim menschen. Berl. Klin. Wochenschr. 50:2083.
5. Dudley, H. W. (1919). Some observations on the active principles of the pituitary gland. J. Pharmacol. Exp. Ther. 14:295.
6. Scharrer, E., and Scharrer, B. (1940). Secretory cells within the hypothalamus. Res. Publ. Assoc. Res. Nerv. Ment. Dis. 20:170.
7. Bargmann, W., and Schaffer, E. (1951). The site of origin of the hormones of the posterior pituitary. Am. Sci. 39:255.
8. Du Vigneaud, V., Ressler, C., Swan, J. M., Roberts, C. W., Katsoyannis, P. G., and Gordon, S. (1954). The synthesis of an octapeptide amide with the hormonal activity of oxytocin. J. Am. Chem. Soc. 75:4870.
9. Du Vigneaud, V., Gish, D. T., and Katsoyannis, A. (1954). A synthetic preparation possessing biological properties associated with arginine vasopressin. J. Am. Chem. Soc. 76:4751.
10. Krisch, B. (1954). Different populations of granules and their distribution in the hypothalamo-neurohypophysial tract of the rat under various

experimental conditions. I. Neurohypophysis, nucleus supraopticus and nucleus paraventricularis. Cell Tiss. Res. 51:117.

11. Morris, J. F., and Dyball, R. E. J. (1974). A quantitative study of the ultrastructural changes in the hypothalamo-neurohypophysial system during and after experimentally-induced hypersecretion. Cell Tiss. Res. 149:525.

12. Pickering, B. T., Jones, C. W., Burford, G. D., McPherson, M., Swann, R. W., Heap, P. F., and Morris, J. F. (1975). The role of neurophysin proteins: suggestions from the study of their transport and turnover. Ann. N. Y. Acad. Sci. 248:15.

13. Norstrom, A. (1975). Axonal transport and turnover of neurohypophyseal proteins in the rat. Ann. N. Y. Acad. Sci. 248:46.

14. Kent, C., and Williams, M. A. (1974). The nature of hypothalamo-neurohypophyseal neurosecretion in the rat: a study by light and electron microscope autoradiography. J. Cell. Biol. 60:554.

15. Heap, P. F., Jones, C. W., Morris, J. F., and Pickering, B. T. (1975). Movement of neurosecretory product through the anatomical compartments of the neural lobe of the pituitary gland: an electron microscopic autoradiographic study. Cell Tiss. Res. 156:483.

16. Pearson, D., Shainberg, A., Osinchak, J., and Sachs, H. (1975). The hypothalamo-neurohypophysial complex in organ culture: morphologic and biochemical characteristics. Endocrinology 96:982.

17. Koizumi, K., and Yamashita, H. (1972). Studies of antidromically identified neurosecretory cells of the hypothalamus by intracellular and extracellular recordings. J. Physiol. (London) 221:683.

18. Dyball, R. E. J. (1971). Oxytocin and ADH secretion in relation to electrical activity in antidromically identified supraoptic and paraventricular units. J. Physiol. (London) 214:245.

19. Hayward, J. N., and Jennings, D. P. (1973). Activity of magnocellular neuroendocrine cells in the hypothalamus of unanesthetized monkeys. II. Osmosensitivity of functional cell types in the supraoptic nucleus and the internuclear zone. J. Physiol. (London) 232:545.

20. Arnauld, E., Vincent, J. D., and Dreifuss, J. J. (1974). Firing patterns of hypothalamic supraoptic neurons during water deprivation in monkeys. Science 185:535.

21. Harris, M. C., Dreifuss, J. J., and Legros, J. J. (1975). Excitation of phasically firing supraoptic neurons during vasopressin release. Nature (London) 258:80.

22. Wakerley, J. B., Poulain, D. A., Dyball, R. E. J., and Cross, B. A. (1975). Activity of phasic neurosecretory cells during hemorrhage. Nature (London) 258:82.

23. Barker, J. L., Crayton, J. W., and Nicoll, R. A. (1971). Supraoptic neurosecretory cells: adrenergic and cholinergic sensitivity. Science 171:208.

24. Moss, R. L., Urban, I., and Cross, B. A. (1972). Microelectrophoresis of cholinergic and aminergic drugs on paraventricular neurons. Am. J. Physiol. 223:310.

25. Nordmann, J. J., Dreifuss, J. J., Baker, P. F., Ravazzola, M., Malaisse-Lagae, F., and Orci, L. (1974). Secretion-dependent uptake of extracellular fluid by the rat neurohypophysis. Nature (London) 250:155.

26. Nakazato, Y., and Douglas, W. W. (1974). Vasopressin release from the isolated neurohypophysis induced by a calcium ionophore, X-537A. Nature (London) 249:279.

27. Russell, J. T., and Thorn, N. A. (1974). Calcium and stimulus-secretion coupling in the neurohypophysis. II. Effects of lanthanum, a varapamil analogue (D600) and prenylamine on 45-calcium transport and vasopressin release in isolated rat neurohypophyses. Acta Endocrinol. (Kbh.) 76:471.

28. Nagasawa, J., Douglas, W. W., and Schulz, R. (1970). Ultrastructural evidence of secretion by exocytosis and of "synaptic vesicle" formation in posterior pituitary glands. Nature (London) 227:407.

29. Dempsey, G. P., Bullivant, S., and Watkins, W. B. (1973). Ultrastructure of the rat posterior pituitary gland and evidence of hormone release by exocytosis as revealed by freeze-fracturing. Z. Zellforsch. Mikrosk. Anat. 143:465.

30. Dreifuss, J. J., Akert, K., Sandri, C., and Moor, H. (1973). The fine structure of freeze-fractured neurosecretory nerve endings in the neurohypophysis. Brain Res. 62:367.

31. Livett, B. G., Uttenthal, L. O., and Hope, D. B. (1971). Localization of neurophysin II in the hypothalamo-neurohypophysial system of the pig by immunofluorescence histology. Phil. Trans. R. Soc. Lond. 261:371.

32. Watkins, W. B., and Evans, J. J. (1972). Demonstration of neurophysin in the hypothalamo-neurohypophysial system of the normal and dehydrated rat by the use of cross-species reactive antineurophysins. Z. Zellforsch. Mikrosk. Anat. 131:149.

33. De Mey, T., Vandesande, F., and Dierickx, K. (1974). Identification of the neurophysin I and the neurophysin II producing neurones in the bovine hypothalamus. Cell Tiss. Res. 153:531.

34. Zimmerman, E. A., Hsu, K. C., Robinson, A. G., Carmel, P. W., Frantz, A. G., and Tonnenbaum, M. (1973). Studies of neurophysin secreting neurons with immunoperoxidase techniques employing antibody to bovine neurophysin. I. Light microscopic findings in monkey and bovine tissues. Endocrinology 92:931.

35. Cheng, K. W., and Friesen, M. G. (1973). Studies of human neurophysin by radioimmunoassay. J. Clin. Endocrinol. Metab. 36:553.

36. Legros, J. J., and Franchimont, P. (1972). Human neurophysin blood levels under normal, experimental and pathological conditions. Clin. Endocrinol. 1:99.

37. Legros, J. J., Reynaert, R., and Peeters, G. (1975). Specific release of bovine neurophysin II during arterial or venous haemorrhage in the cow. J. Endocrinol. 67:297.

38. Zimmerman, E. A., Carmel, P. W., Husain, M. K., Ferin, M., Tannenbaum, M., Frantz, A. G., and Robinson, A. G. (1973). Vasopressin and neurophysin: high concentrations in monkey hypophyseal portal blood. Science 182:925.

39. Valtin, H., Sokol, H. W., and Sunde, D. (1975). Genetic approaches to the study of the regulation and actions of vasopressin. Recent Prog. Horm. Res. 31:447.

40. Goodman, I., and Hiatt, R. B. (1972). Coherin: a new peptide of the bovine neurohypophysis with activity on gastrointestinal motility. Science 178:419.

41. Hayward, J. N. (1975). Neural control of the posterior pituitary gland. Annu. Rev. Physiol. 37:191.

42. Jard, S., and Bockaert, J. (1975). Stimulus-response coupling in neurohypophysial peptide target cells. Physiol. Rev. 55:489.

43. Lauson, H. D. (1974). Metabolism of the neurohypophysial hormones. In

R. O. Greep and E. B. Astwood (eds.), Handbook of Physiology, Section 7: Endocrinology, Vol IV, The Pituitary Gland and its Neuroendocrine Control, Part 1. pp. 287–294. American Physiological Society, Washington, D.C.

44. Leontovich, T. A. (1969). The neurons of the magnocellular neurosecretory nuclei of the dog's hypothalamus. J. Hirnforsch. 11:499.

45. Sloper, J. C., and Bateson, R. G. (1965). Ultrastructure of neurosecretory cells in the supraoptic nucleus of the dog and the rat. J. Endocrinol. 31:139.

46. Zambrano, D., and de Robertis, E. (1966). The secretory cycle of supraoptic neurons in the rat: a structural-functional correlation. Z. Zellforsch. Mikrosk. Anat. 73:414.

47. Kalimo, H. (1971). Ultrastructural studies on the hypothalamic neurosecretory neurones of the rat. I. The paraventricular neurons of the non-treated rat. Z. Zellforsch. Mikrosk. Anat. 122:283.

48. Morris, J. R., and Cannata, M. A. (1973). Ultrastructural preservation of the dense core of posterior pituitary neurosecretory granules and its implications for hormone release. J. Endocrinol. 57:517.

49. La Bella, F. S., Beaulieu, G., and Reiffenstein, R. J. (1962). Evidence for the existence of separate vasopressin and oxytocin-containing granules. Nature (London) 193:173.

50. Pickup, J. C., Johnston, C. I., Nakamura, S., Uttenthal, L. O., and Hope, D. B. (1973). Subcellular organization of neurophysins, oxytocin, (8-lysine)-vasopressin and adenosine triphosphatase in porcine posterior pituitary lobes. Biochem. J. 132:361.

51. Pelletier, G., LeClerc, R., Labrie, F., and Puvianic, R. (1974). Electron microscope immunohistochemical localization of neurophysin in the rat hypothalamus and pituitary. Mol. Cell. Endocrinol. 1:157.

52. Rechardt, L. (1969). Electron microscopic and histochemical observations on the supraoptic nucleus of normal and dehydrated rats. Acta Physiol. Scand. (Suppl.) 329:1.

53. Livingstone, A. (1973). Ultrastructure of the rat neural lobe during recovery from hypertonic saline treatment. Z. Zellforsch. Mikrosk. Anat. 137:361.

54. Cross, B. A., Dyball, R. E. J., Dyer, R. G., Jones, C. W., Lincoln, D. W., Morris, J. F., and Pickering, B. T. (1975). Endocrine neurons. Recent Prog. Horm. Res. 31:243.

55. Ellman, G. L., and Gan, G. L. (1971). Response of the cells of the supra-optic nucleus; kinetic aspects. Exp. Brain. Res. 14:1.

56. Hatton, G. I., and Walters, J. K. (1973). Induced multiple nucleoli, nucleolar margination, and cell size changes in supraoptic neurons during dehydration and rehydration in the rat. Brain Res. 59:137.

57. Daniel, A. R., and Lederis, K. (1966). Effects of ether anaesthesia and haemorrhage on hormone storage and ultrastructure of the rat neurohypophysis. J. Endocrinol. 34:91.

58. Monroe, B. G., and Scott, D. E. (1966). Ultrastructural changes in the neural lobe of the hypophysis of the rat during lactation and suckling. J. Ultrastruct. Res. 14:497.

59. Kalimo, H., and Rinne, U. K. (1972). Ultrastructural studies on the hypothalamic neurosecretory neurons of the rat. II. The hypothalamo-neurohypophysial system in rats with hereditary hypothalamic diabetes insipidus. Z. Zellforsch. Mikrosk. Anat. 134:205.

60. Dyer, R. G., Dyball, R. E. J., and Morris, J. F. (1973). The effect of hypothalamic deafferentation upon the ultrastructure and hormone content of the paraventricular nucleus. J. Endocrinol. 57:509.
61. Palay, S. (1957). The fine structure of the neurohypophysis. In H. Waelsch (ed.), Ultrastructure and Cellular Chemistry of Neural Tissue, pp. 31–44. Hoeber, New York.
62. Olivieri-Sangiacomo, C. (1972). Degenerating pituicytes in the neural lobe of osmotically stressed rats. Experientia 28:1362.
63. Sachs, H., Fawcett, P., Takabatake, Y., and Portanova, R. (1969). Biosynthesis and release of vasopressin and neurophysin. Recent Prog. Horm. Res. 25:447.
64. Pearson, D., Shainberg, A., Malamed, S., and Sachs, H. (1975). The hypothalamo-neurohypophysial complex in organ culture: effects of metabolic inhibitors, biologic and pharmacological agents. Endocrinology 96:994.
65. Sachs, H., Pearson, D., and Nureddin, A. (1975). Guinea pig neurophysin: isolation, developmental aspects, biosynthesis in organ culture. Ann. N. Y. Acad. Sci. 248:36.
66. Cannata, M. A., and Morris, J. F. (1973). Changes in the appearance of hypothalamo-neurohypophysial neurosecretory granules associated with their maturation. J. Endocrinol. 57:531.
67. Vogt, M. (1953). Vasopressor, antidiuretic, and oxytocic activities of extracts of the dog's hypothalamus. Br. J. Pharmacol. 8:193.
68. Dyball, R. E. J., and Henry, J. A. (1975). Relatively greater increase of oxytocin than vasopressin in the supraoptic nucleus of rats after hypophysectomy. J. Endocrinol. 64:125.
69. Norstrom, A., and Sjostrand, J. (1972). Effect of salt-loading, thirst and water-loading on transport and turnover of neurohypophysial proteins of the rat. J. Endocrinol. 52:87.
70. Grainger, F., and Sloper, J. C. (1974). Correlation between microtubular number and transport activity of hypothalamo-neurohypophyseal secretory neurons. Cell Tiss. Res. 153:101.
71. Nordmann, J. J. (1975). Hormone release and Ca uptake in the rat neurohypophysis. In E. Carafoli (ed.), Calcium Transport in Contraction and Secretion, pp. 281–286. North-Holland Publishing Company, New York.
72. Douglas, W. W. (1974). Mechanism of release of neurohypophysial hormones: stimulus-secretion coupling. In R. O. Greep and E. B. Astwood (eds.), Handbook of Physiology, Section 7: Endocrinology, Vol. IV, The Pituitary Gland and Its Neuroendocrine Control, Part 1, pp. 191–224. American Physiological Society, Washington, D.C.
73. Edwards, B. A., Edwards, M. E., and Thorn, N. A. (1973). The release in vitro of vasopressin unaccompanied by the axoplasmic enzymes: lactic acid dehydrogenase and adenylate kinase. Acta Endocrinol. (Kbh.) 72:417.
74. Lederis, K., and Livingstone, A. (1970). Neuronal and subcellular localization of acetylcholine in the posterior pituitary of the rabbit. J. Physiol. (London) 210:187.
75. Dreifuss, J. J. (1975). A review of neurosecretory granules: their contents and mechanisms of release. Ann. N. Y. Acad. Sci. 248:184.
76. Dreifuss, J. J., Kalnins, I., Kelly, J. S., and Ruf, K. B. (1971). Action potentials and release of neurohypophysial hormones in vitro. J. Physiol. (London) 215:805.

77. Ishida, A. (1970). The oxytocin release and the compound action potential evoked by electrical stimulation of the isolated neurohypophysis of the rat. Jap. J. Physiol. 20:84.
78. Nordmann, J. J., and Dreifuss, J. J. (1972). Hormone release evoked by electrical stimulation of rat neurohypophyses in the absence of action potentials. Brain Res. 45:604.
79. Douglas, W. W., and Poisner, A. M. (1964). Stimulus-secretion coupling in a neurosecretory organ: the role of calcium in the release of vasopressin from the neurohypophysis. J. Physiol. (London) 172:1.
80. Dreifuss, J. J., and Nordmann, J. J. (1974). Role du calcium dans la secretion des hormones neurohypophysaires. Bull. Swiss. Acad. Med. Sci. 30:107.
81. Russell, J. T., Hanson, E. L., and Thorn, N. A. (1974). Calcium and stimulus secretion coupling in the neurohypophysis. III. Ca^{++} Ionophore (A-23187)-induced release of vasopressin from isolated rat neurohypophyses. Acta Endocrinol. (Kbh.) 77:443.
82. Dean, P. M. (1974). Neurohypophyseal granules: electrokinetic properties and calcium ion binding. Brain Res. 79:397.
83. Dreifuss, J. J., Nordmann, J. J., Akart, K., Sandri, C., and Moor, H. (1974). Exo-endocytosis in the neurohypophysis as revealed by freeze-fractioning. In F. Knowles and L. Vollrath (eds.), Neurosecretion: The Final Neuroendocrine Pathway, pp. 31–37. Springer-Verlag, New York.
84. Nagasawa, J., Douglas, W. W., and Schulz, R. A. (1971). Micropinocytotic origin of coated and smooth microvesicles ("synaptic vesicles") in neurosecretory terminals of posterior pituitary glands demonstrated by incorporation of horseradish peroxidease. Nature (London) 232:341.
85. Harris, G. W., Manabe, Y., and Ruf, K. B. (1969). A study of the parameters of electrical stimulation of unmyelinated fibres in the pituitary stalk. J. Physiol. (London) 203:67.
86. Wakerley, J. B., and Lincoln, D. W. (1973). The milk-ejection reflex of the rat: a 20- to 40-fold acceleration in the firing of paraventricular neurones during the release of oxytocin. J. Endocrinol. 57:477.
87. Cross, B. A., and Wakerley, J. B. (1974). Reversible blockade of neurosecretory axons in the hypothalamo-neurohypophysial tract with radio-frequency current. J. Physiol. (London) 245:117P.
88. Lincoln, D. W., and Wakerley, J. B. (1974). Electrophysiological evidence for the activation of supraoptic neurones during the release of oxytocin. J. Physiol. (London) 242:533.
89. Lincoln, D. W. (1974). Dynamics of oxytocin secretion. In F. Knowles and L. Vollrath (eds.), Neurosecretion: The Final Neuroendocrine Pathway, pp. 129–133. Springer-Verlag, New York.
90. Dyball, R. E. J. (1975). Potentiation by urethane and inhibition by pentobarbitone of oxytocin release in vitro. J. Endocrinol. 67:453.
91. Bisset, G. W., Clark, B. J., and Haldar, J. (1970). Blood levels of oxytocin and vasopressin during suckling in the rabbit and the problem of their independent release. J. Physiol. (London) 206:711.
92. Legros, J. J., Reynaert, R., and Peeters, J. J. (1974). Specific release of bovine neurophysin I during milking and suckling in the cow. J. Endocrinol. 60:327.
93. Wakerley, J. B., Dyball, R. E. J., and Lincoln, D. W. (1973). Milk ejection in the rat: the result of a selective release of oxytocin. J. Endocrinol. 57:557.

94. Beleslin, D., Bisset, G. W., Haldar, J., and Polak, R. L. (1967). The release of vasopressin without oxytocin in response to haemorrhage. Proc. R. Soc. Lond. B 166:443.
95. Clark, B. J., and Rocha, M., Jr. (1967). An afferent pathway for the selective release of vasopressin in response to carotid occlusion and haemorrhage in the cat. J. Physiol. (London) 191:529.
96. LaBella, F. S. (1968). Storage and secretion of neurohypophyseal hormones. Can. J. Physiol. Pharmacol. 46:335.
97. Orkand, P. M., and Palay, S. L. (1966). The fine structure of the supraoptic nucleus in normal rats compared with that in rats with hereditary diabetes insipidus. Anat. Rec. 154:396 (Abstr.).
98. Sokol, H. W., and Valtin, H. (1967). Evidence for the synthesis of oxytocin and vasopressin in separate neurons. Nature (London) 214:314.
99. Zimmerman, E. A., Defendini, R., Sokol, H. W., and Robinson, A. G. (1975). The distribution of neurophysin-secreting pathways in the mammalian brain: light microscopic studies using the immunoperoxidase technique. Ann. N.Y. Acad. Sci. 248:92.
100. Vandesande, F., and Dierickx, K. (1975). Identification of the vasopressin producing and of the oxytocin producing neurons in the hypothalamine magnocellular-neurosecretory system of the rat. Cell Tiss. Res. 164:153.
101. Swaab, D. F., Nijveldt, F., and Pool, C. W. (1975). Distribution of oxytocin and vasopressin in the rat supraoptic and paraventricular nucleus. J. Endocrinol. 67:461.
102. Le Clerc, R., and Pelletier, G. (1974). Electron microscope immunohistochemical localization of vasopressin in the hypothalamus and neurohypophysis of the normal and Brattleboro rat. Am. J. Anat. 140:583.
103. Rodriguez, E. M. (1971). The comparative morphology of neural lobes of species with different neurohypophysial hormones. Mem. Soc. Endocrinol. 19:263.
104. Lederis, K. (1961). Vasopressin and oxytocin in the mammalian hypothalamus. Gen. Comp. Endocrinol. 1:80.
105. Bisset, G. W., Clark, B. J., and Errington, M. C. (1971). The hypothalamic neurosecretory pathways for the release of oxytocin and vasopressin in the cat. J. Physiol. (London) 217:111.
106. Nibbelink, K. D. W. (1961). Paraventricular nuclei, neurohypophysis and parturition. Am. J. Physiol. 200:1229.
107. Burford, G. D., Dyball, R. E. J., Moss, R. L., and Pickering, B. T. (1974). Synthesis of both neurohypophysial hormones in both the paraventricular and supraoptic nuclei of the rat. J. Anat. 117:261.
108. Sokol, H. W. (1970). Evidence for oxytocin synthesis after electrolytic destruction of the paraventricular nucleus in rats with hereditary diabetes insipidus. Neuroendocrinology 6:90.
109. Bandaranayake, R. C. (1971). Morphology of the accessory neurosecretory nuclei and of the retrochiasmatic part of the synaptic nucleus of the rat. Acta Anat. 80:14.
110. Voloschin, L. M., and Tramezzani, J. H. (1973). The neural input to the milk-ejection reflex in the hypothalamus. Endocrinology 92:973.
111. Bisset, G. W., Errington, M. L., and Richards, C. D. (1973). Distribution of vasopressin and oxytocin in the hypothalamo-neurohypophysial system of the guinea-pig. Br. J. Pharmacol. 48:263.
112. Tindal, J. S., and Knaggs, G. S. (1971). Determination of the detailed

hypothalamic route of the milk-ejection reflex in the guinea-pig. J. Endocrinol. 50:135.

113. Zimmerman, F. A., Robinson, A. G., Huzain, M. K., Acosta, M., Frantz, A. G., and Sawyer, W. H. (1974). Neurohypophysial peptides in the bovine hypothalamus: the relationship of neurophysin I to oxytocin and neurophysin II to vasopressin in supraoptic and paraventricular regions. Endocrinology 95:931.

114. George, J. M., and Jacobowitz, D. M. (1975). Localization of vasopressin in discrete areas of the rat hypothalamus. Brain Res. 93:363.

115. Beyer, C., Mean, F., Packeco, P., and Alcaraz, M. (1962). Effect of central nervous system lesions on lactation in the cat. Fed. Proc. 21:353 (Abstr.).

116. Pickford, M. (1960). Factors affecting milk release in the dog and the quantity of oxytocin liberated by suckling. J. Physiol. (London) 152:515.

117. Cross, B. A., and Harris, G. W. (1952). The role of the neurohypophysis in the milk ejection reflex. J. Endocrinol. 8:148.

118. Yokoyama, A., and Ota, K. (1965). The effect of anaesthesia on milk yield and maintenance of lactation in the goat and rat. J. Endocrinol. 33:341.

119. Folley, S. J., and Knaggs, G. S. (1966). Milk-ejection activity (oxytocin) in the external jugular vein blood of the cow, goat and sow, in relation to the stimulus of milking or suckling. J. Endocrinol. 34:197.

120. McNeilly, A. S. (1972). The blood levels of oxytocin during suckling and hand-milking in the goat with some observations on the pattern of hormone release. J. Endocrinol. 52:177.

121. Cleverley, J. D., and Folley, S. J. (1970). The blood levels of oxytocin during machine milking in cows with some observations on its half-life in the circulation. J. Endocrinol. 46:347.

122. Fox, C. A., and Knaggs, G. S. (1969). Milk-ejection activity (oxytocin) in peripheral venous blood in man during lactation and in association with coitus. J. Endocrinol. 45:145.

123. Cobo, E., Bernal, M. M., Graitan, E., and Quintero, C. A. (1967). Neurohypophyseal hormone release in the human. Am. J. Obstet. Gynecol. 97:519.

124. Fuchs, A. R., and Wagner, G. (1963). Quantitative aspects of release of oxytocin by suckling in anaesthetized rabbits. Acta Endocrinol. (Kbh.) 44:581.

125. Wakerley, J. B., and Lincoln, D. W. (1971). Intermittent release of oxytocin during suckling in the rat. Nature (New Biol.) 233:180.

126. Lincoln, D. W., Hill, A. M., and Wakerley, J. B. (1973). The milk-ejection reflex of the rat: an intermittent function not abolished by surgical levels of anaesthesia. J. Endocrinol. 57:459.

127. Wakerley, J. B., and Deverson, B. M. (1975). Stimulation of the supraoptico-hypophysial tract in the rat during suckling: failure to alter the inherent periodicity of reflex oxytocin release. J. Endocrinol. 66:439.

128. Lincoln, D. W. (1974). Does a mechanism of negative feedback determine the intermittent release of oxytocin during suckling? J. Endocrinol. 60:143.

129. Wakerley, J. B., and Drewett, R. F. (1975). The pattern of sucking in the infant rat during sequences of spontaneous milk ejection. Physiol. Behav. 15:277.

130. Lincoln, D. W., and Wakerley, J. B. (1975). Factors governing the periodic

activation of supraoptic and paraventricular neurosecretory cells during suckling in the rat. J. Physiol. (London) 250:443.

131. Lincoln, D. W., and Wakerley, J. B. (1975). Neurosecretory activation in the rat: correlation of the suckling stimulus with the pulsatile release of oxytocin. J. Physiol. (London) 245:43P.

132. Mena, F., and Grosvenor, C. E. (1968). Effect of number of pups upon suckling induced fall in pituitary prolactin concentration and milk ejection in the rat. Endocrinology 82:632.

133. Cross, B. A., and Dyball, R. E. J. (1974). Central pathways for neurohypophysial hormone release. In R. O. Greep and E. B. Astwood (eds.), Handbook of Physiology, Section 7: Endocrinology, Vol. IV, The Pituitary Gland and Its Neuroendocrine Control, Part I, pp. 269–286. American Physiological Society, Washington, D.C.

134. Zaborsky, L., Leranth, L. S., Makara, G. B., and Palkovits, M. (1975). Quantitative studies on the supraoptic nucleus in the rat. II. Afferent fiber connections. Exp. Brain Res. 23:525.

135. Novin, D., Sundsten, J. W., and Cross, B. A. (1970). Some properties of antidromically activated units in the paraventricular nucleus of the hypothalamus. Exp. Neurol. 26:330.

136. Negoro, H., Vissessuwan, S., and Holland, R. C. (1973). Inhibition and excitation of units in paraventricular nucleus after stimulation of the septum, amygdala and neurohypophysis. Brain Res. 57:479.

137. Novin, D., and Durham, R. (1973). Orthodromic and antidromic activation of the paraventricular nucleus of the hypothalamus in the rabbit. Exp. Neurol. 41:418.

138. Barker, J. L., Crayton, J. W., and Nicoll, R. A. (1971). Noradrenaline and acetylcholine responses of supraoptic neurosecretory cells. J. Physiol. (London) 218:19.

139. Dreifuss, J. J., and Kelly, J. S. (1972). The activity of identified supraoptic neurosecretory neurones and their response to acetylcholine applied by iontophoresis. J. Physiol. (London) 220:105.

140. Fuxe, K., and Hokfelt, T. (1967). The influence of central catecholamine neurons on the hormone secretion from the anterior and posterior pituitary. In F. Stutinsky (ed.), Neurosecretion, pp. 165–177. Springer-Verlag, Berlin.

141. Lindvall, O., and Bjorkland, A. (1974). The organization of the ascending catecholamine neuron systems in the rat brain as revealed by the glyoxylic acid fluorescence method. Acta Physiol. Scand. (Suppl.) 412:1.

142. Shute, C. C. D., and Lewis, P. R. (1966). Cholinergic and monaminergic pathways in the hypothalamus. Br. Med. Bull. 22:221.

143. Cross, B. A., and Findlay, A. L. R. (1966). Comparative and sensory aspects of milk ejection. In M. Reynolds and S. J. Folley (eds.), Lactogenesis: the Initiation of Milk Secretion at Parturition, pp. 245–252. University of Pennsylvania Press, Philadelphia.

144. Eayrs, J. T., and Baddeley, R. M. (1956). Neural pathways in lactation. J. Anat. 90:161.

145. Mena, F., and Beyer, C. (1968). Effect of spinal cord lesions on milk ejection in the rabbit. Endocrinology 83:615.

146. Richard, P., Urban, I., and Denamur, R. (1970). The role of the dorsal tracts of the spinal cord and of the mesencephalic and thalamic leminiscal system in the milk ejection reflex during milking in the ewe. J. Endocrinol. 47:45.

147. Urban, I., Moss, R. L., and Cross, B. A. (1971). Problems in electrical stimulation of afferent pathways for oxytocin release. J. Endocrinol. 51:347.
148. Tindal, J. S., and Knaggs, G. S. (1975). Further studies on the afferent path of the milk-ejection reflex in the brain stem of the rabbit. J. Endocrinol. 66:107.
149. Aulsebrook, L. H., and Holland, R. C. (1969). Central regulation of oxytocin release with and without vasopressin release. Am. J. Physiol. 216:818.
150. Aulsebrook, L. H., and Holland, R. C. (1969). Central inhibition of oxytocin release. Am. J. Physiol. 216:830.
151. Dreifuss, J. J., and Kelly, J. S. (1972). Recurrent inhibition of anti-dromically identified rat supraoptic neurones. J. Physiol. (London) 220:87.
152. Negoro, H., and Holland, R. C. (1972). Inhibition of unit activity in the hypothalamic paraventricular nucleus following antidromic activation. Brain Res. 42:385.
153. Moss, R. L., Dyball, R. E. J., and Cross, B. A. (1972). Excitation of antidromically identified neurosecretory cells of the paraventricular nucleus by oxytocin applied iontophoretically. Exp. Neurol. 34:95.
154. Chard, T. (1973). The posterior pituitary and the induction of labour. Mem. Soc. Endocrinol. 20:61.
155. Boer, K., and Nolten, J. W. C. (1975). Electrical activity of antidromically identified neurosecretory cells in the paraventricular nucleus in relation to uterine contractions of the rat at term. Acta Endocrinol. (Kbh.) (Suppl. 199) 80:183.
156. Folley, S. J., and Knaggs, G. S. (1965). Levels of oxytocin in the jugular vein blood of goats during parturition. J. Endocrinol. 33:301.
157. Gibbens, G. L. D., and Chard, T. (1976). Observations on maternal oxytocin release during human labour and effect of intravenous alcohol administration. Am. J. Obstet. Gynecol. 126:243.
158. Boer, K., Lincoln, D. W., and Swaab, D. F. (1974). Effects of electrical stimulation of the neurohypophysis on labour in the rat. J. Endocrinol. 65:163.
159. Lincoln, D. W. (1971). Labour in the rabbit: effect of electrical stimulation applied to the infundibulum and median eminence. J. Endocrinol. 50:607.
160. Ferguson, J. K. W. (1941). A study of the mobility of the intact uterus at term. Surg. Obstet. Gynecol. 73:359.
161. Roberts, J. S. (1975). Cyclical fluctuations in reflexive oxytocin release during the estrous cycle of the goat. Biol. Reprod. 13:314.
162. Peeters, G., and Houvenaghel, A. (1973). Reflex release of milk-ejection activity by stimulation of organs in the pelvic region in sheep as studied by cross-circulation experiments. J. Endocrinol. 58:53.
163. Roberts, J. S., and Share, L. (1969). Effects of progesterone and estrogen on blood levels of oxytocin during vaginal distension. Endocrinology 84:1076.
164. Moos, R., and Richard, P. (1975). Importance de la liberation d'ocytocine induite par la dilatation vaginale (reflexe de Ferguson) et la stimulation vagale (reflex vago-pituitaire) chez la ratte. J. Physiol. (Paris) 70:307.
165. Fisch, L., Sala, N. L., and Schwarcz, R. L. (1964). Effect of cervical dilatation upon uterine contractility in pregnant women and its relation to oxytocin secretion. Am. J. Obstet. Gynecol. 90:108.

166. Negoro, H., Vasvussen, S., and Holland, R. C. (1973). Reflex activation of paraventricular nucleus units during the reproductive cycle and in ovariectomized rats treated with oestrogen or progesterone. J. Endocrinol. 59:559.

167. McNeilly, A. S., and Ducker, H. A. (1972). Blood levels of oxytocin in the female goat during coitus and in response to stimuli associated with mating. J. Endocrinol. 54:399.

168. Van Demark, N. L., and Moeller, A. N. (1951). Speed of spermatozoan transport in reproductive tract of estrous cow. Am. J. Physiol. 165:674.

169. Morton, D. B., and Fitzpatrick, R. J. (1974). The effect of oxytocin on sperm transport in ovariectomized oestrogen-treated rabbits. J. Endocrinol. 61:139.

170. Sharma, S. C., Fitzpatrick, R. J., and Ward, W. R. (1972). Coitus-induced release of oxytocin in the ram. J. Reprod. Fertil. 31:488.

171. Knight, T. W. (1972). In vivo effects of oxytocin on the contractile activity of the cannulated epididymis and vas deferens in rams. J. Reprod. Fertil. 28:141.

172. Hib, J. (1974). The contractility of the cauda epididymis of the mouse, its spontaneous activity in vitro and the effects of oxytocin. J. Reprod. Fertil. 36:191.

173. Kihlstrom, J. E., and Melin, P. (1963). The influence of oxytocin upon some seminal characteristics in the rabbit. Acta Physiol. Scand. 59:363.

174. Agmo, A. J. (1975). Neurohypophysial hormones and the emission of semen in rabbits. J. Reprod. Fertil. 45:243.

175. Fraser, A. M. (1942). The action of the oxytocic hormone of the pituitary gland on urine secretion. J. Physiol. (London) 101:236.

176. Dicker, S. E., and Heller, H. (1946). The renal action of posterior pituitary extract and its fractions as analysed by clearance experiments on rats. J. Physiol. (London) 104:353.

177. Peters, G., and Roch-Ramel, F. (1972). Renal effects of posterior pituitary peptides and their derivatives. In H. Heller and B. T. Pickering (eds.), Pharmacology of the Endocrine System and Prelated Drugs: the Neurohypophysis, pp. 229–278. Pergamon Press, New York.

178. Verney, E. B. (1947). The antidiuretic hormone and the factors which determine its release. Proc. R. Soc. London B 135:25.

179. Little, J. B., and Radford, E. P. (1964). Bio-assay for antidiuretic activity in blood of undisturbed rats. J. Appl. Physiol. 19:179.

180. Bonjour, J. P., and Malvin, R. L. (1970). Plasma concentrations of ADH in conscious and anaesthetized dogs. Am. J. Physiol. 218:1128.

181. Yoshida, S. K., Motohoshi, K., Ibayashi, H., and Okinaka, S. (1963). Method for the assay of antidiuretic hormone in plasma with a note on the antidiuretic titer of human plasma. J. Lab. Clin. Med. 62:279.

182. Moses, A. M., and Miller, M. (1974). Osmotic influences on the release of vasopressin. In R. O. Greep and E. B. Astwood (eds.), Handbook of Physiology, Section 7: Endocrinology, Vol. IV, The Pituitary Gland and Its Neuroendocrine Control, Part 1, pp. 225–242. American Physiological Society, Washington, D.C.

183. Czaczkes, J. W., Kleeman, C. R., and Koenig, M. (1964). Physiological studies of antidiuretic hormone by its direct measurement in human plasma. J. Clin. Invest. 43:1625.

184. Miller, M., and Moses, A. M. (1972). Radioimmunoassay of urinary antidiuretic hormone in man: response to water load and dehydration in normal subjects. J. Clin. Endocrinol. Metab. 34:537.

185. Saito, T., Yoshida, S., and Nakao, K. (1969). Release of antidiuretic hormone from neurohypophysis in response to haemorrhage and infusion of hypertonic saline in dogs. Endocrinology 85:72.
186. Dunn, F. L., Brennan, T. J., Nelson, A. E., and Robertson, G. L. (1973). The role of blood osmolality and volume in regulating vasopressin secretion in the rat. J. Clin. Invest. 52:3212.
187. Andersson, B., Dallman, M. F., and Olsson, K. (1969). Observations on central control of drinking and of the release of antidiuretic hormone (ADH). Life Sci. 8(I):425.
188. Cross, B. A., and Green, J. D. (1959). Activity of single neurones in the hypothalamus: effect of osmotic and other stimuli. J. Physiol. (London) 148:554.
189. Hayward, J. N., and Vincent, J. D. (1970). Osmosensitive single neurones in the hypothalamus of unanaesthetized monkeys. J. Physiol. (London) 210:947.
190. Dyball, R. E. J., and Poutney, P. S. (1973). Discharge patterns of supraoptic and paraventricular neurones in rats given a 2% NaCl solution instead of drinking water. J. Endocrinol. 56:91.
191. Walters, J. K., and Hatton, G. I. (1974). Supraoptic neuronal activity in rats during five days of water deprivation. Physiol. Behav. 13:661.
192. Dyball, R. E. J. (1974). Single unit activity in the hypothalamo-neurohypophysial system of Brattleboro rats. J. Endocrinol. 60:135.
193. Arnauld, E., Vincent, J. D., and Dreifuss, J. J. (1974). Firing patterns of hypothalamic supraoptic neurones during water deprivation in monkeys. Science 185:535.
194. Wakerley, J. B., and Lincoln, D. W. (1971). Phasic discharge of antidromically identified units in the paraventricular nucleus of the hypothalamus. Brain Res. 25:192.
195. Arnauld, E., Dufy, B., and Vincent, J. D. (1975). Hypothalamic supraoptic neurones: rates and patterns of action potential firing during water deprivation in the unanaesthetized monkey. Brain Res. 100:315.
196. Haskins, J. T., Jennings, D. P., and Rogers, J. M. (1975). Response of supraoptic neuroendocrine cell firing pattern types to measured changes in plasma osmolality. Physiologist 18:240.
197. Brimble, M. J., and Dyball, R. E. J. (1976). Osmotic activation of supraoptic neurosecretory neurons in rats. J. Physiol. (London) (Abstr.) 257:51P.
198. Haberich, F. J. (1968). Osmoreception in the portal circulation. Fed. Proc. 27:1137.
199. Andrews, W. H. H., and Orbach, J. (1975). Effect of osmotic pressure on spontaneous afferent discharge in the nerves of the perfused rabbit liver. Pfluegers Arch. 361:89.
200. Jewell, P. A., and Verney, E. B. (1957). An experimental attempt to determine the site of the neurohypophysial osmoreceptors in the dog. Phil. Trans. R. Soc. Lond. (Biol. Sci.) 240:197.
201. Woods, J. W., Bard, P., and Bleier, R. (1966). Functional capacity of the deafferented hypothalamus: water balance and responses to osmotic stimuli in the decerebrate cat and rat. J. Neurophysiol. 29:751.
202. Eggena, P., and Thorn, N. A. (1970). Vasopressin release from the rat supraoptico-neurohypophysial system in vitro in response to hypertonicity and acetylcholine. Acta Endocrinol. (Kbh.) 65:442.
203. Bridges, T. E., and Thorn, N. A. (1970). The effect of autonomic blocking

agents on vasopressin release *in vivo* induced by osmoreceptor stimulation. J. Endocrinol. 48:265.

204. Vincent, J. D., Arnauld, E., and Bioulac, B. (1972). Activity of osmosensitive single cells in the hypothalamus of the behaving monkey during drinking. Brain Res. 44:371.

205. Milton, A. S., and Paterson, A. T. (1974). A microinjection study of the control of antidiuretic hormone release by the supraoptic nucleus of the hypothalamus in the cat. J. Physiol. (London) 241:607.

206. Kuhn, E. R. (1975). Cholinergic and adrenergic release mechanism for vasopressin in the male rat: a study with injections of neurotransmitters and blocking agents into the third ventricle. Neuroendocrinology 16:255.

207. Bhargava, K. P., Kulshrestha, V. K., and Srivastava, Y. P. (1972). Central cholinergic and adrenergic mechanisms in the release of antidiuretic hormone. Br. J. Pharmacol. 44:617.

208. Share, L. (1961). Acute reduction in extracellular fluid volume and the concentration of antidiuretic hormone in blood. Endocrinology 69:925.

209. Sachs, H., Share, L., Osinchak, J., and Carpi, A. (1967). Capacity of the neurohypophysis to release vasopressin. Endocrinology 81:755.

210. Johnson, J. A., Zehr, J. E., and Moore, W. W. (1970). Effects of separate and concurrent osmotic and volume stimuli on plasma ADH in sheep. Am. J. Physiol. 218:1273.

211. Claybaugh, J. R., and Share, L. (1973). Vasopressin, renin, and cardiovascular responses to continuous slow haemorrhage. Am. J. Physiol. 224:519.

212. Goetz, K. L., Bond, G. C., and Smith, W. E. (1974). Effect of moderate hemorrhage in humans on plasma ADH and renin. Proc. Soc. Exp. Biol. Med. 145:277.

213. Fabian, M., Forsling, M. L., Jones, J. J., and Lee, J. (1969). The release, clearance and plasma protein binding of oxytocin in the anaesthetized rat. J. Endocrinol. 43:175.

214. Shade, R. E., and Share, L. (1975). Volume control of plasma antidiuretic hormone concentration following acute blood volume expansion in the anaesthetized dog. Endocrinology 97:1048.

215. Arnolt, J. O. (1965). Diuresis induced by water infusion into the carotid loop and its inhibition by small haemorrhage. Arch. Geschwulstforch. Physiol. 282:313.

216. Poulain, D. A., Wakerley, J. B., and Dyball, R. E. J. (1977). Electrophysiological differentiation of oxytocin- and vasopressin-secreting neurons. Proc. Roy. Soc. B. 196:367.

217. Dyball, R. E. J., Poulain, D. A., and Wakerley, J. B. (1976). Induction of phasic activity in regularly firing neurosecretory cells of the rat. J. Physiol. (London) 256:108P.

218. Dreifuss, J. J., Harris, M. C., and Tribollet, E. (1976). Excitation of phasically firing hypothalamic supraoptic neurones during carotid occlusion in rats. J. Physiol. (London) 257:337.

219. Share, L. (1974). Blood pressure, blood volume, and the release of vasopressin. *In* R. O. Greep and E. B. Astwood (eds.), Handbook of Physiology, Section 7: Endocrinology, Vol. IV, The Pituitary Gland and Its Neuroendocrine Control, Part I, pp. 243–255.

220. Goetz, K. L., Bond, G. L., and Bloxham, D. D. (1975). Atrial receptors and renal function. Physiol. Rev. 55:157.

221. Share, L., and Levy, M. N. (1962). Cardiovascular receptors and blood titer of antidiuretic hormone. Am. J. Physiol. 203:425.
222. Share, L. (1967). Role of peripheral receptors in the increased release of vasopressin in response to haemorrhage. Endocrinology 81:1140.
223. Share, L., and Levy, M. N. (1966). Carotid sinus pulse pressure, a determinant of plasma antidiuretic hormone concentration. Am. J. Physiol. 211:721.
224. Share, L. (1965). Effects of carotid occlusion and left atrial distension on plasma vasopressin titer. Am. J. Physiol. 208:219.
225. Goetz, K. L., Bond, G. C., Hermreck, A. S., and Trank, J. W. (1970). Plasma ADH levels following a decrease in mean atrial transmural pressure in dogs. Am. J. Physiol. 219:1424.
226. Keil, L. C., Summy-Long, J., and Severs, W. B. (1975). Release of vasopressin by angiotensin II. Endocrinology 96:1063.
227. Shade, R. E., and Share, L. (1975). Vasopressin release during non-hypotensive haemorrhage and angiotensin II infusion. Am. J. Physiol. 228:149.
228. Gainer, H. (1972). Electrophysiological behaviour of an endogenously active neurosecretory cell. Brain Res. 39:403.
229. Silverman, A. J., and Zimmerman, E. A. (1975). Ultrastructural immunocytochemical localization of neurophysin and vasopressin in the median eminence and posterior pituitary of the guinea pig. Cell Tissue Res. 159:291.
230. Meyer, V., and Knobil, E. (1966). Stimulation of growth hormone secretion by vasopressin in the rhesus monkey. Endocrinology 79:1016.
231. Clayton, G. W., Librik, L., Gardner, R. L., and Guillemin, R. (1963). Studies on the circadian rhythm of the pituitary adrenocorticotropic release in man. J. Clin. Endocrinol. Metab. 23:975.
232. Yates, F. E., Russell, S. M., Dallman, M. F., Hedge, G. A., McCann, S. M., and Dhariwal, A. P. S. (1971). Potentiation by vasopressin of corticotropin release induced by corticotropin-releasing factor. Endocrinology 88:3.
233. De Wied, D. (1971). Long term effect of vasopressin on the maintenance of a conditioned avoidance response in rats. Nature (London) 232:58.
234. Van Wimersma Greidanus, T. B., Bohus, B., and De Wied, D. (1973). Effects of peptide hormones on behaviour. In Proceedings of the Fourth International Congress on Endocrinology, Excerpta Med. Int. Congr., Series No. 273. p. 197. Excerpta Medica, Amsterdam.
235. De Wied, D., Bohus, B., and Van Wimersma Greidanus, T. B. (1975). Memory deficit in rats with hereditary diabetes insipidus. Brain Res. 85:152.
236. De Wied, D., Greven, H. M., Lande, S., and Witter, A. (1972). Dissociation of the behavioural and endocrine effects of lysine vasopressin by tryptic digestion. Br. J. Pharmacol. 45:118.

International Review of Physiology
Endocrine Physiology II, Volume 16
Edited by S. M. McCann
Copyright 1977   University Park Press   Baltimore

2
The Hypothalamic Hypophysiotropic Hormones

L. KRULICH and C. P. FAWCETT

Department of Physiology, University of Texas Health Science Center
at Dallas, Dallas, Texas

Research concerning the hypothalamic hypophysiotropic hormones (HHH) is at the present time in a period of explosive growth, which is still gaining momentum. The number of publications related to the many aspects of this field grew at a pace which makes it difficult to keep abreast of all the new developments and impossible to cite them all in this review. The reader will, therefore, often be referred to review articles instead of to the original papers. As rapid as the growth of the field is, still it is uneven. Tremendous advances were achieved with respect to luteinizing hormone-releasing hormone (LRH), thyroid-stimulating hormone-releasing hormone (TRH), and growth hormone release-inhibiting hormone (somatostatin), but the progress in other areas was much slower. These disproportions are also reflected in the present chapter, although an attempt was made to provide a balanced view of the entire field.

There is so far no unanimity with respect to the nomenclature of the HHH; therefore, the simplest nomenclature is considered the best and is used throughout the chapters.

DISTRIBUTION OF HHH

Studies on the distribution of the hypophysiotropic neurohormones in the structures of the central nervous system (CNS) and the related questions of their origin and transport enjoyed a considerable interest and provided many new, unexpected, and valuable data. The main impetus which intensified this line of research was the development of specific radioimmunoassays (RIA) for determination of LRH, TRH, and somatostatin (1–3). This made possible direct determination of these substances in minute quantities and enabled successful use of the nuclear punch technique introduced by Palkovits (4), which in turn made possible isolated removal of individual nuclei and other brain structures. Although these techniques provide a detailed quantitative picture of the gross anatomical distribution of the three neurohormones, they tell nothing about the structural elements with which they are associated. An insight into this problem was obtained by use of the respective antibodies for development of various immunohistological techniques which were applied successfully for direct visualization of the cellular elements involved in the production, transport, and storage of the three neurohormones.

LRH

Studies based on direct determination of LRH by RIA either in thin hypothalamic sections (5) or in the nuclear punches (6) show a relatively simple pattern of distribution. The bulk of LRH, approximately 85% of the total hypothalamic content, is concentrated in the median eminence-arcuate nucleus region. From this amount the median eminence (ME) itself holds 75–80%. Smaller but unmistakable LRH activity is also in the preoptic region in the vicinity of the lamina terminalis (5). These findings are in a good general agreement with the earlier work based on less direct measurements (7–9).

It seems that a large part of the preoptic LRH as found by Wheaton et al. (5) is actually located extrahypothalamically in the organum vasculosum of the lamina terminalis (OVLT), where it was first detected by immunohistology (10) and later determined directly by RIA (11). Smaller but significant quantities of LRH are also in the three remaining periventricular organs (subfornical, subcommisural, and area postrema) (11). There also may be some LRH in the pineal gland and in the brain cortex (12, 13), but there is no universal agreement on this point (14, 15).

Results obtained with immunohistological techniques agree quite well with the pattern of LRH distribution just outlined, but they vary considerably with respect to the LRH-containing structures, which can be visualized. Species differences may be one of the several reasons for the disagreements.

In rat brains, the majority of workers (16–19) detected only LRH-positive nerve fibers in the median eminence and in the OVLT. The fibers in the ME seem to emerge from the retrochiasmatic area or arcuate nucleus; they then appear to form two laterally located bundles and terminate in the external lateral part of the palisade zone of the ME. The nerve terminals are often seen arranged close to the pericapillary spaces of the primary plexus of the portal vessels, and the LRH-positive material in the terminals is packaged in the form of small, dense core vesicles (17). LRH-containing nerve cells were described only by Zimmerman (10) in the arcuate nucleus, and in the preoptic area by Sétáló (20), who, however, had to use special experimental conditions (protracted pentobarbital anesthesia or retrochiasmatic cuts) to make them visible.

In contrast, Barry and associates (21), using guinea pigs, found LRH-containing cell bodies in many structures extending from the septal-preoptic area to the caudal hypothalamus. Many nerve fibers were also detected, some of them forming a preopticoinfundibular pathway, others running to many hypothalamic and extrahypothalamic structures. The perikarya in larger numbers were, however, detectable only if the animals were pretreated with intraventricular injections of drugs, which presumably stopped the axoplasmic flow or inhibited LRH release (colchicine, melotonin). These results, which were heavily criticized, were recently confirmed by Sétáló (20) and by Silverman (22), who was able to detect LRH-positive nerve cells in completely normal animals.

In mouse brains, the LRH nerve terminals were, on the other hand, seen in close association with the tanycytes (15) and, according to other reports, the LRH immunoreactive material was found in the tanycytes themselves (10, 22). In all cases, LRH-positive nerve cells were present in the arcuate nucleus. In primate brains, LRH neurons were concentrated also in the mediobasal hypothalamus and in the preoptic area (23).

TRH

TRH has a far more complex pattern of distribution than LRH. Krulich et al. (8, 24) also found it in high concentrations, aside from the median eminence-arcuate nucleus, in the dorsomedial nucleus and in a larger, less well defined region of the preoptic area. These results were later confirmed and expanded by Brownstein et al. (25) using the nuclear punch technique and RIA, which detected TRH in high concentrations also in the ventral-rostral part of the ventromedial nucleus and in the periventricular nucleus. Lesser concentrations were found in many other locations in the hypothalamus and in the preoptic and septal areas. All four periventricular organs, the pineal and neurohypophysis, contain contain significant amounts of TRH (11, 26).

Most surprising were, however, the reports from several laboratories that TRH is not confined to the hypothalamus and preoptic area, but that it can be detected in most other brain structures (for review see ref. 27). The physiological significance of the extrahypothalamic TRH is unknown, and recently Jeffcoate and White (28) questioned its authenticity.

Immunohistological studies are so far very rare and showed only TRH-positive fibers in most of the TRH-rich hypothalamic structures (29).

Somatostatin

Growth hormone release-inhibiting activity was first detected by Krulich et al. (30) in the median eminence and in lesser amounts also in the suprachiasmatic area in rat brains. Later work based on RIA (31) showed that somatostatin, not unlike TRH, is found not only in the hypothalamus but in many other sites in the CNS. Among the hypothalamic structures with high concentrations of somatostatin, not counting the median eminence, are the arcuate, ventromedial, ventral premammillary, and the periventricular nucleus. Somatostatin is also in the periventricular organs and in the pineal gland (11, 31).

These findings correlate well with immunohistological studies, which show somatostatin-positive nerve fibers in the median eminence, where their course differs from the LRH fibers, and in the hypothalamic nuclei, which were shown to contain high concentrations of somatostatin by RIA (32). In contrast, somatostatin-positive cell bodies were detected only in the area of the periventricular nucleus (32, 33). Somatostatin was further detected in the substantia gelatinosa of the dorsal horns of the spinal cord, and scattered cells also were found in the spinal ganglia (32).

The distribution of somatostatin is, however, not limited to the CNS structures. Both direct determination by RIA and immunohistology showed large amounts of somatostatin in the wall of the stomach, duodenum, upper jejunum, and in the pancreas (32, 34, 35). In the pancreas, somatostatin is contained in the argentophylic D-cells of the islets of Langerhans (32). It has not been established whether all this material is identical with the hypothalamic tetradecapeptide or whether it is a different but immunologically related peptide.

Others

In contrast to this wealth of data on the distribution of LRH, TRH, and somatostatin, our present knowledge of the distribution of the remaining neurohormones in very limited. Krulich et al. (30), using bioassay and thin hypothalamic sections, detected growth hormone-releasing activity in the ventromedial nucleus and the adjacent lateral region. The same authors (36) also found prolactin-releasing activity in the median eminence and in the basal portion of the anterior hypothalamus, whereas the lateral portions of the anterior hypothalamus exhibited a prolactin release-inhibiting activity. However, since prolactin release in in vitro systems can be influenced by catecholamines, TRH, somatostatin, and possibly γ-aminobutyric acid, it is difficult to decide whether these activities were due to genuine prolactin-releasing factor (PRF) and prolactin release-inhibiting factor (PIF) or to some other factors. Taleisnik et al. (37) reported the presence of a melanocyte-stimulating hormone (MSH)-releasing factor in the paraventricular nucleus, whereas supraoptic nucleus has MSH release-inhibiting activity. Quite recently, Krieger et al. (38) demonstrated very high corticotropin-releasing factor (CRF) activity in the median eminence and smaller but still substantial activity in the arcuate, ventromedial, dorsomedial, and periventricular nuclei, but no activity either in preoptic and septal areas or in other cerebral structures, with a possible exception of the thalamus.

ORIGIN OF HHH

The localization studies, especially the immunohistological techniques, demonstrated conclusively that the HHH are true neurosecretions. They are produced in specialized nerve cells, presumably conveyed in their axons by axoplasmic flow to the terminals, where they are stored before being released. The multiplicity of the hypothalamic and extrahypothalamic sites in which the individual neurohormones can be detected brings up an important question: which of these sites are production sites, which are storage sites and, more specifically, which of the production sites feed their product to the median eminence and thus participate in the regulation of adenohypophysial secretions?

LRH

This problem was so far best studied in the case of LRH. The current evidence indicates that LRH in the median eminence is derived both from the arcuate nuclei and preoptic area.

Despite the fact that it is difficult to find LRH-positive nerve cells in the arcuate nuclei in the rat, there is little doubt that arcuate nucleus is producing LRH, which is involved in the regulation of gonadotropin secretion. Elimination of anterior hypothalamus by lesions (39) as well as complete or partial surgical isolation of the mediobasal hypothalamus (40–43) have only a relatively small and variable effect on the basal gonadotropin levels, and they do not eliminate the control of gonadotropin secretion by negative feedback of gonadal steroids, although they may impede it to a variable extent.

There is also, however, good evidence for the participation of the preoptic LRH. It was shown first by Schneider et al. (44) that lesions in the suprachiasmatic area reduced bioassayable LRH in the median eminence. More recently, complete deafferentation of mediobasal hypothalamus (MBH) or even frontal retrochiasmatic cuts were reported to reduce the LRH content in the median eminence by 60–90% (42, 43, 45, 46). According to Kalra (42) and Kalra et al. (43), there is a concomitant increase of the LRH content in the rostral areas (in front of the cut), which is presumably due to accumulation of LRH because of the interruption of its transport to the caudal hypothalamus. These results seem to indicate

that the preoptic LRH is actually a major source of the LRH in the median
eminence and that it also plays a major role in the overall LRH economy and in
the regulation of gonadotropin secretion. It is, however, questionable whether
the degree of LRH depletion in the ME following placements of the cuts is
directly proportional to the contribution by the preoptic LRH. Interruption of
nervous inputs which may influence synthesis of LRH in the arcuate region,
together with an increased drain put on it by the operation of the negative
feedback, may be responsible for an incalculable part of the depletion.

TRH

The present information on the site or sites of origin of TRH is still limited.
Mitnick and Reichlin (47) reported that fragments of hypothalamic tissue
obtained either from the mediobasal or dorsomedial hypothalamus synthesize
TRH in vitro from the precursor amino acids. Similarly, Knigge et al. (48) found
TRH synthesis in hypothalamic tissue in an area extending from the pericomis-
sural region to the caudal hypothalamus. These findings indicated that TRH
might be produced at many different sites. This work was, however, criticized on
several accounts (49, for review see ref. 27), and its validity is doubtful.

In contrast, it has been shown repeatedly that lesions in the anterior
hypothalamus, especially in the area of the paraventricular nuclei, impair thyroid
function and depress serum thyroid-stimulating hormone (TSH) levels presumably by impairing TRH release (for references see 24, 50). Mess (51) reported a
complete disappearance of bioassayable TRH from the mediobasal hypothalamus following electrolytic destruction of the paraventricular or suprachiasmatic
nucleus; more recently, a large decrease of immunoassayable TRH in the MBH
was found in rats subjected to frontal retrochiasmatic cuts (52). These findings
suggest that TRH in the structures of the MBH is mostly derived from anterior
hypothalamus or preoptic area. In contrast, Hefco et al. (53, 54) concluded from
the effects of different types of hypothalamic deafferentations on TSH secretion
that most of the TRH which is involved in the regulation of TSH secretion is
produced in the arcuate nucleus.

Somatostatin

Somatostatin-positive cell bodies have been found so far only in the periventricular nuclei, whereas in other somatostatin-rich hypothalamic areas only nerve
fibers were detected. The obvious implication that somatostatin is produced by
the nerve cells of the periventricular nuclei and conveyed to the other structures
finds support in a recent demonstration that a complete deafferentation of the
MBH leads to a drastic reduction of somatostatin content inside the hypothalamic island (55).

In contrast, the same operation increased the CRF content in the deafferented island (38), which may mean that CRF is produced in the structures of
the mediobasal hypothalamus, whereas its release is controlled by inputs from
the outside.

INTRACEREBRAL TRANSPORT OF HHH

There is no doubt that the HHH reach the pituitary by way of the hypophysial portal vessels. This is supported by extensive indirect evidence as well as by detection of several of the neurohormones in pituitary stalk blood. There is, however, less unanimity with respect to the mechanism by which the neurohormones get into the blood in the capillaries of the primary plexus.

The more generally accepted view is that they diffuse into it across the pericapillary spaces after having been released from their respective nerve terminals. Although this very process has not been directly demonstrated, the anatomical organization of the nerve terminals in the proximity of the capillaries makes it very likely.

According to the alternative hypothesis, concurrently with this process the neurohormones are also released into the cerebrospinal fluid of the ventricles and reabsorbed from it by specialized ependymal cells, tanycytes, lining the floor of the third ventricle. They are subsequently released into the pericapillary spaces from the processes of the tanycytes, which penetrate the median eminence. It is sometimes suggested that this indirect transport may play a role also for the neurohormones released from the nerve terminals in the median eminence.

This view originated from morphological studies of the structure of the tanycytes (56, 57) but was later adopted by some workers on functional grounds (48, 58–60) which are briefly listed below.

LRH and TRH were found in considerable quantities in rat cerebrospinal fluid (CSF) by Knigge and co-workers (61–63), and TRH was also found in human CSF (64). However, Cramer and Barraclough (65) failed to detect LRH in rat CSF. LRH and TRH injected into the ventricular CSF can reach the pituitary via the hypophysial portal system and stimulate release of luteinizing hormone (LH) or TSH, respectively (66, 67). Involvement of the tanycytes in this process is indicated by findings that labeled neurohormones injected into the ventricles are later found in the tanycytes (68, 69).

Although many of these observations are quite suggestive, it is impossible to determine at the present time whether this mechanism plays a physiological role and how important it might be with respect to the transport by diffusion from the nerve terminals. The source of the LRH and TRH in CSF is unclear. They may perhaps arise from circumventricular organs such as the OVLT.

EFFECTS OF HHH

LRH

LRH is certainly the best studied member of the entire neurohormone family. A large amount of early work was done with semipurified hypothalamic preparations; after the synthetic product became available, it was tested extensively both in animals and humans in a large variety of conditions (for review see refs. 9, 70–74).

It has been conclusively demonstrated that either the highly purified natural product or the synthetic decapeptide stimulates secretion of LH as well as of follicle-stimulating hormone (FSH) both in vivo and in vitro (75, 76). There are, however, significant differences between the two gonadotropins.

LH responds to even a brief pulse of LRH produced by intravenous injection of a small dose of the neurohormone. The secretory response is so rapid that an elevation of serum LH levels is detectable within 2 min after the injection and attains peak values within 10–12 min. The responses are dose-related–in the rat, for instance, over a range from 1 to 50 ng/animal (77, 78). In order to stimulate FSH secretion, the elevated levels of LRH have to be maintained for prolonged periods of time, either by continuous infusion of LRH or by subcutaneous administration of larger doses (76, 79). The FSH-releasing mechanism has a lower sensitivity than the LH mechanism even if the time factor is eliminated (80, 81), dose-related responses are more difficult to establish, and the dynamics of the secretory responses is also different from the dynamics of LH (79). These differences and other physiological evidence still leave some doubt whether the regulation of the secretion of both gonadotropins can be explained by LRH only, as has been postulated by Schally et al. (82).

An appropriate dose of LRH given at an appropriate time was shown to induce ovulation in hamsters, rabbits, rats, or women (78, 83, 84). In in vitro conditions, LRH stimulates not only release of both gonadotropins but also their synthesis. The effect can be demonstrated more readily in long-term cultures of pituitary cells (85, 86) than in short-term incubations, which produced positive (87) as well as negative results (88, 89). It is, however, not clear whether the stimulation of synthesis is an effect independent from the release of gonadotropins or a secondary process induced by it. There is no indication that LRH acts on other pituitary hormones, at least not in normal individuals (90).

TRH

The effects of TRH on the secretion of TSH resemble in general the effects of LRH on LH secretion to the extent that it would be redundant to describe them in any detail (91–94; for review see refs. 73, 74, 95). In addition to TSH, TRH stimulates secretion of prolactin and under certain conditions the secretion of growth hormone (GH).

The effect of TRH on the secretion of prolactin was first described by Tashjian (96) in in vitro conditions, but it was shown subsequently in vivo in several species, including humans (97–100). There are, however, large differences in the responsiveness of the lactotrophs among the different species. In lactating cows, the prolactin response is larger than the TSH response (99); in humans both systems respond approximately equally (101), whereas in rats, with a partial exception of females in proestrus, the thyrotrophs are much more sensitive than the lactotrophs (100, 102). Females in general respond more than males (100, 101, 103), most probably because of a sensitization of the lacto- trophs by estrogen (100, 104).

It has been suggested that TRH is a physiological regulator of prolactin secretion and that it actually might be the rather elusive PRF (101). This assumption seems unwarranted because the secretion of both hormones, under physiological conditions, is more often dissociated than associated. In humans, nursing or stress stimulates prolactin secretion but does not affect TSH (105, 106). In rats, stress also stimulates prolactin, but actually inhibits TSH (107). Similar dissociation can be induced in rats by exposure to either cold or heat (108, 109). Conversely, there are several reports claiming the existence of a PRF distinct from TRH.

Somatostatin

The discovery of growth hormone release-inhibiting factor (GIF) in purified sheep hypothalamic extracts was based on the property of this substance to inhibit GH release from rat pituitaries in vitro (110, 111). The same property was later used for its complete purification, which led to the elucidation of its structure by Brazeau et al. (112), who renamed it somatostatin.

It was subsequently shown that in in vitro systems somatostatin inhibits basal release of GH as well as release stimulated by cyclic AMP or theophylline (113, 114). The inhibition lasts as long as somatostatin is present in the system, but it is followed by an increased release after somatostatin has been removed (115). The magnitude of the rebound is proportional to the magnitude of the inhibition, so that no net inhibition results if both phases are taken into account (116).

Inhibition of growth hormone secretion in vivo was demonstrated in several animal species, as well as in humans, under a great variety of experimental conditions (for review see refs. 114, 117). The inhibitory effects are dose-re- lated, but very short-lived if somatostatin is administered as a single bolus. In order to obtain sustained effects, the neurohormone has to be given in a continuous infusion. Upon discontinuation of the infusion, GH secretion is rapidly resumed and a rebound increase of secretion is often seen.

After synthetic somatostatin became available, it was soon discovered that it inhibits many other secretory processes, the list of which is still growing. In addition to GH, somatostatin consistently inhibits TRH-stimulated TSH secre- tion, but not basal release of TSH. In in vitro systems, it also inhibits basal release of prolactin (118, 119), but no effects were found in vivo (120) and, therefore, the significance of the effect of somatostatin on the secretion of prolactin is uncertain.

The most surprising discovery, however, was that somatostatin inhibits secretion of insulin and glucagon in humans and other species (121–123) by a direct effect on the islets of Langerhans (124, 125).

The physiological significance of this effect is unknown, but it is highly probable that somatostatin is involved in the regulation of secretion of the pancreatic hormones. For this possibility speak the facts that somatostatin is produced by the D-cell of the islets and that the volume density and number of these cells are increased in juvenile diabetics as well as in rats made experimentally diabetic by Streptozotocin (126).

In addition to these effects on the endocrine pancreas, somatostatin also inhibits secretion of gastrin (127), hydrochloric acid (128), secretin (129) and cholecystokinin-pankreozymin (130). By these actions it may influence gastric and pancreatic secretions as well as the motility of the stomach and gallbladder (131). The physiological significance of these effects is unknown, but again probable because of the presence of somatostatin in stomach, duodenum, and jejunum.

Others

The knowledge of the effects of the remaining neurohormones is much more limited in scope and in most instances does not go beyond demonstration that they stimulate or inhibit the secretion of the corresponding pituitary hormones in vivo or in vitro. Therefore, only a partial list of references is given where the pertinent information can be found: GRF effects in vitro (132), in vivo (133, 134), PIF in vitro (135, 136), in vivo (137), PRF (138–140), CRF (141), melanocyte-stimulating hormone release-inhibiting factor (MIF) and melanocyte-stimulating hormone-releasing factor (MRF) (142).

REGULATION OF SECRETION AND EFFECTS OF HHH

The hypothalamo-adenohypophysial pituitary systems obviously can be divided into two categories with respect to the basic principles of their regulation. In the case of the hypothalamo-gonadotropic, -thyrotropic, and adrenocorticotropic systems, the basic regulation rests on the negative feedback exerted by the respective target hormones. It is now becoming clear that the feedback effects of the target hormones rest in turn on a simultaneous modulation of the effects as well as of the release of the corresponding hypothalamic releasing hormones. The regulation of the secretion of growth hormone, prolactin, and possibly MSH has, in contrast, the character of an open loop system. It seems that in this instance the stability as well as flexibility of the secretion of these hormones is safeguarded by two hypothalamic neurohormones for each pituitary hormone, which have opposite effects on their secretion. Unfortunately, with the exception of somatostatin, our knowledge of the properties of these neurohormones and of the working of these systems is still rather elementary.

LRH and Gonadotropins

Modulation of Effects and Secretion of LRH by Negative Feedback of Gonadal Steroids   It has been shown by several workers (143–145) that estrogens or testosterone inhibits secretion of gonadotropins by a direct effect on the pituitary gonadotrophs. It is now becoming clear that this effect is mainly due to a decrease of responsiveness of the gonadotrophs to LRH. The gonadotropin secretory response to exogenous LRH is conspicuously decreased or completely suppressed in normal or castrated male rats treated with testosterone (146, 147), in ovariectomized female rats treated with estrogen (148, 149), and in normal women with artificially elevated estrogen levels (150, 151). The inhibitory effect of gonadal steroids can also be demonstrated on pituitaries incubated in vitro (152, 153, 154).

In contrast, the responsiveness to LRH is enhanced in subjects with hypogonadism (151), and a small increase was seen also in rats following castration (155).

The effect of progesterone on the pituitary responsiveness to LRH is controversial. According to some reports, progesterone reduced pituitary responsiveness (156, 157), but other workers failed to see any effect (158, 159).

There is at the present time little doubt that the gonadal steroids also inhibit the release of LRH from the hypothalamus. This was indicated by several earlier studies, based on indirect indices, that intrahypothalamic implants of estrogen or testosterone inhibit gonadotropin secretion, presumably by inhibiting release of LRH (for review see ref. 160). More recently it was shown that intra-hypothalamic implants of testosterone or systemic injection of estradiol increases the hypothalamic content of LRH, possibly by reducing its release (145, 161), and injection of small quantities of estradiol into the third ventricle lowered LH levels in ovariectomized female rats without affecting their pituitary responsiveness to exogenous LRH (162).

In contrast, there is conclusive evidence that LRH release is enhanced following castration. This is documented by demonstration of an increased concentration of bioassayable LRH in portal blood (163, 164) and of radio-immunoassayable LRH in systemic circulation (165, 166). It has also been conclusively shown by direct determination of LRH in portal blood of ovariec-tomized monkeys that the increase of LRH secretion occurs in the form of secretory pulses of low frequency but very large amplitude (167).

This pulsatile release of LRH explains in all likelihood the large periodic fluctuations of serum LH levels, the so-called circhoral rhythm, described in ovariectomized monkeys, rats, and sheep (168–170). The mechanism which generates these pulses is not known. It resides in the medial-basal hypothalamus since it is not abolished by complete deafferentation of this region (171, 172), and it is related to the activity of the central neurotransmitter systems because it is modified by drugs which affect the activity of the noradrenergic, dopa-minergic, and cholinergic systems, respectively (173, 174).

Regulation of Gonadotropin Secretion by Positive Feedback   In contrast to the negative feedback regulation which operates in both sexes and is exerted by both types of gonadal steroids, the positive feedback, in its full extent and under physiological conditions, operates only in females and is primarily induced by elevated levels of estrogen. As is the case with negative feedback, it also has a pituitary and a central component (for review see refs. 175, 176).

The pituitary manifestations of the positive feedback are, phenomenologically, the reverse of the negative feedback and appear as an enhancement of the pituitary responsiveness to LRH. A conspicuous augmentation of LH secretory response to injection of an LRH-containing hypothalamic extract was first demonstrated by Ramirez and McCann (177) in spayed rats given a large dose of estrogen and progesterone. The enhancement of the secretory responses of both gonadotropins to exogenous LRH following administration of estrogen was subsequently documented in females of several species, including humans (158, 178). The effect can be induced in normal as well as in spayed animals, and much smaller doses of estrogen than those used originally by Ramirez and McCann (177) are effective. Progesterone has no effect either alone or in combination with estrogen (158).

In contrast to the inhibitory effect of estrogen which appears rapidly, the augmented effect appears with a latency of several hours. Therefore, administration of a single dose of estrogen has a biphasic effect, first inducing an inhibition of the pituitary responsiveness, which is later superseded by the augmented responsiveness (159, 179).

Central Component of Positive Feedback   Administration of estrogen to normal or ovariectomized females is followed within several to many hours, depending upon the species and arrangement of the experiment, by a massive release of gonadotropins, which resembles the spontaneous preovulatory surge. There is conclusive evidence that this effect of estrogen is mediated by the hypothalamus and preoptic area (for review see 175, 176). The details of the mechanism of this effect are only incompletely understood. It is likely that estrogen, acting on estrogen-sensitive neurons, facilitates neural inputs which eventually enhance release of LRH, which in combination with the simultaneously augmented pituitary responsiveness and the self-priming effect of LRH (see below) brings about the gonadotropin surge.

Self-priming Effect of LRH   It has been shown first by Aiyer et al. (180) and confirmed later by Castro-Vazques and McCann (181) that if two doses of LRH, separated by 60 min, are administered to rats in the afternoon of proestrus, the LH secretory response to the second injection is much larger than the response to the first one. During the other stages of the estrous cycle, this effect is small or absent. FSH secretion also participates in this effect although in a less striking manner than LH (182). It has been further shown that this self-potentiating effect can be reproduced by release of endogenous LRH induced by electrical stimulation of the preoptic area and that it occurs regardless of whether LRH is administered in separate injections or in a continuous infusion (183). Recently, this phenomenon was demonstrated in normal women at midcycle (151).

The self-potentiating effect is induced in the rat by the elevated levels of estrogen on the morning of proestrus, because it is abolished by ovariectomy on diestrus day 2 and restored by administration of estrogen (184). The importance of estrogen is further documented by findings that the self-priming effect can also be obtained in neonatally androgenized rats (181) which have elevated levels of estrogen.

The mechanism of the LRH self-potentiation is not clear. It appears to depend upon de novo RNA-directed protein synthesis (185) and may involve LRH receptors, since a positive cooperativity between LRH and its pituitary receptors was found (186). An increased availability of releasable LH may be another factor (187).

LRH Effects and Secretion During Ovarian Cycle According to present concepts, it seems that ovarian cycles result basically from the alternations of the negative and positive feedback effects of estrogen. The low gonadotropin levels encountered throughout most of the cycle are undoubtedly an expression of the negative feedback effect of the relatively low levels of estrogen, whereas the preovulatory surge is due to the positive feedback effect of the rapidly rising estrogen levels which precede it.

The alternations of the negative and positive effects are clearly shown by the cyclic variability of the pituitary responsiveness to exogenous LRH. In the rat, the responsiveness to LRH increases during proestrus, attaining an abrupt maximum on the afternoon of proestrus (184, 188, 189). It seems that a large part of this conspicuous and sudden increase of pituitary responsiveness is actually caused by a preceding priming of the pituitary with endogenous LRH rather than by an increased responsiveness of the gonadotrophs per se. To this effect points the fact that administration of pentobarbital at approximately 1:30 p.m., which blocks release of LRH, greatly reduces the responsiveness (190, 191). Similar cyclic variability of the pituitary responsiveness was also described in other species, which include the ewe, monkey, and woman at midcycle (192–194).

There is no doubt that the enhanced responsiveness combined with the self-priming effect of LRH plays a major part in the mechanism of the preovulatory surge, but recent observations suggest that the release of LRH is also enhanced at the same time.

Elevated or, more exactly, detectable levels of LRH were found in plasma of normal women at midcycle (195, 196), but negative results were also reported (13). Similarly, a higher incidence of detectable or even elevated levels of LRH was reported in rats killed by decapitation in the afternoon of proestrus (166, 197). In a recent work (198), consistently elevated LRH levels were found on the afternoon of proestrus in pituitary stalk blood of female rats anesthetized with Althesin, an anesthetic which does not block the proestrus gonadotropin surge. Similar findings were also reported in monkeys (Neil et al. cited by Sarkar in ref. 198). The difficulties in detecting elevated levels of LRH in peripheral blood of nonanesthetized serially sampled sheep or rats during the preovulatory gonadotropin surge (165, 166, 199, 200) may simply reflect the fact that the changes of LRH in peripheral blood are too small to be measured due to the high degree of dilution of pituitary blood in systemic circulation.

Modulation of TRH Effects and
Secretion by Negative Feedback of Thyroid Hormones

The basic characteristics of the regulation of TSH secretion are very similar to those of the negative feedback regulation of gonadotropins (for review see refs. 50, 201).

Thyroid hormones, T_3 being approximately 5 times more potent than T_4, inhibit the TSH-releasing effect of TRH by a direct action on the pituitary thyrotrophs, as has been shown in several experiments in vivo and in vitro (202–204). Similarly, the TSH secretory responses to exogenous TRH are diminished or completely suppressed in hyperthyroid human subjects, whereas they are exaggerated in patients with primary hypothyroidism (205, 206). The feedback modulation of the TRH effects is very delicate, so that changes of thyroid hormone levels, which are still in the range of physiological variability, markedly influence TSH responses to exogenous TRH in human subjects (207, 208). Similar observations were recently reported also in rats (209).

It is not clear at the present time whether the thyroid hormones also modulate release of TRH. Injections or implants of thyroxine into the anterior hypothalamus (210, 211) or to the immediate vicinity of the paraventricular nucleus (212) were reported to inhibit thyroid activity. Conversely, a decrease of bioassayable TRH was found in the hypothalami of thyroidectomized rats, perhaps resulting from an increased release (213).

Although these results seem to indicate that elevated levels of thyroid hormones inhibit TRH release and vice versa, recent results based on direct determinations of TRH by RIA are rather confusing. Reichlin et al. (201) proposed a hypothesis according to which thyroid hormones inhibit TRH effect at the pituitary level but stimulate its release from the hypothalamus. This hypothesis was based on observations that thyroxin stimulated synthesis of TRH in hypothalamic tissue in vitro and on the observation that rats treated with thyroxine excrete more TRH in urine than controls (214). However, doubts were voiced about the validity of the results concerning the in vitro synthesis of TRH (49) as well as about the identity of the TRH-like activity in urine (215). In contrast, several other workers (216–218) failed to find any changes in hypothalamic or plasma levels of TRH in animals made experimentally hyper- or hypothyroid.

Effect of Cold and Heat on Secretion of TRH   It has been known for a long time that exposure to low ambient temperature activates the pituitary thyroid system, and it was assumed from indirect evidence that this activation is caused by an increased release of TRH (for review see refs. 201, 219). This assumption was recently confirmed by demonstration of elevated TRH levels in systemic circulation of rats exposed to cold (217, 220), although negative results were also reported (218).

Exposure to heat, on the contrary, leads to a very marked reduction of serum TSH levels (108). It is probable that this effect is due to a reduced release of TRH since the TSH levels are low despite an increased pituitary responsiveness to exogenous TRH (108). It should be noted that, in contrast to rats, exposure to cold or heat has no effect on serum TSH in normal human subjects (221, 222).

Modulation of Effects of TRH by Somatostatin Soon after somatostatin became available it was found that, in addition to its many other effects, it also inhibits TRH-stimulated TSH release in animals (223) and in humans, although it has no effect on the basal secretion of TSH (224). The inhibitory effect is also readily demonstrable in in vitro experiments on cultured pituitary cells (115, 204, 223). The inhibitory effect has a noncompetitive character, and the inhibition takes place beyond the TRH-TRH receptor interaction (225). Several recent reports indicate that in the rat this effect of somatostatin may have physiological significance, since neutralization of endogenous somatostatin by injection of antisomatostatin antibodies elevated basal levels of TSH and enhanced TSH response either to exogenous TRH or to exposure to cold (226–228).

However, the rat is so far the only known species which reacts to stress, including the stress of exposure to cold, with an enhanced release of somatostatin and it is, therefore, premature to make any general conclusions.

Modulation of Effects of CRF and its Secretion by Negative Feedback of Cortical Steroids and by Stress

The regulation of the secretion of ACTH is a rather complex affair because the negative feedback regulation by adrenal glucocorticoids is countered by the effects of stress, which activates ACTH release through release of hypothalamic CRF (for reviews see refs. 229, 230).

Glucocorticoids, as do the other target hormones in the feedback regulated systems, exert their effect mainly by inhibiting the ACTH-releasing effect of CRF on the corticotrophs (231, 232), although they probably also inhibit synthesis of ACTH (233). The feedback effects can also be readily demonstrated in vitro. Pituitaries removed from animals treated with corticoids release less ACTH and respond less to a CRF preparation than pituitaries from control animals, whereas pituitaries from adrenalectomized rats show opposite changes (234, 235). Corticoids added to the in vitro system inhibit both the basal as well as CRF-stimulated ACTH release and probably also synthesis of ACTH (233, 235, 236).

Recent evidence further indicates that corticoids, in addition to their effects at the pituitary level, also modulate release of CRF from the hypothalamus. It has been shown that the release of CRF from synaptosomes prepared from hypothalami of rats treated with corticoids was reduced with respect to controls. Corticoids had an inhibitory effect also upon addition to the synaptosomes in vitro (237). Conversely, hypothalami removed from adrenalectomized rats released more CRF in vitro than controls (238) and systemic administration of corticoids reduced the CRF content in isolated hypothalamic islands (38).

There is little doubt that stress activates CRF release from the hypothalamus. This is borne out by findings that lesions in the median eminence prevent the stress-induced activation of adrenocortical secretion (239). Stress also leads to marked changes of the CRF content in the median eminence, which are characterized by an almost instantaneous increase, followed by a decline during the ensuing 10–20 min which might be followed by another increase 60 min later if an intense stress is used (240, 241).

Since stress activates the secretion of corticoids, which, in turn, inhibit both the release and effects of CRF, it was natural to search for the mutual interplay of these two effects.

It has been shown that administration of corticoids can inhibit the reaction to stress, although some types of stress (laparotomy with intestinal traction) are rather corticoid-resistant (242). It further seems that the inhibitory effect of corticoids is due to two different mechanisms. One type of inhibition is almost instantaneous, but transient, and it is related to the rate of increase of serum corticoid levels, but not to their absolute levels (243). The second type of inhibition has a latency of approximately 1 hr, lasts for many hours, and is related to the corticoid levels.

It seems that both types of inhibition are exerted by endogenous corticoids released during stress. Pointing in this direction are the findings that adrenalectomy, which at the same time elicits stress but eliminates corticoid release, leads to a larger and longer lasting elevation of serum ACTH levels than a sham operation (244). Simultaneous monitoring of hypothalamic CRF levels and of serum levels of ACTH and corticoids in sham-operated and adrenalectomized rats, either nontreated or given corticoids, indicated that the initial rise of serum corticoids in stressed animals inhibits CRF release, whereas the elevated levels at the later times inhibit CRF synthesis (241, 245).

Somatostatin and GRF in Regulation of GH Secretion The respective roles of somatostatin and GRF in the regulation of GH secretion are only very poorly understood (for review see ref. 117). One problem is the lack of techniques for determination of either neurohormone in plasma; another complication is the pulsatile character of GH secretion. This feature is very prominent in the rat (246), whereas in humans the pulsatile pattern is strongly expressed mainly during the initial stages of sleep. A further complication is the existence of large differences in the general reactivity of the system among different species. Whereas primates react to many stressful stimuli (hypoglycemia, exercise, vasopressin, emotional stress) by increased secretion of GH, in dogs stress has no influence; in rats, it inhibits GH secretion.

Although somatostatin has been shown to inhibit basal secretion and any type of stimulated GH secretion, the physiological relevance of these effects is still virtually unknown. Only recently two reports were published (247, 248) which indicate that in the rat stress-induced inhibition of GH secretion is probably due to an increased release of somatostatin because it could be partially prevented by administration of an antiserum to somatostatin prior to the application of stress. It is not known whether a similar mechanism operates also in primates. The only indication that it might is contained in Brown's report that the GH secretory response to stress is enhanced in monkeys with lesions in either premammillary nuclei or anterior hypothalamus, both of which contain high concentrations of somatostatin (249).

It seems that the neural inputs for the release of somatostatin are transmitted through the medial preoptic area because its electrical stimulation inhibited GH secretion in the rat (250), whereas its destruction by lesions reversed the effect of stress on GH secretion (251). There might be a slight tonic inhibition even during stress-free states because antiserum to somatostatin increased the amplitude of GH secretory pulses and somewhat elevated their baseline without, however, affecting their frequency (228). In this direction also point observations that frontal cuts through the anterior hypothalamus or complete deafferentation of the MBH increase growth in the rat and are associated in some cases with increased plasma GH levels (252–254). However, the inhibitory influence is obviously working against a background of a positive hypothalamic drive because transection of the pituitary stalk or lesions in the median eminence lead to permanently low levels of GH.

Since there is no evidence that elimination of the inhibitory effect of somatostatin by itself enhances secretion of GH, activation of GH secretion must be due, by exclusion, to some stimulatory influence—most probably to release of GRF. This possibility is documented by several lines of circumstantial evidence. GRF activity was found in the ventromedial nuclei (VMN) (30). Ventromedial nuclei and median eminence are the only hypothalamic sites from which an enhanced GH secretion can be elicited by electrical stimulation (255, 256). In contrast, lesions of the VMN decrease serum GH levels (257), abolish the pulsatile secretion (246), and abolish the GH-releasing effect of electrical stimulation of the basolateral amygdala (250). Finally, activation of GH secretion was seen after direct microinjection of norepinephrine into the ventromedial nuclei (258).

PIF and PRF in Regulation of Prolactin Secretion It has been well established that the low prolactin levels seen in resting conditions are due to a tonic inhibitory influence exerted by the hypothalamus on the secretory activity of the pituitary lactotrophs (for review see refs. 136, 259). Disconnection of the hypothalamo-pituitary linkage either by pituitary stalk section or by transplantation of the pituitary to a site distant from the hypothalamus results in enhanced prolactin secretion. Similar effects are produced by lesions in the median eminence (39). Until recently, it was generally assumed that the tonic inhibition was carried out by hypothalamic PIF, the release of which was in turn activated by the tuberoinfundibular dopaminergic system. It was also assumed that the enhanced release of prolactin observed in lactating females during suckling, in animals exposed to stress, or in animals given drugs which inhibit the activity of the dopaminergic system was due to a decreased release of PIF. In contrast, agents which depress prolactin secretion were assumed to activate PIF release. This contention was supported by data that in the first instance the increased secretion of prolactin was associated with a decrease of the PIF activity in the median eminence, whereas the inhibitory agents were associated with an increase of hypothalamic PIF and in some cases with appearance of PIF activity in peripheral circulation (for review see ref. 136). This rather simple view is being modified at the present time. Several workers raised claims that the PIF activity is actually directly due to dopamine. This would not fundamentally change the basic concept of the inhibitory role of the hypothalamus on prolactin secretion, but there is also growing evidence for the existence of a PRF. If this turns out to be the case, many of the findings concerning the changes of hypothalamic PIF would have to be reevaluated because the assays used in these studies might have measured the net sum of both PIF and PRF activities and might not give a reliable assessment of changes of the PIF alone.

Control of MSH Secretion   As in the case of prolactin, the secretion of MSH appears to be also under a tonic inhibitory influence from the hypothalamus. This notion is supported by findings that pituitary transplantation or hypothalamic lesions (260–262) are associated with changes of pituitary MSH indicative of its increased secretion. Lesions in the paraventricular nuclei were particularly effective and were shown to cause a measurable increase of circulating MSH levels (263). It is usually assumed that the hypothalamic inhibitory influence is due to release of MIF, and the changes seen following hypothalamic lesions are, therefore, explained by removal of the MIF inhibition. It is, however, also possible, at least in some animal species, that the inhibition is carried out directly by dopaminergic nerve fibers which innervate the neurointermediate lobe (264). Several stimuli, such as suckling, copulation, or ingestion of hypertonic saline solution, were reported to stimulate MSH secretion (265, 266), as judged from changes of pituitary MSH concentration, but it is difficult to decide whether these changes were caused by inhibition of MIF or by activation of MRF secretion. Increased release of MRF may be responsible for the increased serum MSH levels in female rats in the morning of proestrus since they were correlated with an increased activity of the hypothalamic MRF-producing enzymes (267). It should be noted that rats secrete α-MSH produced in the neurointermediate lobe, and results obtained in this species are not applicable to humans, who secrete β-MSH produced possibly in the same cell as ACTH (268, 269). The functional role of MSH is mammals is unknown.

ROLE OF CENTRAL NEUROTRANSMITTERS
IN REGULATION OF SECRETION OF HHH

There is little doubt that the release of the HHH and, through them, the secretion of the corresponding pituitary hormones are controlled by the central neurotransmitter systems, which, according to present concepts, include the

dopaminergic (DA), noradrenergic (NE) and possibly adrenergic (E), serotoninergic (SER), and cholinergic systems, although other systems, for instance,
histamine and GABA-ergic systems, were also considered.

This view is documented by copious experimental data on the effects of the
individual transmitters or of drugs which inhibit or mimic their action, on the
secretion of the pituitary hormones, or, in some instances, on the release of the
neurohormones themselves. It is further corroborated by recent research on the
distribution of the neurotransmitters in the CNS, which shows that they are in
high concentrations in certain hypothalamic areas which also contain high
concentrations of the neurohormones (for review see refs. 28, 270).

There is, however, still a considerable confusion and uncertainty about the
roles of the individual transmitters in the release of the individual neurohormones, and many conflicting results have been published. This confusion results
mainly from the complexity of the system, which seems to grow ever greater the
more we know about it and which is not matched by the presently available
research techniques.

It is also true that many experiments, discussed later, are of purely pharmacological character. They only indicate that a certain mechanism might be
operative, but they tell very little about whether the mechanism operates under
physiological conditions and what its role is.

LRH and Gonadotropins

A considerable effort was spent in attempts to elucidate the role of the central
catecholamines in the regulation of LRH release, but the issue still remains
controversial (for review see refs. 29, 271, 272).

Dopamine was found to stimulate LRH release from hypothalami in vitro
(273–275), but negative results were also reported (276). According to the
original work of Schneider and McCann (277, 278) and Kamberi et al. (279,
280), injection of DA into the third ventricle stimulated LRH release in the rat,
whereas NE was effective only if applied in large doses. However, according to
more recent reports based on the same technique, DA had only weak effects
(281), no effect (282, 283), or, in certain situations, inhibited LH release (282),
whereas NE stimulated LH release (281, 283, 284).

The importance of the central NE system in the regulation of gonadotropin
secretion is further emphasized by experiments with drugs which interfere with
its activity. Selective blockade of NE synthesis prevented the postcastration rise
of serum gonadotropins (285, 286), depressed their elevated levels in castrated
animals (174, 287), and prevented the proestrus LH surge (288) or the LH
release induced by progesterone in spayed estrogen-primed rats (289). Blockade
of α receptors has similar effects as inhibition of NE synthesis (289). It seems
that the NE inputs are conveyed to the hypothalamus by the ventral noradrenergic pathway (290).

In contrast to the NE system, activation of the central SER system inhibited
LRH release. Intraventricular injections of serotonin and melatonin depressed

gonadotropin levels in castrated rats (276, 291) and inhibited preovulatory gonadotropin surge and ovulation in rats and ewes (292, 293). However, a certain level of activity of the SER system seems necessary for the operation of the positive feedback because inhibition of SER synthesis with p-chlorophenyl-alanine prevented the estrogen-induced LH surges in ovariectomized rats (294).

There is certainly a cholinergic input into the regulation of LRH release, but its role is also uncertain. Blockade of the muscarinic receptors with atropine inhibited the proestrus surge, as well as the postcastration rise of gonadotropins (295). However, activation of the same receptors with pilocarpine strongly inhibited LH secretion in ovariectomized rats (296), and activation of nicotinic receptors with nicotine inhibited the proestrus surge (297). In contrast, acetylcholine applied to hypothalami in vitro was reported to stimulate LRH release (298).

TRH and TSH   There is growing evidence that the release of TRH is activated by the central NE system as originally suggested by Grimm and Reichlin (299). Increased secretion of TSH was described following administration of the α receptor agonist clonidine (300, 301), whereas selective inhibition of NE syntheses or blockade of α receptors strongly depressed serum TSH levels (300, 302). NE system is almost certainly involved in the cold-induced release of TRH (300, 302, 303).

In contrast, stimulation of the DA receptors with apomorphine inhibited basal- or cold-stimulated secretion of TSH (300, 302, 304), but, since blockade of the DA receptors had no effect, the physiological role of the DA system in the regulation of TRH release is unknown.

The role of the central SER system is also unknown, and the reports available so far are conflicting. Activation of the SER system by a large dose of tryptophan conspicuously inhibited TSH secretion (305), whereas administration of 5-OH-tryptophan, another serotonin precursor, had no effect (305). However, a strong inhibition of TSH secretion was also seen following blockade of serotonin synthesis with p-chlorophenylalanine (306). All these results were obtained in rats. Similar pharmacological interventions in humans had no effect on TSH secretion (307, 308).

GH   In humans and other primates, activation of central NE system, acting via α adrenergic mechanism, stimulates secretion of GH. This is documented by observations that GH secretion can be stimulated by systemic administration of the α receptor agonist clonidine in humans and monkeys (308, 309) or by microinjection of NE into the ventromedial nuclei in baboons (258). Conversely, blockade of α receptors prevents stimulation of GH secretion by hypoglycemia, exercise, or vasopressin (310, 311). In contrast, activation of β receptors appears to inhibit GH secretion as might be assumed from the observation that blockade of β receptors enhances the stimulating effect of hypoglycemia or vasopressin (310, 311).

Contrary to several other hormonal systems, the central DA system possibly also activates GH secretion in humans. This was first inferred from the GH-stimulating effects of systemic administration of L-3,4-dihydroxyphenylalanine (L-dopa) (312) and more recently confirmed by the use of dopamine receptor agonist apomorphine (313, 314). However, in monkeys, apomorphine in subemetic doses had no effect (309).

Stimulation of GH secretion is also seen following activation of the central SER system by administration of 5-OH-tryptophane (309, 315). SER system possibly plays a physiological role because blockade of serotonin receptors prevented activation of GH secretion by hypoglycemia (316).

In the rat, the situation is quite different. The role of the adrenergic receptors seems to be reversed, and activation of the DA system has an inhibiting effect (292, 317). However, activation of the SER system seems to stimulate GH secretion in the rat, as it does in primates (292).

At the present time it is impossible to resolve all these effects in terms of changes of secretion of somatostatin and GRF.

Prolactin   The most conspicuous feature of the transmitter regulation of the secretion of prolactin is its tonic inhibition by the activity of the tuberoinfundibular DA system. This has been amply documented by many pharmacological experiments in rats which show that depletion of central DA or blockade of the DA receptors leads to a conspicuous elevation of serum prolactin, whereas activation of DA receptors following intraventricular injection of dopamine or systemic injection of L-dopa or apomorphine inhibits secretion of prolactin (292, 318–321; for review see refs. 136, 272, 322). Similar effects can be induced in humans (for review see ref. 323).

It seems that the main physiological role of the DA system is to keep prolactin secretion low during resting states. The activation of prolactin secretion by stress or suckling is not caused by an inhibition of the DA system since both stimuli still activated prolactin release after the influence of the DA system had been eliminated by reserpine, pimozide, or α-methyl-p-tryosine (324–326).

The role of the NE system in the regulation of prolactin secretion is not clear. Stimulation of prolactin secretion was observed following intraventricular injection of α receptor blockers, but also following injection of NE or clonidine (281, 321, 327), whereas systemic injection of α and β receptor blockers inhibited periodic prolactin surges in ovariectomized rats treated with estrogen (328).

In contrast, there is considerable evidence that activation of the central SER system very effectively stimulates prolactin secretion. Stimulation of prolactin secretion was described following intraventricular injection of serotonin or melatonin (291) and following systemic administration of serotonin precursors, tryptophane, and 5-OH-tryptophane, both in rats and humans (329, 330).

The mechanism of the serotoninergic activation of prolactin secretion is unknown, but it seems to play a physiological role in the activation of prolactin secretion by stress, suckling, or by the positive feedback effect of progesterone because all these interventions become ineffective following blockade of serotonin receptors (324, 331, 332).

Activation of the cholinergic system via either muscarinic or nicotinic receptors inhibits prolactin secretion (296, 333, 334). The effect of stimulation of the muscarinic receptors is probably indirect and is mediated by the DA system (335).

CRF-ACTH   Ganong and co-workers (for review see ref. 336) accumulated considerable evidence that depletion of central NE increases the activity of the adenopituitary system and enhances the effects of stress, whereas increased NE activity has opposite effects. They, therefore, concluded that central NE system inhibits CRF release.

However, not everybody agrees. Intrahypothalamic implants or injections of NE stimulated adrenocortical secretion (337, 338); neither depletion nor elevation of central NE stores had any effect on the basal or stress-activated secretion of corticoids (338); and, similarly, neither L-dopa nor clonidine affected the basal adrenocortical secretion or its activation by 5-OH-tryptophane in monkeys (309).

The DA system does not seem to play any role in the regulation of CRF release (336, 309), but there is relative unanimity that the SER system activates CRF release. This was observed following hypothalamic implants of serotonin in rats (337, 339), as well as following systemic administration of 5-OH-tryptophane in monkeys (309) and humans (315). A similar unanimity also reigns with respect to the activating role of the cholinergic system (268, 340, 341).

Recently, Hillhouse and associates (342, 343) demonstrated in an in vitro system that CRF release is stimulated by acetylcholine, predominantly via a nicotinic receptor and also by serotonin. The effect of serotonin seems to be indirect and to involve a cholinergic interneuron. In contrast, NE inhibits both the basal release and release stimulated by acetylcholine.

MSH   It seems that the tonic inhibition of MSH secretion is exerted, as in the case of prolactin, by the central DA system. Therefore, blockade of DA receptors leads to an increase of MSH secretion (344, 345), whereas stimulation of DA receptors inhibits it (346). These effects may be mediated through changes in the release of MIF, but they may be due to direct innervation by dopaminergic fibers (264) of the neurointermediate lobe, which has been shown to respond to direct application of catecholamines or DA receptor agonists and blockers (347). Taleisnik et al. (348) provided evidence that the central NE and SER systems also play a role in the regulation of MSH secretion, but their relation to MIF and MRF release is so far indecipherable.

EFFECT OF PROSTAGLANDINS ON SECRETION OF HHH

Prostaglandins are ubiquitous substances which display a great variety of effects on almost all the systems and functions of the body. The mechanism of their action is not well understood, but it seems that in cells with secretory functions they are involved in some stage of the stimulus-secretion coupling process. It is, therefore, not very surprising that they affect both the release of the HHH and the secretion of the pituitary hormones. There are, however, large differences in the responsiveness of the individual hormonal systems (for review see ref. 349).

Certain prostaglandins are very potent activators of the release of LRH. If they are injected into the third ventricle, they cause a marked and rapid elevation of serum LH levels, accompanied by an elevation of LRH titers in systemic circulation as well as in portal blood (350–352). The strongest effect is obtained with PGE_2, although $PGF_{2\alpha}$ and $PFG_{2\beta}$ are also quite effective, whereas compounds of the PGE_1 series and other types have only a weak activity or none at all (350, 353). It seems that the active prostaglandins stimulate LRH neurons directly, because their effect is not abolished by blockade of any of the transmitter systems which may be involved in LRH release (354). This notion is further supported by findings that microimplants of PGE_2 activate LRH release only if they are placed in the median eminence, arcuate nucleus, or the medial preoptic area (355), sites which contain LRH.

A physiological role of prostaglandins in the release of LRH is indicated by reports that blockade of prostaglandin synthesis with aspirin blocked ovulation in the rat (356), whereas indomethacin, another inhibitor of prostaglandin synthesis, prevented the postcastration rise of the gonadotropins in rats, lowered the LH levels of castrated animals, and blocked the LR surge following administration of estrogen or progesterone (357).

In contrast to LRH, there is no evidence that prostaglandins stimulate TRH release since they failed to alter serum TSH levels following either intraventricular or systemic injection (353, 358).

Prostaglandins of the E series are powerful stimulators of GH secretion from the pituitary as has been shown both in vivo and in vitro (359, 360); however, a hypothalamic mechanism may also operate because increased GH secretion was seen following implantation of PGE_1 into the median eminence (361).

Intraventricular injection of PGE_1 stimulated prolactin secretion in ovariectomized rats, whereas PGE_2 and $PGF_{2\alpha}$ were effective in normal males (362, 353). These effects might be due to interference with the inhibitory action of DA systems (363). Systemic injection of PGE_1 had no effect on prolactin secretion in the rat, but PGEs and PGFs were effective, as was $PGF_{2\alpha}$ in cattle and humans (364, 365). Since prostaglandins do not affect prolactin secretion by a direct effect on the pituitary (353, 366), it is probable that the systemically injected prostaglandins act through a hypothalamic mechanism.

CENTRAL EFFECTS OF HHH

The presence of the HHH in many hypothalamic and extrahypothalamic structures suggests that the neurohormones may have some direct influence on the activity of the CNS and may possibly play a role in physiological processes unrelated to the regulation of pituitary secretions. There is growing evidence that this may indeed be the case, but in most instances the mechanism of these central effects and their physiological relevance are unknown.

So far, the most clear-cut example of a central action of the HHH is the effect of LRH on the mating behavior in female rats. Moss and McCann (367) were the first to demonstrate that systemic injection of synthetic LRH induces mating behavior in ovariectomized rats primed with estrogen. This effect can be obtained also in hypophysectomized-ovariectomized animals (368), and it has been shown by intracerebral infusion of LRH that the responsive sites are within the arcuate nucleus and preoptic area (369). It is possible to assume that the enhanced activity of the LRH system during the spontaneous proestrus surge may be instrumental in facilitating the subsequent mating behavior.

A variety of effects was obtained with TRH (for review see refs. 370, 371). It has been shown to strongly antagonize the CNS-depressive effects of pentobarbital and alcohol (372, 373), but to enhance the excitatory effects of strychnine (373). Another consistent finding is that TRH potentiates the behavioral effects of L-dopa. Intraventricular injection was reported to increase spontaneous motor activity in rat (375), to induce rotational movements in rats treated with apomorphine or reserpine (376), and to decrease body temperature in cats (377). In humans, TRH was seen to ameliorate symptoms of depression by some workers (378), but also to be without effect by others (379).

Intraventricular injection of somatostatin also induced a peculiar motor activity, described as "barrel rotation" (380), paraplegia, and clonic-tonic seizures (375). In contrast to TRH, it potentiates the effect of pentobarbital but diminishes the effect of strychnine (373).

MIF-I (α-prolyl-1-leucylglycine amide) also potentiates the behavioral effects of L-dopa and very effectively inhibits the Parkinson-like symptoms induced by oxotremorine (381, 382).

The mechanism of all these effects is obscure so far. Many of them hint at an association with the central neurotransmitter systems, especially with the DA system, but so far no direct proof has been obtained in the brain; it has been shown, however, that TRH counteracts the effects of dopamine agonists on prolactin release from pituitaries in vitro (383). On the other hand, microiontophoretic application of TRH, LRH, or somatostatin directly to individual neurons in different brain areas affected their spontaneous activity (for review see ref. 384), which speaks for a general type of influence on the CNS.

CHEMICAL AND BIOCHEMICAL ASPECTS

Progress in this area has been significant but not earthshaking, as many investigators (perhaps too many) have directed their resources toward reaping the rewards made possible by the availability of synthetic versions of the three hypophysiotropic hormones—TRH, LRH, and somatostatin. Two major and unexpected trends have resulted from this direction of effort, each a blow to the original hypothesis of neuroendocrine control of the anterior pituitary. One is the realization that each of the three peptides can regulate the release of more than one pituitary hormone, and the other is that each may also have important extrapituitary function. Whereas isolation, chemical characterization, and synthesis of the original factors permitted the demonstration of these new phenomena, the ball is now very much in the court of the endocrine physiologist, who must evaluate their true significance, while the chemically and biochemically oriented workers return to their extracts, homogenates, columns, and test tubes.

Unidentified Hypophysiotropic Factors

PIF and PRF   Little information has appeared that would suggest that the characterization of a PIF or PRF of genuine physiological significance is imminent. A series of brief reports has documented the progress toward isolation of no less than four PIF-like components (385) from half a million hypothalamic fragments. As well as illustrating the sheer tenacity required for this type of work, the results also illustrate the potential hazards involved since the active agents identified thus far, catecholamines (386) and γ-aminobutyric acid (387), are certainly not universally accepted as physiologically important factors. Independent evidence for the existence of a peptide form of PIF appears to have been obtained (388), although during the isolation work less than approximately 100 ng survived a 14-stage purification procedure which consumed 80,000 hypothalamic fragments (389). It is a little surprising that in the above endeavors no PRF activity was encountered during the screening of column fractions. Two other groups who have succeeded in detecting and partially purifying this factor do not appear to have been dealing with the same entity, as judged by the gel filtration characteristics of their active materials (390, 391).

CRF   Some progress toward the characterization of CRF has been reported which may aid in its eventual identification. Intriguing evidence has been obtained which suggests that CRF consists of two dissociable moieties, apparently of quite different size, by the procedure of assaying recombined gel filtration fractions. This was carried out on a modest scale, and it illustrates the value of conducting small scale pilot experiments prior to a major commitment to "bucket scale" isolation work (392). Slightly complicating this information, however, are the reports of the detection of two CRF-like entities by separation on Sephadex of material emanating from hypothalamic tissue which had been stimulated in vitro by 5-hydroxytryptophan (393, 394). In this context, it now seems definite that the claim that pressinoic acid exhibited high ACTH-releasing activity was erroneous (395). It is to be hoped that the extended struggle to isolate and identify a true CRF will be facilitated by the ability to estimate ACTH by radioimmunoassay.

GRF   The progress of the characterization of GRF illustrates a classic combination of pitfalls and side steps. Following on the heels of the realization that "porcine GRF" had the same sequence as the NH_2-terminal portion of the β chain of porcine hemoglobin and the discovery that neither the natural nor the synthetic version stimulated the release of immunoassayable GH in several species, yet another unphysiological "GRF" has been identified as myelin basic protein which showed activity in vitro but not in vivo (396). In an attempt to substantiate the existence of a true GRF, re-examination of GH-releasing activity in Sephadex-separated fractions of porcine hypothalamic extracts with the aid of the more physiological but cumbersome portal vessel infusion procedure revealed two distinct GH-releasing entities. Each of these was active at dose equivalent to 0.02 hypothalamic fragment, a level of activity which suggests that the agents responsible may indeed be of physiological significance (397). The second of these activities in order of elution appears to have the same elution position as another GRF which was detected by means of its ability to release immunoassayable GH in vitro. In this case, support for physiological significance of the GRF might be seen in the ability of this material to elevate pituitary cyclic GMP (cGMP) and GH release simultaneously and rapidly (398). Reminiscent of this rapid action is the report that the synthetic porcine hemoglobin terminal peptide, although previously scorned as a physiological GRF, will induce short-term release of immunoassayable GH after portal vessel infusion concomitant with electron microscopically detected exocytosis of pituitary cell granules (399). As the peptide has also been shown to stimulate GH release in vitro from cloned rat pituitary cells of tumor origin (400), one wonders if we are to be subjected to another cycle of confusion regarding the true nature of GRF.

Identified Hypophysiotropic Hormones

TRH Studies of TRH chemistry and biochemistry range from physical chemistry to enzymology and encompass investigations of its conformation by nuclear magnetic resonance (401), Raman spectroscopy (402), calculations (403), investigation of its binding to cultured pituitary cell membranes by means of fluorescence quenching (404), and its apparent subcellular compartmentalization by ultracentrifugation (405). An example of how classical biochemical studies may reveal potentially important information to the physiologist may be seen in a recent reinvestigation of the enzymological degradation of TRH. The TRH-amidase and pyroglutamyl peptidase enzymes from hamster hypothalami have been found to be inhibited (in vitro) by TSH and hydrocortisone, respectively (406). Another recent study of TRH degradation suggests the need for a cofactor requirement by the rat hypothalamic "peptidase," although the nature of the specific cleavage was not defined in this study (407). At the pituitary level, interesting studies with the GH_3 clonal strain of pituitary cells indicate that, during long-term incubation with TRH, not only does the peptide have the ability to regulate the number of its own receptors (408), but it also undergoes degradation by the cell, with subsequent incorporation of its amino acids into protein (409).

The synthesis of analogs of TRH in order to find an inhibitor has not been very rewarding. Cyclopentyl-histidyl-pyrrolidine, a molecule having the same tricyclic skeleton as TRH, has been reported to inhibit the TRH-induced increase in circulating ^{131}I in vivo (410). Reliable inhibition was not obtained, however, when this compound was tested in vitro. In the latter system, cyclopentyl-thienylalanyl-pyrrolidine was claimed to be a better antagonist. It is of interest that neither analog was able to inhibit the TRH-induced release of prolactin in monkeys (411).

The interest in TRH biosynthesis stimulated by a claim that it occurred via a nonribosomal mechanism (412) has subsided somewhat following unsuccessful attempts to repeat the work (413, 414). These developments illustrate only too well the pitfalls in studies on peptide biosynthesis in that not only does the presence of peptidase activity tend to negate desired de novo synthesis but also incomplete purification of labeled products can lead to quite erroneous conclusions. While some ability to add labeled Pro to pGlu His, possibly via a reverse peptidase reaction, has been demonstrated in hypothalamic preparations (414), the only satisfactory demonstration of de novo TRH biosynthesis in vitro has been accomplished in cultures of hypothalamic tissue fragments with the aid of a six-stage purification procedure which proved that the labeled product was indeed TRH (415). Further studies with these cultures have revealed that unfortunately after about 3 days the neuronal elements degenerate in parallel with a loss of the ability to incorporate label into TRH (416).

Somatostatin   Much of the interest and effort in the area of the chemistry and biochemistry of somatostatin and its activities has centered around its potential extrapituitary importance in general and its occurrence in the D-cells of the pancreas in particular. This exciting area has somewhat overshadowed efforts directed toward the evaluation of the true role of this peptide in regulating the release of GH and, in some circumstances, TSH and even PRL (prolactin).

The preparation of analogs of somatostatin has been aimed at obtaining a peptide with prolonged and possibly more selective activity. The introduction of a single amino acid having the unnatural D configuration enhances its ability to inhibit the release of GH in vitro as well as its inhibitory effect on insulin and glucagon release in vivo. This may well be due to the reduced susceptibility of the analog to enzymatic inactivation (417). A somatostatin-cleaving enzyme has been described which has an endopeptidase rather than an amino- or carboxy-peptidase type of action (418); however, this may or may not be similar to the plasma enzymes presumed responsible for the short half-life of somatostatin. Most of the testing of somatostatin analogs has been performed in vivo by using as indices of activity the reversal or prevention of pharmacologically induced elevation of circulating GH levels (419, 420). Removal of its NH_2-terminal Ala^1-Gly^2 residues produces differential effects on the various activities of somatostatin. Although its ability to inhibit GH release is reduced by 90%, inhibition of insulin release is unaffected even though inhibition of glucagon release is lost altogether (421). Acyl derivatives of this des-Ala—Gly peptide had been reported as possessing longer acting characteristics (419); however, it now seems that this desirable property is not consistently demonstrable (422). The poor aqueous solubility of these compounds may contribute to this variability due to the resulting injection of preparations which are part solution and part microsuspension. At present, only the use of a protamine-zinc injection vehicle has been able to bring about significant prolongation of the actions of somatostatin although it seems possible that the preparation of more of the hormonogen type of analog (peptides bearing additional amino acids on the NH_2-terminus) may yield a more useful compound, particularly if a D-amino acid is included near the center of the peptide (423, 424).

LRH   Only the highlights of the many recent advances in the physiological chemistry of LRH are covered here as complete coverage of the subject would require at least a chapter of its own. The LRH molecule must by now have become one of the most intensively studied of all the known peptide hormones. Its conformation has been examined in various solvents by nuclear magnetic resonance (425, 426), circular dichroism, optical rotatory dispersion, and fluorescence spectroscopy (427). These studies indicate that the molecule has no preferred conformation, although the optical studies provided some evidence for an ordered structure in trifluorethanol. The use of these sophisticated biophysical techniques represents one end of the spectrum of approaches now compiling information which, it is hoped, will lead to the design of an ideal inhibitor for use in contraception or analogs suitable for treatment of infertility. At the other end of this spectrum, studies on enzymatic cleavage of LRH by neural tissue have provided a possible biochemical basis for the increased activity of analogs containing a D-amino acid and an ethylamide substituent at the COOH terminus (428, 429). Apparently, inactivation at the neural level is relevant to the inactivation mechanism in the blood and at the pituitary level. These studies may help clarify the significance of the rather nonspecific hypothalamic LRH-inactivating enzymes for which a regulatory role has been suggested (430, 431).

Several reports have appeared of the existence in various hypothalamic extracts of LRH-like immunoactive components which are chromatographically distinguishable from the decapeptide. At present no physiological significance can be assigned to these entities although suggestions have been made as to their nature and role which range from biosynthetic precursors to artifacts (432–436).

On the question of the existence of an FSHRF (follicle-stimulating hormone releasing factor) in extracts of hypothalamic tissue, confirmation has been obtained of the earlier detection (437) of an entity capable of releasing more FSH than LH from the pituitaries of immature female rats. Because this factor was inactive in vivo, it has been held to be physiologically insignificant and indeed a massive resurvey of hypothalamic extracts and fractions failed to yield any sign of a distinct, genuine FSHRF (438).

Studies on the action of LRH at the pituitary level have largely been directed toward elucidating the involvement of cyclic AMP (cAMP). A recent review describes the actions of LRH, TRH, and somatostatin entirely in terms of observed changes in tissue cAMP content (439); however, reports linking cGMP to the action of hypophysiotropic hormones (440, 441) suggest that further experimentation using simultaneous measurement of both cyclic nucleotides will be required before this aspect of the mechanism of release is clear.

Another avenue being explored in connection with LRH action concerns the mechanism whereby two or more doses of the hormone result in successively greater quantities of LH being released from the pituitary. This has been referred to as a self-potentiating or priming effect. Several groups have shown that the increased response to a second dose of LRH or the later phase of the response to continual stimulation is dependent upon protein synthesis as indicated by a sensitivity to cycloheximide, actinomycin D, and puromycin (442–445). Elucidation of the mechanism whereby the overall response of the gonadotroph to LRH is controlled appears to have the makings of a biochemical tour de force. Not only has it also been shown that both the inhibitory and augmentative effects of estradiol may be dependent upon protein synthesis (446), but also the steroid milieu appears to be capable of modulating the nature of LRH binding to the gonadotroph (447, 448). A further fascinating piece of information bearing on the action of LRH concerns its ability to stimulate the incorporation of glucosamine, but not amino acids, into LH (449).

The search for an antagonist of LRH for use as a fertility control agent has led to the synthesis and screening of a host of LRH peptide analogs. By combining observations on the properties of singly substituted peptides, several groups have converged toward the deduction that D-amino acid substitution at positions 2, 3, and 6 of the decapeptide would produce a reasonable inhibitor with little agonistic activity. Milligram quantities of such peptides have indeed been demonstrated to have ovulation-inhibiting action in small animals (450–452).

This coverage of recent progress in releasing hormone chemistry and biochemistry is brief and, therefore, rather selective. Some of the gaps may be filled by consulting other reviews (453–455), but there remain several exciting areas in which pioneering steps are being taken, particularly those in which techniques from the biochemistry and cell biology laboratories are being adapted to the peculiar requirements necessary for the investigation of the function of the hypothalamo-adenohypophysial system at the molecular level.

REFERENCES

1. Nett, T. M., Akbar, A. M., Niswender, G. D., Hedlund, M. T., and White, W. F. (1973). A radioimmunoassay for gonadotropin-releasing hormone (Gn-RH) in serum. J. Clin. Endocrinol. 36:880.
2. Bassiri, R. M., and Utiger, R. D. (1972). The preparation of specific antibody to thyrotropin-releasing hormone. Endocrinology 90:722.
3. Arimura, A., Sato, H., Coy, D. H., and Schally, A. V. (1975). Radioimmunoassay for GH-release inhibiting hormones. Proc. Soc. Exp. Biol. Med. 148:784.
4. Palkovits, M. (1973). Isolated removal of hypothalamic or other brain nuclei of the rat. Brain Res. 59:449.
5. Wheaton, J. E., Krulich, L., and McCann, S. M. (1975). Localization of luteinizing hormone-releasing hormone in the preoptic area and hypothalamus of the rat using radioimmunoassay. Endocrinology 97:30.
6. Palkovits, M., Arimura, A., Brownstein, M., Schally, A. V., and Saavedra, J.

M. (1974). Luteinizing hormone-releasing hormone (LH-RH) content of the hypothalamic nuclei in the rat. Endocrinology 95:554.
7. Crighton, D. B., Schneider, H. P. G., and McCann, S. M. (1970). Localization of LH-releasing factor in the hypothalamus and neurohypophysis as determined by an *in vitro* method. Endocrinology 87:323.
8. Quijada, M., Krulich, L., Fawcett, C. P., Sundberg, D. K., and McCann, S. M. (1971). Localization of TSH-releasing factor (TRF), LH-RF and FSH-RF in rat hypothalamus. Fed. Proc. 30:197.
9. McCann, S. M. (1962). A hypothalamic luteinizing-hormone releasing factor. Am. J. Physiol. 202:395.
10. Zimmerman, E. A., Hsu, K. C., Ferin, M., and Kozlowski, G. P. (1972). Localization of gonadotropin-releasing hormone (Gn-RH) in the hypothalamus of the mouse by immunoperoxidase technique. Endocrinology 95:1.
11. Kizer, J. S., Palkovits, M., and Brownstein, M. J. (1976). Releasing factors in the circumventricular organs of the rat brain. Endocrinology 98:311.
12. White, W. F., Hedlund, M. T., Wilber, G. F., Rippel, R. H., Johnson, E. S., and Wilber, J. F. (1974). The pineal gland: a supplemental source of hypothalamic-releasing hormones. Endocrinology 94:1422.
13. Jonas, H. A., Burger, H. G., Cumming, I. A., Findlay, J. K., and DeKretser, D. M. (1975). Radioimmunoassay for luteinizing hormone-releasing hormone (LH-RH): its application to the measurement in ovine and human plasma. Endocrinology 96:384.
14. Araki, S., Ferin, M., Zimmerman, E. A., and Vande Wiele, R. L. (1975). Ovarian modulation of immunoreactive gonadotropins releasing hormone (Gn-RH) in the rat brain: evidence for a different effect on the anterior and midhypothalamus. Endocrinology 96:644.
15. Gross, D. (1976). Distribution of gonadotropin-releasing hormone in the mouse brain as revealed by immunohistochemistry. Endocrinology 98:1408.
16. Kordon, C., Kerdelhué, B., Pattou, E., and Jutisz, M. (1974). Immunocytochemical localization of LH-RH in axons and nerve terminals of the rat median eminence. Proc. Soc. Exp. Biol. Med. 147:122.
17. Pelletier, G., Labrie, F., Puviani, R., Arimura, A., and Schally, A. V. (1974). Immunohistochemical localization of luteinizing hormone-releasing hormone in the rat median eminence. Endocrinology 95:314.
18. King, J. C., Parsons, J. A., Erlandsen, S. G., and Williams, T. H. (1974). Luteinizing hormone-releasing hormone (LH-RH) pathway of the rat hypothalamus revealed by the unlabeled antibody peroxidase-antiperoxidase method. Cell Tissue Res. 153:211.
19. Baker, B. L., Dermody, W. C., and Reel, J. R. (1975). Distribution of gonadotropin-releasing hormone in the rat brain as observed with immunocytochemistry. Endocrinology 97:125.
20. Sétáló, G., Vigh, S., Schally, A. V., Arimura, A., and Flerkó, B. (1975). Immunohistological study of the origin of LH-RH containing nerve fibers of the rat hypothalamus. Brain Res. 103:597.
21. Barry, J., Dubois, M. P., and Doulain, P., (1973). LRF producing cells of the mammalian hypothalamus: a fluorescent antibody study. Z. Zellforsch. 146:351.
22. Silverman, A. J. (1976). Distribution of luteinizing hormone-releasing hormone (LH-RH) in the guinea pig brain. Endocrinology 99:30.

23. Barry, J. (1976). Histophysiological studies of LH-RH neurons in the primates. Sixth International Congress of Endocrinology, p. 19 (Abstr.). Hamburg, Germany.
24. Krulich, L., Quijada, M., Hefco, E., and Sundberg, D. K. (1974). Localization of thyrotropin-releasing factor (TRF) in the hypothalamus of the rat. Endocrinology 59:9.
25. Brownstein, M. J., Palkovits, M., Saavedra, J. M., Bassiri, R., and Utiger, R. D. (1974). Thyrotropin-releasing hormone in specific nuclei of rat brain. Science 185:267.
26. Jackson, I. M. D., and Reichlin, S. (1974). Thyrotropin-releasing hormone (TRH): distribution in hypothalamic and extrahypothalamic tissues of mammalian and submammalian chordates. Endocrinology 95:854.
27. Reichlin, S., Saperstein, R., Jackson, I. M. D., Boyd, A., and Patel, Y. (1976). Hypothalamic hormones. Ann. Rev. Physiol. 38:389.
28. Jeffcoate, S. L., and White, N. (1975). Is there any thyrotrophin-releasing hormone in mammalian extrahypothalamic brain tissue? J. Endocrinol. 67:42(P).
29. Fuxe, K., Hökfelt, T., Löfström, A., Johansson, O., Aquatil, L., Everitt, B., Goldstein, M., Jeffcoate, S., White, N., Emroth, P., Qustafsson, J. A., and Skett, P. (1976). On the role of neurotransmitters and hypothalamic hormones and their interactions in hypothalamic and extrahypothalamic control of pituitary function and sexual behavior. In F. Naftolin, K. J. Ryan, and I. J. Davies (eds.), Subcellular Mechanisms in Reproductive Neuroendocrinology, pp. 193–246. Elsevier, Amsterdam.
30. Krulich, L., Illner, P., Fawcett, C. P., Quijada, M., and McCann, S. M. (1971). Dual hypothalamic regulation of growth hormone secretion. In A. Pecile and E. E. Müller (eds.), Growth and Growth Hormone, pp. 306–316. Excerpta Medica, Amsterdam.
31. Brownstein, M., Arimura, A., Sato, H., Schally, A. V., and Kizer, J. S. (1975). The regional distribution of somatostatin in the rat brain. Endocrinology 96:1456.
32. Hökfelt, T., Efendić, S., Hellerström, C., Johansson, O., Luft, R., and Arimura, A. (1975). Cellular localization of somatostatin in endocrine-like cells and neurons of the rat with special references to the A_1-cells of the pancreatic islets and to the hypothalamus. Acta Endocrinol. (Suppl.) 800:1.
33. Alpert, L. C., Brawer, J. R., Patel, Y. C., and Reichlin, S. (1976). Somatostatinergic neurons in anterior hypothalamus: immunohistochemical localization. Endocrinology 98:255.
34. Leclerc, R., Pelletier, G., Puviani, R., Arimura, A., and Schally, A. V. (1976). Immunohistochemical localization of somatostatin in endocrine cells of the rat stomach. Mol. Cell Endocrinol. 4:257.
35. Arimura, A., Sato, H., DuPont, A., Nishi, A., and Schally, A. V. (1975). Abundance of immunoreactive GH-release inhibiting hormone in the stomach and pancreas of rat. Science 189:1009.
36. Krulich, L., Quijada, M., and Illner, P. (1971). Localization of prolactin-inhibiting factor (PIF), P-releasing factor (PRF), growth hormone releasing factor (GRF) and GIF activities in the hypothalamus of the rat. Program of the 53rd Meeting of the Endocrine Society, No. 82 (Abstr.).
37. Taleisnik, S., and Tomatis, M. E. (1967). Melanocyte-stimulating hormone-releasing and inhibiting factors in two hypothalamic extracts. Endocrinology 81:819.

38. Krieger, D. T., Liotta, A., and Brownstein, M. J. (1977). Corticotrophin releasing-factor distribution in normal and Brattleboro rat brain and effect of deafferentation, hypophysectomy and steroid treatment in normal animals. Endocrinology 100:227.

39. Bishop, W., Fawcett, C. P., Krulich, L., and McCann, S. M. (1972). Acute and chronic effects of hypothalamic lesions on the release of FSH, LH and prolactin in intact and castrated rats. Endocrinology 91:643.

40. Halasz, B., and Gorski, R. A. (1967). Gonadotropic hormone secretion in female rats after partial or total interruption of neural afferents to the medial basal hypothalamus. Endocrinology 80:608.

41. Blake, C. A., Weiner, R. I., Gorski, R. A., and Sawyer, C. H. (1972). Secretion of pituitary luteinizing hormone and follicle stimulating hormone in female rats made persistently estrous or diestrous by hypothalamic deafferentation. Endocrinology 90:855.

42. Kalra, S. P. (1976). Tissue levels of luteinizing hormone-releasing hormone in the preoptic area and hypothalamus and serum concentrations of gonadotropins following anterior hypothalamic deafferentation and estrogen treatment of the female rat. Endocrinology 99:101.

43. Kalra, S. P., Kalra, P. S., and Mitchell, E. O. (1977). Differential response of luteinizing hormone-releasing hormone in the basal hypothalamus and the preoptic area following anterior hypothalamic deafferentation and/or castration in male rats. Endocrinology 100:201.

44. Schneider, H. P. G., Crighton, D. B., and McCann, S. M. (1969). Suprachiasmatic LH-releasing factor. Neuroendocrinology 5:271.

45. Weiner, R. I., Pattou, E., Kerdelhué, B., and Kordon, C. (1975). Different effects of hypothalamic deafferentation upon luteinizing hormone-releasing hormone in the median eminence and organum vasculosum of the lamina terminalis. Endocrinology 97:1597.

46. Brownstein, M. J., Arimura, A., Schally, A. V., Palkovits, M., and Kizer, J. S. (1976). The effect of surgical isolation of the hypothalamus on its luteinizing hormone-releasing hormone content. Endocrinology 98:662.

47. Mitnick, M., and Reichlin, S. (1972). Enzymatic synthesis of thyrotropin-releasing hormone (TRH) by hypothalamic TRH synthetase. Endocrinology 91:1145.

48. Knigge, K. M., Joseph, S. A., Schock, D., Silverman, A. J., Ching, M. C. H., Scott, D. E., Zeman, D., and Krobish-Dudley, G. (1974). Role of the ventricular system in neuroendocrine processes: synthesis and distribution of thyrotropin-releasing factor (TRF) in the hypothalamus and third ventricle. Can. J. Neurol. Sci. 1(1):74.

49. Bauer, K., and Lipmann, F. (1976). Attempts towards biosynthesis of the thyrotropin-releasing hormone and studies on its breakdown in hypothalamic tissue preparation. Endocrinology 99:230.

50. Florsheim, W. H. (1974). Control of thyrotropin secretion. Handbook of Physiology, Sec. 7, Vol. IV, pp. 449–468. Am. Physiol. Soc., Washington, D.C.

51. Mess, B. (1970). Intrahypothalamic localization and onset of production of thyrotropin-releasing factor (TRF) in the albino rat. Hormones 1:332.

52. Brownstein, M. J., Utiger, R. D., Palkovits, M., and Kizer, J. S. (1975). Effect of hypothalamic deafferentation on thyrotropin-releasing hormone levels in rat brain. Proc. Natl. Acad. Sci. U. S. A. 72:4177.

53. Hefco, E., Krulich, L., and Aschenbrenner, J. E. (1975). Effect of hypothalamic deafferentation on the secretion of thyrotropin in resting conditions in the rat. Endocrinology 97:1226.

54. Hefco, E., Krulich, L., and Aschenbrenner, J. E. (1975). Effect of hypothalamic deafferentation on the secretion of thyrotropin during thyroid blockade and exposure to cold in the rat. Endocrinology 97:1234.
55. Brownstein, M. J., Arimura, A., Fernandez-Durango, R., Schally, A. V., Palkovits, M., and Kizer, J. S. (1977). The effect of hypothalamic deafferentation on somatostatin-like activity in the rat brain. Endocrinology 100:246.
56. Löfgren, F. (1959). The infundibular recess, a component in the hypothalamo-adenohypophyseal system. Acta Morphol. Neerl. Scand. 3:55.
57. Knowless, F. W. G., and Kumar, T. C. A. (1969). Structural changes related to reproduction in the hypothalamus and in the pars tuberalis of the rhesus monkey. Part 1, The hypothalmus; Part 2, The pars tuberalis. Philos. Trans. R. Soc. Lond. 256:357.
58. Porter, J. C., Mical, R. S., Tippit, P. R., and Drane, J. W. (1970). Effect of selective surgical interruption of the anterior pituitary's blood supply on ACTH release. Endocrinology 86:590.
59. Knigge, K. M., Joseph, S. A., Scott, D. E., and Jacobs, J. J. (1971). Observations on the architecture of the arcuate-median eminence region after deafferentation, with reference to the organization of hypothalamic RF-producing elements. In Mack, Sherman (eds.), The Neuroendocrinology of Human Reproduction, pp. 6–22. Thomas, Springfield.
60. Porter, J. C., Ben-Jonathan, N., Oliver, C., and Eskay, R. L. (1975). Secretion of releasing hormones and their transport from CSF to hypophysial portal blood. In K. M. Knigge and D. E. Scott (eds.), Brain Endocrine Interactions II, pp. 285–305. Karger, Basel.
61. Knigge, K. M., and Joseph, S. A. (1976). Thyrotropin-releasing factor (TRF) in cerebrospinal fluid of the 3rd ventricle of rat. Acta Endocrinol. (Kbh.) 76:209.
62. Joseph, S. A., Sorrentino, S., Jr., and Sundberg, D. K. (1975). Releasing hormones LRF and TRF in the cerebrospinal fluid of the third ventricle. In K. M. Knigge and D. E. Scott (eds.), Brain Endocrine Interactions II, pp. 306–312. Karger, Basel.
63. Morris, M., Tandy, B., Sundberg, D. K., and Knigge, K. M. (1975). Modification of brain and CSF LH-RH following deafferentation. Neuroendocrinology 18:131.
64. Oliver, C., Charvet, J. L., Codaccioni, J. L., Vogue, J., and Porter, J. C. (1974). TRH in human CSF. Lancet 1:873.
65. Cramer, O. M., and Barraclough, C. A. (1975). Failure to detect luteinizing hormone-releasing hormone in third ventricle cerebral spinal fluid under a variety of experimental conditions. Endocrinology 96:913.
66. Ondo, J. G., Eskay, R. L., Mical, R. S., and Porter, J. C. (1973). Release of LH by LRF injected into CSF: a transport role for median eminence. Endocrinology 93:231.
67. Oliver, C., Ben-Jonathan, N., Mical, R. S., and Porter, J. C. (1975). Transport of thyrotropin-releasing hormone from cerebro-spinal fluid to hypophysial portal blood and the release of thyrotropin. Endocrinology 97:1138.
68. Joseph, S. A., Scott, D. E., Vaala, S. S., and Knigge, K. M. (1974). Localization and content of thyrotropin-releasing factor (TRF) in median eminence of the hypothalamus. Acta Endocrinol. (Kbh.) 79:215.
69. Kobayashi, H., (1975). Absorption of cerebrospinal fluid by ependymal cells of the median eminence. In K. M. Knigge and D. E. Scott (eds.), Brain Endocrine Interactions II, pp. 109–122. Karger, Basel.

70. McCann, S. M., and Ramirez, D. V. (1964). The neuroendocrine regulation of hypophyseal luteinizing-hormone secretion. Recent Prog. Horm. Res. 20:131.

71. McCann, S. M., and Porter, J. C. (1969). Hypothalamic pituitary stimulating and inhibiting hormones. Physiol. Rev. 49:240.

72. Gual, C. (1973). Clinical effects and uses of hypothalamic releasing and inhibiting factors. In W. F. Ganong and L. Martin (eds.), Frontiers in Neuroendocrinology, pp. 89–132. Oxford University Press, New York.

73. Besser, G. M., and Mortimer, C. H. (1975). Clinical neuroendocrinology. In L. Martin and W. F. Ganong (eds.), Frontiers in Neuroendocrinology, pp. 227–254. Oxford University Press, New York.

74. Hall, R., and Gomez-Pan, A. (1976). The hypothalamic regulatory hormones and their clinical applications. Adv. Clin. Chem. 18:173.

75. Schally, A. V., Redding, T. W., Matsuo, H., and Arimura, A. (1972). Stimulation of FSH and LH release in vitro by natural and synthetic LH and FSH releasing hormone. Endocrinology 90:1561.

76. Arimura, A., Debeljuk, L., and Schally, A. V. (1972). Stimulation of FSH release in vivo by prolonged infusion of synthetic LH-RH. Endocrinology 91:529.

77. Gay, V. L., Niswender, G. D., and Midgley, A. R., Jr. (1970). Response of individual rats and sheep to one or more injections of hypothalamic extract as determined by radioimmunoassay of plasma LH. Endocrinology 86:1305.

78. Humphrey, R. R., Dermody, W. C., Brink, H. O., Bonsley, F. G., Schoffin, N. H., Sakowski, R., Vaithus, J. W., Veloso, H. T., and Reel, T. R. (1973). Induction of luteinizing hormone (LH) release and ovulation in rats, hamsters and rabbits by synthetic luteinizing hormone-releasing factor (LRF). Endocrinology 92:1515.

79. Zeballos, G., and McCann, S. M. (1974). The effect of subcutaneous administration of synthetic luteinizing-hormone releasing factor on plasma gonadotropins and prolactin in the rat. Proc. Soc. Exp. Biol. Med. 145:415.

80. Watson, J. T., Krulich, L., and McCann, S. M. (1971). Effect of crude rat hypothalamic extract on serum gonadotropin and prolactin levels in normal and orchidectomized male rats. Endocrinology 89:1412.

81. Ondo, J. G., Eskay, R. L., Mical, R. S., and Porter, J. C. (1973). Effect of synthetic LRF infused into hypophysial portal vessel on gonadotropin release. Endocrinology 93:205.

82. Schally, A. V., Arimura, A., Kastin, A. J., Matsuo, H., Baba, Y., Redding, T. W., Nair, R. M. G., and Debeljuk, L. (1971). Gonadotropin-releasing hormone: one polypeptide regulates secretion of luteinizing and follicle stimulating hormones. Science 173:1036.

83. Arimura, A., Matsuo, H., Baba, Y., and Schally, A. V. (1971). Ovulation induced by synthetic luteinizing hormone-releasing hormone in the hamster. Science 179:511.

84. Zarate, A., Canales, E. S., Schally, A. V., Valdes, L. A., and Kastin, A. J. (1972). Successful induction of ovulation with synthetic luteinizing hormone-releasing hormone in anovulatory infertility. Fertil. Steril. 23:672.

85. Redding, T. W., Schally, A. V., Arimura, A., and Matsuo, H. (1972). Stimulation of release and synthesis of luteinizing hormone (LH) and follicle stimulation hormone (FSH) in tissue cultures of rat pituitaries in

response to natural and synthetic LH and FSH releasing hormone. Endocrinology 90:764.

86. Labrie, F., Pelletier, G., Lemay, A., Borgeat, P., Borden, N., Dupont, A., Savary, M., and Côté Boucher, J. R. (1973). Control of protein synthesis in anterior pituitary gland. Acta Endocrinol. (Suppl.) 180:301.

87. Apfelbaum, M. E., and Taliesnik, S. (1976). Interaction between oestrogen and gonadotrophin-releasing hormone on the release and synthesis of luteinizing hormone and follicle stimulating hormone from incubated pituitaries. J. Endocrinol. 68:127.

88. Wakabayashi, K., and McCann, S. M. (1970). In vitro responses of anterior pituitary glands from normal, castrated and androgen-treated male rats to LH-releasing factor (LRF) and high potassium medium. Endocrinology 87:771.

89. Nakano, H., Fawcett, C. P., and McCann, S. M. (1976). Enzymatic dissociation and short-term culture of isolated rat anterior pituitary cells for studies on the control of hormone secretion. Endocrinology 98:278.

90. Wagner, H., Böchel, K., Hrubesch, M., Grote, G., and Hauss, W. H (1972). On the effect of synthetic LH-releasing hormone on the blood levels of LH, FSH, HGH, TSH, ACTH, insulin and blood sugar in man. Horm. Metab. Res. 4:403.

91. Martin, J. B., and Reichlin, S. (1972). Plasma thyrotropin (TSH) response to hypothalamic electrical stimulation and to injection of synthetic thyrotropin-releasing hormone (TRH). Endocrinology 90:1079.

92. Azizi, F., Vagenakis, A. G., Bollinger, J., Reichlin, S., Bush, J. E., and Braverman, L. E. (1972). The effect of a single large dose of thyrotropin-releasing hormone on various aspects of thyroid function in the rat. Endocrinology 95:1769.

93. Vale, W., Burgus, R., Dunn, T. F., and Guillemin, R. (1970). Release of TSH by oral administration of synthetic peptide derivatives with TRF activity. J. Clin. Endocrinol. 30:148.

94. Snyder, P. J., and Utiger, R. D. (1972). Response to thyrotropin-releasing hormone (TRH) in normal man. J. Clin. Endocrinol. 34:380.

95. Blackwell, R. E., and Guillemin, R. (1973). Hypothalamic control of adenohypophysial secretions. Ann. Rev. Physiol. 35:357.

96. Tashjian, A. H., Barowsky, N. J., and Jensen, D. K. (1971). Thyrotropin-releasing hormone: direct evidence for stimulation of prolactin production by pituitary cells in culture. Biochem. Biophys. Res. Commun. 43:516.

97. Bowers, C. Y., Friesen, H. G., Hwang, P., Guyda, H. J., and Folkers, K. (1971). Prolactin and thyrotropin release in man by synthetic pyroglutamy L-histidy L-prolinamide. Biochem. Biophys. Res. Commun. 45:1033.

98. Debeljuk, L., Arimura, A., Redding, T., and Schally, A. V. (1973). Effect of TRH and triiodothyronine on prolactin release in sheep. Proc. Soc. Exp. Biol. Med. 142:421.

99. Kelly, P. A., Bedirian, K. N., Baker, R. D., and Friesen, H. C. (1973). Effect of synthetic TRF on serum prolactin, TSH and milk production in the cow. Endocrinology 92:1289.

100. Mueller, G. P., Chen, H. J., and Meites, J. (1973). *In vivo* stimulation of prolactin release in the rat by synthetic TRH. Proc. Soc. Exp. Biol. Med. 144:613.

101. Bowers, C. Y., Friesen, H. C., and Folkers, K. (1973). Further evidence

that TRH is also a physiological regulator of PRL secretion in man. Biochem. Biophys. Res. Commun. 51:512.

102. Lu, K. H., Shaar, C. J., Kortright, K. H., and Meites, J. (1972). Effects of synthetic TRH on *in vitro* and *in vivo* prolactin release in the rat. Endocrinology 91:1540.

103. Jacobs, L. S., Snyder, P. J., Utiger, R. D., and Daughaday, W. H. (1973). Prolactin response to thyrotropin-releasing hormone in normal subjects. J. Clin. Endocrinol. Metab. 36:1069.

104. Ojeda, S. R., Castro-Vasquez, A., and Jameson, H. E. (1977). Prolactin release in response to blockade of dopaminergic receptors and to TRH injection in developing and adult rats: role of estrogen in determining sex differences. Endocrinology 100:427.

105. Gautwick, K. M., Weintraub, B. D., Graeber, C. T., Maloof, F., Zuckerman, J. E., and Tashjian, A. H., Jr. (1973). Serum prolactin and TSH: effect of nursing and pyro-Glu-His-Pro-NH$_2$ administration in postpartum woman. J. Clin. Endocrinol. 37:135.

106. Frantz, A. G., Kleinberg, D. L., and Noel, G. (1972). Studies on prolactin in man. Recent Prog. Horm. Res. 28:1972.

107. Mueller, G. P., Twohy, C. P., Chen, H. T., Advis, J. P., and Meites, J. (1976). Effects of 1-tryptophane and restraint stress on hypothalamic and brain serotonin turnover and pituitary TSH and prolactin release in rats. Life Sci. 18:715.

108. Krulich, L., Hefco, E., and Illner, P. (1976). Effect of exposure to cold or heat on the activity of the pituitary thyroid system. Isr. J. Med. Sci. 12:1090.

109. Jobin, M., Ferland, L., and Labrie, F. (1976). Effect of pharmacological blockade on ACTH and TSH secretion on the acute stimulation of prolactin release by exposure to cold and ether stress. Endocrinology 99:146.

110. Krulich, L., Dhariwal, A. P. S., and McCann, S. M. (1968). Stimulatory and inhibitory effects of purified hypothalamic extracts on growth hormone release from rat pituitary *in vitro*. Endocrinology 83:783.

111. Dhariwal, A. P. S., Krulich, L., and McCann, S. M. (1969). Purification of a growth hormone-inhibiting factor (GIF) from sheep hypothalamus. Neuroendocrinology 4:282.

112. Brazeau, P., Vale, W., Burgus, R., Ling, N., Butcher, M., Rivier, J., and Guillemin, R. (1973). Hypothalamic polypeptide that inhibits the secretion of immunoreactive pituitary growth hormone. Science 179:77.

113. Vale, W., Brazeau, P., Grant, G., Nussey, A., Burgus, R., Rivier, J., Ling, N., and Guillemin, R. (1972). Premières observations sur le mode d'action de la somatostatine, un facteur hypothalamique qui inhibe la sécrétion de l'hormone de croissance. C. R. Acad. Sci. (Paris) 275:2913.

114. Vale, W., Brazeau, P., Riviere, C., Brown, M., Boss, B., Rivier, J., Burgus, R., Ling, N., and Guillemin, R. (1975). Somatostatin. Prog. Horm. Res. 31:365.

115. Carlson, H. E., Mariz, I. K., and Daughaday, W. H. (1972). Thyrotropin-releasing hormone stimulation and somatostatin inhibition of growth hormone secretion from perfused rat adenohypophyses. Endocrinology 94:1709.

116. Stachura, M. E. (1976). Influence of synthetic somatostatin upon growth hormone release from perfused rat pituitaries. Endocrinology 99:678.

117. Martin, J. B. (1976). Brain regulation of growth hormone secretion. *In* L.

Martini and W. F. Ganong (eds.), Frontiers in Neuroendocrinology, pp. 129–168. Raven Press, New York.

118. Vale, W., Rivier, C., Brazeau, P., and Guillemin, R. (1972). Effects of somatostatin on the secretion of thyrotropin and prolactin. Endocrinology 95:968.

119. Grant, N. H., Sarantakis, D., and Yardley, J. P. (1972). Action of growth hormone release inhibitory hormone on prolactin release in rat pituitary cell cultures. J. Endocrinol. 61:163.

120. Siler, T. M., Yen, S. S. C., Vale, W., and Guillemin, R. (1974). Inhibition by somatostatin on the release of TSH induced in man by thyrotropin-releasing factor. J. Clin. Endocrinol. Metab. 38:742.

121. DeVane, G. W., Siler, T. M., and Yen, S. S. C. (1973). Acute suppression of insulin and glucose levels by synthetic somatostatin in normal human subjects. J. Clin. Endocrinol. 38:913.

122. Koerker, D. J., Ruch, W., Chideckel, E., Palmer, J., Goodner, C. J., Ensinck, J., and Gale, C. C. (1972). Somatostatin: hypothalamic inhibitor of the endocrine pancreas. Science 184:482.

123. Sakurai, H., Dobbs, R., and Unger, R. H. (1972). Somatostatin-induced changes in insulin and glucagon secretion in normal and diabetic dogs. J. Clin. Invest. 54:1395.

124. Johnson, D. G., Ensinck, J. W., Koerker, D., Palmer, J., and Goodner, C. J. (1975). Inhibition of glucagon and insulin secretion by somatostatin in the rat pancreas perfused in situ. Endocrinology 96:370.

125. Fujimoto, W. Y., Ensinck, J. W., and Williams, R. H. (1974). Somatostatin inhibits insulin and glucagon release by monolayer cell cultures of rat endocrine pancreas. Life Sci. 15:1999.

126. Orci, L., Baetens, D., Rufener, C., Amherdt, M., Ravazzola, M., Studer, P., Malaisse-Lagae, F., and Unger, R. H. (1976). Hypertrophy and hyperplasia of somatostatin-containing D-cells in diabetes. Proc. Natl. Acad. Sci. U. S. A. 73:1338.

127. Bloom, S. R., Mortimer, C. H., Thorner, M. O., Besser, G. H., Hall, R., Gomez-Pan, A., Roy, V. M., Russell, R. C. G., Coy, D. H., Kastin, A. J., and Schally, A. V. (1974). Inhibition of gastrin and gastric acid secretion by growth hormone release-inhibiting hormone. Lancet 2:1106.

128. Albinus, M., Blair, E. L., Grund, E. R., Reed, J. D., Sanders, D. J., Gomez-Pan, A., Schally, A. V., and Besser, G. M. (1975). The mechanism whereby growth hormone-release inhibiting hormone (somatostatin) inhibits food stimulated gastric acid secretion in the cat. Agents Actions 5:4.

129. Boden, G., Sivitz, M. C., and Owen, O. E. (1975). Somatostatin suppresses secretin and pancreatic exocrine secretion. Science 190:163.

130. Konturek, S. J., Tasler, J., Obtulowicz, W., Coy, D. H., and Schally, A. V. (1976). Effect of growth hormone-release inhibiting hormone on hormones stimulating exocrine pancreatic secretion. J. Clin. Invest. 58:1.

131. Bloom, S. R., Jaffe, S. N., and Polak, J. M. (1975). Effect of somatostatin on pancreatic and biliary function. Gut 16:10.

132. Stachura, M. E., Dhariwal, A. P. S., and Frohman, L. A. (1972). Growth hormone synthesis and release in vitro: effects of partially purified ovine hypothalamic extract. Endocrinology 91:1071.

133. Smith, G. W., Katz, S., Root, A. W., Dhariwal, A. P. S., Bongiovanni, A., Eberlein, W., and McCann, S. M. (1968). Growth hormone-releasing activity of crude ovine SME extracts in Rhesus monkeys. Endocrinology 83:25.

134. Malacara, J. M., and Reichlin, S. (1972). Elevation of plasma radioim-munoassayable growth hormone in the rat induced by porcine hypo-thalamic. extract. *In* A. Pecile and E. E. Müller (eds.), Growth and Growth Hormone, pp. 299–305. Excerpta Medica, Amsterdam.

135. Talwalker, P. K., Ratner, A., and Meites, J. (1963). *In vitro* inhibition of pituitary prolactin synthesis and release by hypothalamic extracts. Am. J. Physiol. 205:213.

136. Meites, J., Lu, K. H., Wuttke, W., Welsch, C. W., Nagasawa, H., and Quadri, S. K. (1972). Recent studies on function and control of prolac-tin secretion in rats. Recent Prog. Horm. Res. 28:471.

137. Kühn, E., Krulich, L., Fawcett, C. P., and McCann, S. M. (1976). The ability of hypothalamic extracts to lower blood prolactin levels in lactating rats. Proc. Soc. Exp. Biol. Med. 146:104.

138. Nicoll, C. S., Fiorindo, R. P., McKennee, C. T., and Parsons, J. A. (1970). Assay of hypothalamic factors which regulate prolactin secretion. *In* J. Meites (ed.), Hypophysiotropic Hormones of the Hypothalamus: Assay and Chemistry, p. 115. Williams and Wilkins, Baltimore.

139. Valverde, C., Chieffo, V., and Rechlin, S. (1972). Prolactin-releasing factor in porcine and rat hypothalamic tissue. Endocrinology 91:982.

140. Szabo, M., and Frohman, L. A. (1976). Dissociation of prolactin-releasing activity from thyrotropin-releasing hormone in porcine stalk median eminence. Endocrinology 98:1451.

141. Vernikos-Danellis, J., and Marks, B. H. (1970). Assay of CRF. *In* J. Meites (ed.), Hypophysiotropic Hormones of the Hypothalamus: Assay and Chemistry, pp. 74–89. Williams and Wilkins, Baltimore.

142. Kastin, A. J., Viosca, S., and Schally, A. V. (1971). Assay of mammalian MSH release-regulating factor(s). *In* J. Meites (ed.), Hypophysiotropic Hormones of the Hypothalamus: Assay and Chemistry, p. 171. Williams and Wilkins, Baltimore.

143. Bogdanove, E. M. (1963). Direct gonad-pituitary feedback: analysis of the effects of intracranial estrogenic depots on gonadotropin secretion. En-docrinology 73:696.

144. Ramirez, V. D., Abrams, R., and McCann, S. M. (1964). Effect of estradiol implants in the hypothalamo-hypophysial region of the rat on secretion of LH. Endocrinology 75:243.

145. Kamberi, I. A., and McCann, S. M. (1972). Effects of implants of testoster-one in the median eminence and pituitary on FSH secretion. Neuroendo-crinology 9:20.

146. Debeljuk, L., Arimura, A., and Schally, A. V. (1972). Effects of testoster-one and estradiol on the LH and FSH release by LH-releasing hormone (LH-RH) in intact male rats. Endocrinology 90:1578.

147. Debeljuk, L., Vilchez-Martinez, J. A., Arimura, A., and Schally, A. V. (1974). Effect of gonadal steroids on the response to LH-RH in intact and castrated male rats. Endocrinology 94:1519.

148. Negro-Vilar, A., Orias, R., and McCann, S. M. (1973). Evidence for a pituitary site of action for the acute inhibition of LH release by estrogen in the rat. Endocrinology 92:1680.

149. Cooper, K. J., Fawcett, C. P., and McCann, S. M. (1974). Inhibitory and facilitatory effects of estradiol 17-β on pituitary responsiveness to a luteinizing hormone-follicle stimulating hormone-releasing factor (LH-RH/FSH-RF) preparation in ovariectomized rat. Proc. Soc. Exp. Biol. Med. 145:1422.

150. Keye, W. R., and Jaffe, R. B. (1974). Modulation of pituitary gonadotropin response to gonadotropin-releasing hormone by estradiol. J. Clin. Endocrinol. Metab. 38:805.
151. Yen, S. S. C., Lasley, B. L., Wang, C. F., Leblanc, H., and Siler, T. M. (1975). The operating characteristics of the hypothalamic-pituitary system during the menstrual cycle and observations of biological action of somatostatin. Recent Prog. Horm. Res. 31:321.
152. Schally, A. V., Redding, T. W., and Arimura, A. (1973). Effect of sex steroids on pituitary response to LH and FSH-releasing hormone in vitro. Endocrinology 93:893.
153. Tang, L. K. L., and Spies, H. G. (1975). Effect of gonadal steroids on the basal and LRF induced gonadotropin secretion by cultures of rat pituitary. Endocrinology 96:349.
154. Drouin, J., and Labrie, F. (1976). Selective effects of androgens on LH and FSH release in anterior pituitary cells in culture. Endocrinology 98:1528.
155. Cooper, K. J., Fawcett, C. P., and McCann, S. M. (1975). Augmentation of pituitary responsiveness to luteinizing hormone/follicle stimulating hormone-releasing factor (LH-RF) as a result of acute ovariectomy in the four-day cyclic rat. Endocrinology 96, 1123.
156. Arimura, A., and Schally, A. V. (1970). Progesterone suppression of LH-releasing hormone-induced stimulation of LH release in rats. Endocrinology 87:653.
157. Greeley, G. H., Allen, M. B., and Mahesh, V. (1975). Potentiation of luteinizing-hormone release by estradiol at the level of the pituitary. Neuroendocrinology 18:233.
158. Libertun, C., Cooper, K. J., Fawcett, C. P., and McCann, S. M. (1974). Effects of ovariectomy and steroid treatment on hypophysial sensitivity to purified LH-releasing factor (LRF). Endocrinology 94:518.
159. Libertun, C., Orias, R., and McCann, S. M. (1974). Biphasic effect of estrogen on the sensitivity of the pituitary of luteinizing hormone-releasing factor (LRF). Endocrinology 94:1094.
160. Davidson, J. M. (1969). Feedback control of gonadotropin secretion. In W. L. Ganong and L. Martini (eds.), Frontier in Neuroendocrinology, p. 343. Oxford Press, New York.
161. Ajika, K., Krulich, L., Fawcett, C. P., and McCann, S. M. (1972). Effects of estrogen on plasma and pituitary gonadotropin and prolactin and on hypothalamic releasing and inhibiting factors. Neuroendocrinology 9:304.
162. Orias, R., Negro-Vilar, A., Libertun, C., and McCann, S. M. (1974). Inhibitory effect on LH release of estradiol injected into the third ventricle. Endocrinology 94:852.
163. Burger, H. G., Fink, G., and Lee, V. W. K. (1972). Luteinizing hormone-releasing factor in ultrafiltrates of blood collected from the pituitary stalk of ovariectomized rats and rats subjected to electrical stimulation of the preoptic area. J. Endocrinol. 54:227.
164. Ben-Jonathan, N., Mical, R. S., and Porter, J. C. (1973). Superfusion of hemipituitaries with portal blood. I. LRF secretion in castrated and diestrous rat. Endocrinology 93:497.
165. Nett, T. M., Akbar, A. M., and Niswender, G. D. (1974). Serum levels of luteinizing hormone and gonadotropin-releasing hormone in cycling, castrated, and anestrous ewes. Endocrinology 94:713.

166. Wheaton, J. E., and McCann, S. M. (1976). Luteinizing hormone-releasing hormone in peripheral plasma and hypothalamus of normal and ovariectomized rats. Neuroendocrinology 21:296.
167. Carmel, P. W., Araki, S., and Ferin, M. (1976). Pituitary stalk portal blood collection in Rhesus monkeys: evidence for pulsatile release of gonadotropin-releasing hormone (GnRH). Endocrinology 99:243.
168. Dierschke, D. J., Bhattacharya, A. N., Atkinson, L. E., and Knobil, E. (1970). Circhoral oscillations of plasma LH levels in the ovariectomized Rhesus monkey. Endocrinology 87:850.
169. Gay, V. L., and Sheth, N. A. (1972). Evidence for a periodic release of LH in castrated male and female rats. Endocrinology 90:158.
170. Buttler, W. R., Malven, P. V., Willett, L. B., and Bolt, D. J. (1972). Patterns of pituitary release and cranial output of LH and prolactin in ovariectomized ewes. Endocrinology 91:793.
171. Blake, C. A., and Sawyer, C. H. (1972). Effects of hypothalamic deafferentation on the pulsatile rhythm in plasma concentration of luteinizing hormone in ovariectomized rats. Endocrinology 94:730.
172. Krey, L. C., Buttler, W., and Knobil, E. (1975). Surgical disconnections of the medial basal hypothalamus and pituitary functions in the Rhesus monkey. I. Gonadotropin secretion. Endocrinology 96:1073.
173. Bhattacharya, A. N., Dierske, D. J., Yamaji, T., and Knobil, E. (1972). The pharmacologic blockade of the circhoral mode of LH secretion in the ovariectomized monkey. Endocrinology 90:778.
174. Gnodde, H. P., and Schuiling, G. A. (1976). Involvement of catecholaminergic and cholinergic mechanisms in the pulsatile release of LH in the long-term ovariectomized rat. Neuroendocrinology 20:212.
175. McCann, S. M. (1974). Regulation of secretion of follicle stimulating and luteinizing hormone. Handbook of Physiology, Vol. IV, Sec. 7, pp. 489–517. American Physiological Society, Washington.
176. Barraclough, C. A. (1973). Sex steroid regulation of reproductive neuroendocrine processes. Handbook of Physiology, Vol. II, Sec. 7, pp. 29–56, American Physiological Society, Washington.
177. Ramirez, V. D., and McCann, S. M. (1963). A highly sensitive test for LH-releasing activity: the ovariectomized, estrogen progesterone-blocked rat. Endocrinology 73:193.
178. Reeves, J. J., Arimura, A., and Schally, A. V. (1971). Changes in pituitary responsiveness to luteinizing hormone-releasing hormone (LH-RH) in anestrous ewes pretreated with estradiol benzoate. Biol. Reprod. 4:88.
179. Vilchez-Martinez, J. A., Arimura, A., Debeljuk, L., and Schally, A. V. (1974). Biphasic effect of estradiol benzoate on the pituitary responsiveness to LH-RH. Endocrinology 94:1300.
180. Aiyer, M. S., Chiappa, S. A., and Fink, G. (1974). A priming effect of luteinizing hormone-releasing factor on the anterior pituitary gland in the female rat. J. Endocrinol. 62:573.
181. Castro-Vazques, A., and McCann, S. M. (1975). Cyclic variations in the increased responsiveness of the pituitary to luteinizing hormone-releasing hormone (LH-RH) induced by LH-RH. Endocrinology 97:13.
182. Aiyer, M. S., Sood, M. C., and Brown-Grant, K. (1976). The pituitary response to exogenous luteinizing hormone-releasing factor in steroid-treated gonadectomized rat. J. Endocrinol. 69:255.
183. Fink, G., Chiappa, S. A., and Aiyer, M. S. (1976). Priming effect of luteinizing hormone-releasing factor elicited by preoptic stimulation and

by intravenous infusion and multiple injections of the synthetic decapeptide. J. Endocrinol. 69:359.

184. Aiyer, M. S., and Fink, G. (1973). The role of sex steroid hormones in modulating the responsiveness of the anterior pituitary gland to luteinizing hormone-releasing factor in the female rat. J. Endocrinol. 62:553.

185. Pickering, A. J. M. C., and Fink, G. (1976). Priming effect of luteinizing hormone-releasing hormone factor: *in vitro* and *in vivo* evidence consistent with its dependence upon protein and RNA synthesis. J. Endocrinol. 69:373.

186. Zolman, J., and Valenta, L. (1976). Positive cooperativity in the gonadotropin-releasing hormone (GnRH)-receptor interaction. Sixth International Congress of Endocrinology, p. 21 (Abstr.), Hamburg.

187. Pickering, A., and Fink, G. (1976). Priming effect of luteinizing hormone-releasing factor: *in vitro* studies with raised potassium concentration. J. Endocrinol. 69:453.

188. Cooper, K. J., Fawcett, C. P., and McCann, S. M. (1973). Variations in pituitary responsiveness to luteinizing hormone-releasing factor during the rat estrous cycle. J. Endocrinol. 57:187.

189. Martin, J. E., Tyrey, L., Everett, J. W., and Fellows, R. E. (1974). Variations in responsiveness to synthetic LH-releasing factor (LRF) in proestrous and diestrous-3 rats. Endocrinology 94:556.

190. Gordon, J. H., and Rechlin, S. (1974). Changes in pituitary responsiveness to luteinizing hormone-releasing factor during the rat estrous cycle. Endocrinology 74: 974.

191. Aiyer, M. S., Fink, G., and Greig, F. (1974). Changes in the sensitivity of the pituitary gland to luteinizing hormone-releasing factor during the estrous cycle in the rat. J. Endocrinol. 60:47.

192. Howley, R. D., Baxter, R. W., Chamley, W. A., Cumming, I. A., Jonas, H. A., and Findlay, J. K. (1974). FSH and LH response to gonadotropin-releasing hormone during the ovine estrous cycle and following progesterone administration. Endocrinology 95:937.

193. Ferin, M., Warren, M., Dyrenfurth, I., Vandewiele, R. L., and White, W. F. (1974). Responses of Rhesus monkeys to LRH throughout the ovarian cycle. J. Clin. Endocrinol. Metab. 38:231.

194. Yen, S. S. C., Vandenberg, G., Rebar, R., and Ehara, Y. (1972). Variations of pituitary responsiveness to synthetic LRF during different phases of the menstrual cycle. J. Clin. Endocrinol. Metab. 35:931.

195. Malacara, J. M., Seyler, E. L., Jr., and Reichlin, S. (1972). Luteinizing hormone-releasing factor activity in peripheral blood from women during mid-cycle luteinizing hormone ovulatory surge. J. Clin. Endocrinol. 34:271.

196. Arimura, A., Kastin, A. J., and Schally, A. V. (1974). Immunoreactive LH-releasing hormone in plasma: mid-cycle elevation in women. J. Clin. Endocrinol. Metab. 38:510.

197. Fraser, H. M., Jeffcoate, S. L., Holland, D. T., and Gunn, A. (1973). Detection of luteinizing hormone-releasing hormone in the peripheral blood of the rat on the afternoon of proestrus. J. Endocrinol. 59:375.

198. Sarkar, D. K., Chiappa, S. A., and Fink, G. (1976). Gonadotropin-releasing hormone surge in proestrous rat. Nature (Lond.) 264:461.

199. Fink, G., Greig, F., Chiappa, S., and Henderson, S. R. (1974). Peripheral plasma luteinizing hormone-releasing factor and spontaneous and reflex release of luteinizing hormone in the rat. J. Endocrinol. 63:33P.

200. Foster, J. P., Jeffcoate, S. L., Crighton, D. B., and Holland, D. T. (1976). Luteinizing hormone and luteinizing hormone-releasing hormone like immunoreactivity in the jugular venous blood of sheep at various stages of the oestrous cycle. J. Endocrinol. 68:409.

201. Reichlin, S., Martin, J. B., Mitnick, M., Boshans, R. L., Grimm, Y., Bollinger, J., Gordon, J., and Malacara, J. (1972). The hypothalamus in pituitary thyroid regulation. Recent Prog. Horm. Res. 28:229.

202. Guillemin, R., Yamazaki, E., Jutisz, M., and Sakiz, E. (1962). Présence dans un extrait de tissus hypothala migues d'une substance stimulant la secrétion de l'hormone hypophysaire thyréotrophe (TSH). Premiére purification par filtration sur gel sephadex. C. R. Acad. Sci. (Paris) 55:1018.

203. Vale, W., Burgus, R., and Guillemin, R. (1967). Competition between thyroxine and TRF at the pituitary level in the release of TSH. Proc. Soc. Exp. Biol. Med. 125:210.

204. Eto, S., and Fleisher, N. (1976). Regulation of thyrotropin (TSH) release and production in monolayer cultures of transplantable TSH producing mouse tumors. Endocrinology 98:114.

205. Shenkeman, L., Mitsuma, T., Suphavai, A., and Hollander, C. S. (1972). Response to thyrotropin releasing hormone in man: feedback inhibition by thyroid hormone. Ann. J. Med. Sci. 263:426.

206. Hershman, J. M., and Pittman, J. A., Jr. (1970). Response to synthetic thyrotropin-releasing hormone in man. J. Clin. Endocrinol. Metab. 31: 457.

207. Snyder, P. J., and Utiger, R. D. (1972). Inhibition of thyrotropin response to thyrotropin-releasing hormone by small quantities of thyroid hormones. J. Clin. Invest. 57:2077.

208. Saberi, M., and Utiger, R. D. (1975). Augmentation of thyrotropin responses to thyrotropin-releasing hormone following small decreases in serum thyroid hormone concentration. J. Clin. Endocrinol. Metab. 40: 435.

209. Garcia, M. D., Escobar del Rey, F., and Morreale de Escobar, G. (1976). Thyrotropin-releasing hormone and thyroid hormone interactions on thyrotropin secretion in the rat: lack of inhibiting effects of small doses of triiodothyronine in the hypothyroid rat. Endocrinology 98:203.

210. Yamada, T., and Greer, M. A. (1959). Studies on the mechanism of hypothalamic control of thyrotropine secretion: effect of thyroxine injection into the hypothalamus or the pituitary on thyroid hormone release. Endocrinology 64:559.

211. Knigge, K. M., and Joseph, S. A. (1971). Neural regulation of TSH secretion: sites of thyroxine feedback. Neuroendocrinology 8:273.

212. Chambers, W. F., and Sobel, R. J. (1971). Effect of thyroxine-agar tube application to the rat hypothalamus. Neuroendocrinology 7:37.

213. Sinha, D., and Meites, J. (1966). Effect of thyroidectomy and thyroxine on hypothalamic concentration of thyrotropin-releasing factor, and pituitary content of thyrotropin in rats. Neuroendocrinology 1:4.

214. Jackson, I. M. D., Gagel, R., and Popapetrou, P. (1974). Pituitary hypothalamic and urinary thyrotropin-releasing hormone (TRH) concentration in altered thyroid states of rat and man. Clin. Res. 23:342a.

215. Vagenakis, A. G., Roti, E., Mannix, J., and Braverman, L. E. (1975). Problems in the measurement of urinary TRH. J. Clin. Endocrinol. Metab. 41:801.

216. Bassiri, R. M., and Utiger, R. D. (1974). Thyrotropin-releasing hormone in the hypothalamus of the rat. Endocrinology 94:188.
217. Montoya, E., Seibel, M. J., and Wilber, J. F. (1975). Thyrotropin-releasing hormone secretory physiology: studies by radioimmunoassay and affinity chromatography. Endocrinology 96:1413.
218. Emerson, C. H., and Utiger, R. D. (1975). Plasma thyrotropin-releasing hormone concentrations in the rat: effect of thyroid excess and deficiency and cold exposure. J. Clin. Invest. 56:1564.
219. Hefco, E., Krulich, L., Illner, P., and Larsen, P. R. (1975). Effect of acute exposure to cold on the activity of the hypothalamic-pituitary-thyroid system. Endocrinology 97:1185.
220. Eskay, R. L., Oliver, C., Warberg, J., and Porter, J. C. (1976). Inhibition of degradation and measurement of immunoreactive thyrotropin-releasing hormone in rat blood and plasma. Endocrinology 98:269.
221. Hershman, T. M., Read, P. G., Bailey, A. L., Norman, V. D., and Gibson, T. B. (1970). Effect of cold exposure on serum thyrotropin. J. Clin. Endocrinol. 30:430.
222. Fisher, R. A., and Odell, W. D. (1971). Effect of cold on TSH secretion in man. J. Clin. Endocrinol. 33:859.
223. Vale, W., Rivier, C., Brazeau, P., and Guillemin, R. (1974). Effects of somatostatin on the secretion of thyrotropin and prolactin. Endocrinology 95:968.
224. Hall, R., Besser, G. M., Schally, A. V., Coy, D. H., Evered, D., Goldie, D. J., Kastin, A. J., McNeilly, A. S., Mortimer, C. H., Phenekos, C., Tunbridge, W. H. G., and Weightman, D. (1973). Action of growth-hormone release inhibitory hormone in healthy men and in acromegaly. Lancet 2:581.
225. Drouin, J., DeLéan, A., Rainville, D., Lachance, R., and Labrie, F. (1976). Characteristics of the interaction between thyrotropin releasing hormone and somatostatin for thyrotropin and prolactin release. Endocrinology 98:514.
226. Arimura, A., and Schally, A. V. (1976). Increase in basal and thyrotropin-releasing hormone (TRH) stimulated secretion of thyrotropin (TSH) by passive immunization with antiserum to somatostatin in rats. Endocrinology 98:1069.
227. Florsheim, W. H., and Kozbur, X. (1976). Physiological modulation of thyrotropin secretion by somastatin and thyroliberin. Biochem. Biophys. Res. Commun. 72:603.
228. Ferland, L., Labrie, F., Jobin, M., Arimura, A., and Schally, A. V. (1976). Physiological role of somatostatin in the control of growth hormone and thyrotropin secretion. Biochem. Biophys. Res. Commun. 68:149.
229. Yates, F. E., and Maran, J. W. (1974). Stimulation and inhibition of adrenocorticotropin release. Handbook of Physiology, Vol. IV, Sec. 7, Part 2, pp. 367–404. American Physiological Society, Washington.
230. Kendall, J. W., Tang, L., and Cook, D. M. (1975). Sites of feedback control in the pituitary-adrenocortical system. In E. Stumpf and L. D. Grant (eds.), Anatomical Neuroendocrinology, pp. 276–283. Karger, New York.
231. Kendall, J. W., and Allen, C. (1968). Studies on the glucocorticoid feedback control of ACTH secretion. Endocrinology 82:397.
232. Gonzales-Lugue, A., L'age, M., Dhariwal, A. P. S., and Yates, F. E. (1970). Stimulation of corticotropin release by corticotropin releasing factor

(CRF) or by vasopressin following intrapituitary infusion in unanesthetized dogs: inhibition of the responses by dexamethasone. Endocrinology 86:1134.

233. Kendall, J. W., Stott, A. V., Allen, C. F., and Greer, M. A. (1966). Evidence for ACTH secretion and ACTH suppressibility in hypophysectomized rats with multiple heterotropic pituitaries. Endocrinology 78:533.

234. Sayers, G., and Portanova, R. Secretion of ACTH by isolated anterior pituitary cells: kinetics of stimulation by corticotropin-releasing factor and inhibition by corticosterone. Endocrinology 94:1723.

235. Yasuda, N., Takebe, K., and Greer, M. A. (1976). Studies on ACTH dynamics in cultured adenohypophysial cells: effect of adrenalectomy or dexamethasone in vivo. Endocrinology 98:717.

236. Fleisher, N., and Rawls, W. (1970). ACTH synthesis and release in pituitary menolayer culture: effects of dexamethasone. Ann. J. Physiol. 219:445.

237. Edwardson, J. A., and Bennett, G. W. (1974). Modulation of corticotrophin releasing-factor release from hypothalamic synaptosomes. Nature (Lond.) 251:425.

238. Hillhouse, E. W., and Jones, M. T. (1976). Effect of bilateral adrenalutomy and corticosteroid therapy on the secretion of corticotropin-releasing factor activity from the hypothalamus of the rat in vitro. J. Endocrinol. 71:21.

239. Porter, J. C., Dhariwal, A. P. S., and McCann, S. M. (1967). Response of anterior pituitary-adrenocortical axis to purified CRF. Endocrinology 80:679.

240. Hiroshige, T., Sato, T., and Abe, K. (1971). Dynamic changes in the hypothalamic content of corticotropin-releasing factor following noxious stimuli: delayed response in early neonates in comparison with biphasic response in adult rats. Endocrinology 89:1287.

241. Sato, T., Sato, M., Shinsako, J., and Dallman, M. F. (1975). Corticosterone-induced changes in hypothalamic corticotropin-releasing factor (CRF) content after stress. Endocrinology 97:265.

242. Dallman, M. F., and Yates, F. E. (1968). Anatomical and functional mapping of central neural input and feedback pathways of the adrenocortical system. Mem. Soc. Endocrinol. 17:39.

243. Dallman, M. F., and Yates, F. E. (1969). Dynamic asymmetrics in the corticosteroid feedback path and distribution-metabolism-binding elements of the adrenocortical system. Ann. N. Y. Acad. Sci. 156:696.

244. Dallman, M. F., Jones, M. T., Vernikos-Danellis, J., and Ganong, W. F. (1972). Corticosteroid feedback control of ACTH secretion: rapid effects of bilateral adrenalectomy on plasma ACTH in the rat. Endocrinology 91:961.

245. Sakakura, M., Saita, Y., Takebe, K., and Ishui, K. (1976). Studies on the fast feedback mechanism by endogenous glucocorticoids. Endocrinology 98:954.

246. Martin, J. B., Renaud, L. P., and Brazeau, P. (1974). Pulsatile growth hormone secretion: suppression by hypothalamic ventromedial lesions and by long-acting somatostatin. Science 186:538.

247. Arimura, A., Smith, W. D., and Schally, A. V. (1976). Blockade of the stress induced decrease in blood GH by anti-somatostatin serum in rats. Endocrinology 98:540.

248. Terry, L. C., Willoughby, J. O., Brazeau, P., and Martin, J. B. (1976).

Antiserum to somatostatin prevents stress-induced inhibition of growth hormone secretion in the rat. Science 192:565.

249. Brown, G. M., Schalch, D. S., and Reichlin, S. (1971). Hypothalamic mediation of growth hormone and adrenal stress response in the squirrel monkey. Endocrinology 89:694.

250. Martin, J. B. (1974). The role of hypothalamic and extrahypothalamic structures in the control of GH secretion. In S. Raiti (ed.), Advances in Human Growth Hormone Research, No. 74-612, pp. 223–249. NIH Publication, Washington.

251. Rice, R. W., and Critchlow, V. (1976). Extrahypothalamic control of stress induced inhibition of growth hormone secretion in the rat. Endocrinology 99:970.

252. Mitchell, J., Smyrl, R., Hutchins, M., Schindler, W. J., and Critchlow, V. (1972). Plasma growth hormone levels in rats with increased naso-anal lengths to hypothalamic surgery. Neuroendocrinology 10:31.

253. Collu, R., Jéquier, J.-C., Letarte, J., Leboeuf, G., and Ducharme, J. R. (1973). Effect of stress and hypothalamic deafferentation on the secretion of growth hormone in the rat. Neuroendocrinology 11:183.

254. Kato, Y., Chihara, K., Ohgo, W., and Imura, A. (1974). Effect of hypothalamic surgery and somatostatin on chlorpromazine-induced growth hormone release in rats. Endocrinology 95:1608.

255. Frohman, L. A., Bernardis, L. L., and Kant, K. (1968). Hypothalamic stimulation of growth hormone secretion. Science 162:580.

256. Martin, J. B. (1972). Plasma growth hormone (GH) response to hypothalamic or extrahypothalamic electrical stimulation. Endocrinology 91:107.

257. Frohman, L. A., and Bernardis, L. L. (1968). Growth hormone and insulin levels in weanling rats with ventromedial hypothalamic lesions. Endocrinology 82:1125.

258. Toivola, P. T. K., and Gale, C. C. (1972). Stimulation of growth hormone release by microinjection of norepinephrine into hypothalamus of baboons. Endocrinology 90:895.

259. Neill, J. D. (1974). Prolactin: its secretion and control. Handbook of Physiology, Vol. IV, Sec. 7, pp. 469–488. American Physiological Society, Washington.

260. Kastin, A. J., and Ross, G. T. (1965). Melanocyte-stimulating activity in pituitaries of frogs with hypothalamic lesions. Endocrinology 77:45.

261. Guardabassi, A. (1961). The hypophysis of Xenopus laevis after removal of anterior hypothalamus. Gen. Comp. Endocrinol. 1:348.

262. Taleisnik, S., Olmos, J., Orias, R., and Tomatis, M. D. (1967). Effect of hypothalamic lesions on pituitary meanocyte stimulating hormone. J. Endocrinol. 39:555.

263. Thody, A. J. (1974). Plasma and pituitary MSH levels in the rat after lesions of the hypothalamus. Neuroendocrinology 16:323.

264. Tilders, F. J. H., Mulder, A. H., and Smelik, P. G. (1975). On the presence of a MSH-release inhibiting system in the rat neurointermediate lobe. Neuroendocrinology 18:125.

265. Taleisnik, S., Celis, M. S., and Tomatis, M. E. (1974). Release of melanocyte-stimulating hormone by several stimuli through the action of a 5-hydroxytryptamine-mediated inhibiting neuronal mechanism. Neuroendocrinology 13:327.

266. Howe, A., and Thody, A. J. (1969). The effect of hypothalamic lesions on the melanocyte-stimulating hormone content and histology of the pars intermedia of the rat pituitary gland. J. Physiol. 203:159.

267. Celis, M. E. (1975). Serum MSH levels and hypothalamic enzymes involved in the formation of MSH-RF during the estrus cycle in the rat. Neuroendocrinology 18:256.
268. Abe, K., Nicholson, W. E., Liddle, G. W., Orth, D. N., and Island, D. D. (1969). Normal and abnormal regulation of β-MSH in man. J. Clin. Invest. 48:1580.
269. Phifer, R. F., Orth, D. N., and Spicer, S. S. (1974). Specific demonstration of the human hypophyseal adrenocortico-melanotropic (ACTH/MSH) cell. J. Clin. Endocrinol. 39:689.
270. Brownstein, J. J., Palkovits, M., Saavedra, J. M., and Kizer, J. S. (1976). Distribution of hypothalamic hormones and neurotransmitters within the diencephalon. In L. Martini and W. F. Ganong (eds.), Frontiers in Neuroendocrinology, p. 123. Raven Press, New York.
271. McCann, S. M., and Moss, R. L. (1975). Putative neurotransmitters involved in discharging gonadotropin-releasing neurohormones and the action of LH-releasing hormone on the CNS. Life Sci. 16:833.
272. McCann, S. M., and Ojeda, S. R. The role of brain monoamines, acetylcholine and prostaglandins in the control of anterior pituitary function. In L. Martini (ed.), Metabolic Basis of Endocrinology, in press.
273. Kamberi, I. A., Schneider, H. P. G., and McCann, S. M. (1970). Action of dopamine to induce release of FSH-releasing factor (FRF) from hypothalamic tissue in vitro. Endocrinology 86:278.
274. Schneider, H. P. G., and McCann, S. M. (1969). Possible role of dopamine as transmitter to promote discharge of LH-releasing factor. Endocrinology 85:121.
275. Rotszstein, W. H., Charli, J. L., Pattou, E., Epelbaum, J., and Kordon, C. (1976). In vitro release of lutenizing hormone-releasing hormone (LHRH) from rat mediobasal hypothalamus: effects of calcium, potassium and dopamine. Endocrinology 99:1663.
276. Quijada, M., Illner, P., Krulich, L., and McCann, S. M. (1973/4). The effect of catecholamines on hormone release from anterior pituitaries and ventral hypothalami incubated in vitro. Neuroendocrinology 13:151.
277. Schneider, H. P. G., and McCann, S. M. (1970). Mono- and indoleamines and control of LH secretion. Endocrinology 86:1127.
278. Schneider, H. P. G., and McCann, S. M. (1970). Release of LH releasing factor (LRF) into peripheral circulation of hypophysectomized rats by dopamine and its blockade by estradiol. Endocrinology 87:249.
279. Kamberi, I. A., Mical, R. S., and Porter, J. C. (1970). Effect of anterior pituitary perfusion and intraventricular injection of catecholamines and indoleamines on LH release. Endocrinology 87:1.
280. Kamberi, I. A., Mical, R. S., and Porter, J. C. (1969). Luteinizing hormone releasing activity in hypophyseal stalk blood and elevation of dopamine. Science 166:388.
281. Vijayan, E., and McCann, S. M. Re-evaluation of the role of catecholamines in control of gonadotropin and prolactin release. Neuroendocrinology (submitted for publication).
282. Cramer, O. M., and Porter, J. C. (1973). Input to releasing factor cells. Prog. Brain Res. 39:73.
283. Krieg, R. J., and Sawyer, C. H. (1976). Effects of intraventricular catecholamines on luteinizing hormone release on ovariectomized steroid-primed rats. Endocrinology 99:411.
284. Bacha, J. C., and Donoso, A. O. (1974). Enhanced luteinizing hormone

release after noradrenaline treatment in 6-hydroxydopamine treated rats. J. Endocrinol. 62:169.

285. Ojeda, S. R., and McCann, S. M. (1973). Evidence for participation of a catecholaminergic mechanism in the postcastration rise in plasma gonadotropins. Neuroendocrinology 12:295.

286. Cocchi, D., Fraschini, F., Jalanbo, H., and Müller, E. E. (1974). Role of brain catecholamines in the postcastration rise in plasma LH of prepuberal rats. Endocrinology 95:1649.

287. Donoso, A. O., Bishop, W., Fawcett, C. P., Krulich, L., and McCann, S. M. (1971). Effects of drugs that modify brain monoamine concentrations on plasma gonadotropin and prolactin levels in the rat. Endocrinology 89:774.

288. Kalra, S. P., and McCann, S. M. (1974). Effect of drugs modifying catecholamine synthesis on plasma LH and ovulation in the rat. Neuroendocrinology 15:79.

289. Kalra, P. S., Kalra, S. P., Krulich, L., Fawcett, C. P., and McCann, S. M. (1972). Involvement of norepinephrine in transmission of the stimulatory influence of progesterone on gonadotropin release. Endocrinology 90:1168.

290. Martinovic, J. V., and McCann, S. M. Effect of lesions in the ventral noradrenergic tract produced by microinjection of 6-hydroxydopamine on gonadotropin release in the rat. Endocrinology 100:1206.

291. Kamberi, I. A., Mical, R. S., and Porter, J. C. (1971). Effects of melatonin and serotonin on the release of FSH and prolactin. Endocrinology 88:1288.

292. Collu, R., Fraschini, F., and Martini, L. (1973). Role of indoleamines and catecholamines in the control of gonadotrophin and growth hormone secretion. Prog. Brain Res. 39:289.

293. Domański, E., Przekop, F., Skubiszewski, B., and Wolińskia, E. (1975). The effect and site of action of indoleamines on the hypothalamic centers involved in the control of LH release and ovulation in sheep. Neuroendocrinology 17:265.

294. Héry, M., Laplante, C., and Kordon, C. (1976). Participation of serotonin in phasic release of LH. I. Evidence from pharmacological experiments. Endocrinology 99:496.

295. Libertun, C., and McCann, S. M. (1973). Blockade of the release of gonadotropins and prolactin by subcutaneous or intraventricular injection of atropine in male and female rats. Endocrinology 92:1714.

296. Libertun, C., and McCann, S. M. (1974). Further evidence for cholinergic control of gonadotropin and prolactin secretion. Proc. Soc. Exp. Biol. Med. 147:498.

297. Blake, C. A., Scaramuzzi, R. J., Norman, R. L., Kanematsu, S., and Sawyer, C. H. (1972). Nicotine delays the ovulatory surge of luteinizing hormone in the rat. Proc. Soc. Exp. Biol. Med. 141:1014.

298. Fiorindo, R. P., and Martini, L. (1975). Evidence for a cholinergic component in the neuroendocrine control of luteinizing hormone (LH) secretion. Neuroendocrinology 18:322.

299. Grimm, Y., and Reichlin, S. (1973). Thyrotropin-releasing hormone (TRH): neurotransmitter regulation of secretion by mouse hypothalamic tissue in vitro. Endocrinology 93:626.

300. Krulich, L., Giachetti, A., Marchlewska-Koj, A., Hefco, E., and Jameson, H. E. (1977). On the role of the central noradrenergic and dopaminergic

systems in the regulation of TSH secretion in the rat. Endocrinology 100:496.

301. Scapagnini, U., Raxas, M., D'Agata, R., Annuziato, L., and Preziosi, P. (1976). Chronic depletion of brain catecholamines (CA) and thyrotropin secretion. Fifth International Congress of Endocrinology, p. 330. Excerpta Medica, Amsterdam.

302. Tuomisto, J., Ranta, T., Männistö, P., Saarinen, A., and Leppäluoto, J. (1975). Neurotransmitter control of thyrotropin secretion in the rat. Eur. J. Pharmacol. 30:221.

303. Onaya, T., and Hashizume, K. (1976). Effects of drugs that modify brain biogenic amine concentration on thyroid activation induced by exposure to cold. Neuroendocrinology 20:47.

304. Mueller, G. P., Simpkins, J., Meites, J., and Moore, K. E. (1976). Differential effects of dopamine agonists and haloperidol on release of prolactin, thyroid stimulating hormone, growth hormone and luteinizing hormone in rats. Neuroendocrinology 20:121.

305. Mueller, G. P., Twohy, C. P., Chen, H. T., Advis, J. P., and Meites, J. (1976). Effect of L-tryptophane and restraint stress on hypothalamic and brain turnover, and pituitary TSH and prolactin release in rats. Life Sci. 18:715.

306. Shopsin, B., Shenkemean, L., Saughoi, I., and Hollander, C. S. (1974). Toward a relationship between the hypothalamic-pituitary-thyroid axis and the synthesis of serotonin. Adv. Biochem. Psychopharmacol. 10:279.

307. Woolf, P. D., Lee, L. A., and Schalch, D. S. (1972). Adrenergic manipulation and thyrotropin-releasing hormone (TRH)-induced thyrotropin (TSH) release. J. Clin. Endocrinol. Metab. 35:616.

308. Lal, S., Talis, G., Martin, J. B., Brown, G. M., and Guyda, H. (1975). Effects of clonidine on growth hormone, prolactin, luteinizing hormone, follicle stimulating hormone and thyroid stimulation hormone in the serum of normal man. J. Clin. Endocrinol. Metab. 41:703.

309. Chambers, J. W., and Brown, G. M. (1976). Neurotransmitter regulation of growth hormone and ACTH in the rhesus monkey: effects of biogenic amines. Endocrinology 98:420.

310. Blackard, W. G., and Heidingsfelder, S. A. (1968). Adrenergic receptor control mechanism for growth hormone secretion. J. Clin. Invest. 47:1407.

311. Hansen, A. P. (1972). The effect of alpha and beta blocking agents on exercise induced growth hormone release in normal subjects and juvenile diabetes. Fourth International Congress of Endocrinology, p. 31. Excerpta Medica, Amsterdam.

312. Boyd, A. E., Lebovitz, H. E., and Pfeiffer, J. B. (1970). Stimulation of human GH secretion by L-Dopa. N. Engl. J. Med. 283:1425.

313. Maany, I., Frazer, A., and Mendels, J. (1975). Apomorphine: effect on growth hormone. J. Clin. Endocrinol. 40:162.

314. Lal, S., de La Vega, C. E., Sourkes, T. L., and Friesen, H. G. (1973). Effect of apomorphine on growth hormone, prolactin, luteinizing hormone and follicle-stimulating hormone levels in human serum. J. Clin. Endocrinol. Metab. 37:719.

315. Imura, H., Nakai, I., and Hoshimi, T. (1973). Effect of 5-hydroxy-tryptophane (5-HTP) on growth hormone and ACTH release in man. J. Clin. Endocrinol. Metab. 36:204.

316. Bivens, C. H., Lebovitz, H. E., and Feldman, J. M. (1973). Inhibition of hypoglycemia-induced growth hormone secretion by the serotonin antagonists cyproheptadine and methysergide. N. Engl. J. Med. 289:236.

317. Kato, Y., Dupre, J., and Beck, J. C. (1973). Plasma growth hormone in the anesthetized rat: effect of dibutyryl cyclic AMP, prostaglandin E, adrenergic agents, vasopressin, chlorpromazine, amphetamine and L-Dopa. Endocrinology 93:135.

318. Lu, K. H., and Meites, J. (1971). Inhibition by L-Dopa and monoamine oxidase inhibitors of pituitary prolactin release, stimulation by methyldopa and d-amphetamine. Proc. Soc. Exp. Biol. Med. 137:480.

319. Kamberi, I. A., Mical, R. S., and Porter, J. C. (1971). Effect of anterior pituitary perfusion and intraventricular injection of catecholamines on prolactin release. Endocrinology 88:1012.

320. Ojeda, S. R., Harms, P. G., and McCann, S. M. (1974). Effect of blockade of dopaminergic receptors on prolactin and LH release: median eminence and pituitary sites of action. Endocrinology 94:1650.

321. Lawson, D. M., and Gala, R. R. (1975). The influence of adrenergic, dopaminergic, cholinergic and serotoninergic drugs on plasma prolactin levels on ovariectomized, estrogen treated rats. Endocrinology 96:313.

322. MacLeod, R. M. (1976). Regulation of prolactin secretion. In L. Martini and W. F. Ganong (eds.), Frontiers in Neuroendocrinology, pp. 169–194. Raven Press, New York.

323. Frantz, A. G. (1973). Catecholamines and the control of prolactin secretion in humans. Prog. Brain Res. 39:311.

324. Marchlewska-Koj, A., and Krulich, L. (1975). The role of central monoamines in the stress induced prolactin release in the rat. Fed. Proc. 39:252.

325. Valverde, R., Chieffo, V., and Reichlin, S. (1973). Failure of reserpine to block ether-induced release of prolactin: physiological evidence that stress induced prolactin release is not caused by acute inhibition of PIF secretion. Life Sci. 12:327.

326. Voogt, J. L., and Carr, L. A. (1975). Potentiation of suckling-induced release of prolactin by inhibition of brain catecholamine synthesis. Endocrinology 97:891.

327. Gala, R. R., Janson, P. A., and Kuo, E. Y. (1972). The influence of neural blocking agents injected into the third ventricle of the rat brain and hypothalamic electrical stimulation on serum prolactin. Proc. Soc. Exp. Biol. Med. 140:569.

328. Subramanian, M. G., and Gala, R. R. (1976). The influence of cholinergic, adrenergic and serotoninergic drugs on the afternoon surge of plasma prolactin in ovariectomized, estrogen treated rats. Endocrinology 98:892.

329. Lu, K. H., and Meites, J. (1973). Effects of serotonin precursors and melatonin on serum prolactin release in rats. Endocrinology 93:152.

330. MacIndoe, J. H., and Turkington, R. W. (1973). Stimulation of human prolactin secretion by intravenous infusion of L-tryptophan. J. Clin. Invest. 52:1972.

331. Gallo, R. V., Rabii, J., and Moberg, G. P. (1975). Effect of methysergide, a blocker of serotonin receptors, on plasma prolactin levels in lactating and ovariectomized rats. Endocrinology 97:1096.

332. Caligaris, L., and Taleisnik, S. (1974). Involvement of neurons containing 5-hydroxytryptamine in the mechanism of prolactin release induced by estrogen. J. Endocrinol. 62:25.

333. Grandison, E., Gelato, M., and Meites, J. (1974). Inhibition of prolactin secretion by cholinergic drugs. Proc. Soc. Exp. Biol. Med. 145:1236.

334. Blake, C. A., Norman, R. L., Scaramuzzi, R. J., and Sawyer, C. H. (1973). Inhibition of proestrus surge of prolactin in the rat by nicotine. Endocrinology 92:1334.

335. Grandison, L., and Meites, J. (1976). Evidence for adrenergic mediation of cholinergic inhibition of prolactin release. Endocrinology 99:775.

336. VanLoon, G. R. (1973). Brain catecholamines and ACTH secretion. In W. F. Ganong and L. Martini (eds.), Frontiers in Neuroendocrinology, pp. 209–248. Oxford University Press, New York.

337. Krieger, H. P., and Krieger, D. T. (1970). Chemical stimulation of the brain: effect on adrenal cortical release. Am. J. Physiol. 218:1632.

338. Abe, K., and Hiroshige, T. (1974). Changes in plasma corticosterone and hypothalamic CRF levels following intraventricular injection or drug-induced changes of brain biogenic amines in the rat. Neuroendocrinology 14:195.

339. Naumenko, E. V. (1968). Hypothalamic chemoreactive structures and the pituitary adrenal function: effect of local injections of norepinephrine, carbachol and serotonin into the brain of guinea pigs with intact brains and after mesencephalic transection. Brain Res. 11:1.

340. Hedge, G. A., and deWied, D. (1971). Corticotropin and vasopressin secretion after hypothalamic implantation of atropine. Endocrinology 88:1257.

341. Suzuki, T., Ikeda, H., Narita, S., Shibata, O., Waki, S., and Egashira, K. (1973). Adrenal cortical secretion in response to nicotine in conscious and anesthetized dogs. Q. J. Exp. Physiol. 58:139.

342. Hillhouse, E. W., Burden, J., and Jones, M. T. (1975). The effects of various putative neurotransmitters on the release of corticotrophin releasing hormone from the hypothalamus of the rat in vitro. I. The effect of acetylcholine and noradrenaline. Neuroendocrinology 17:1.

343. Jones, M. T., Hillhouse, E. W., and Burden, J. (1975). Effect of various putative neurotransmitters on the secretion of corticotrophin-releasing hormones from the rat hypothalamus in vitro: a model of the neurotransmitters involved. J. Endocrinol. 69:1.

344. Scott, G. T., and Stillings, W. A. (1972). Evidence for the release of MSH by phenothiazine ataractics. Endocrinology 90:1972.

345. Usategni, R., Oliver, C., Vaudry, H., Lombardi, G., Rozenberg, I., and Mourre, A. M. (1976). Immunoactive α-MSH and ACTH levels in rat plasma and pituitary. Endocrinology 98:189.

346. Smith, A. F. (1975). The effect of apomorphine and ergocriptine on the release of MSH by the pars intermedia of Rana pipiens. Neuroendocrinology 19:363.

347. Bower, A., Hadley, Mac A., and Hruby, V. J. (1974). Biogenic amines and control of melanophore stimulating hormone release. Science 184:70.

348. Taleisnik, S., Tomatis, M. E., and Celis, M. E. (1972). Role of catecholamines in the control of melanocyte-stimulating hormone secretion in rats. Neuroendocrinology 10:235.

349. McCann, S. M., Ojeda, S. R., Harms, P. G., Wheaton, J. E., Sundberg, D. K., and Fawcett, C. P. (1976). Control of adenohypophyseal hormone secretion by prostaglandins. In F. Naftolin, K. J. Ryan, and I. J. Davies (eds.), Subcellular Mechanisms in Reproductive Neuroendocrinology, pp. 407–422. Elsevier, Amsterdam.

350. Harms, P. G., Ojeda, S. R., and McCann, S. M. (1974). Prostaglandin

induced release of pituitary gonadotropins: central nervous system and pituitary sites of action. Endocrinology 94:1459.

351. Ojeda, S. R., Wheaton, J. E., and McCann, S. M. (1975). Prostaglandin E_2-induced release of luteinizing hormone-releasing factor (LRF). Neuroendocrinology 17:283.

352. Eskay, R. L., Warberg, J., Mical, R. S., and Porter, J. C. (1975). Prostaglandin E_2-induced release of LHRH into hypophysial portal blood. Endocrinology 97:816.

353. Warberg, J., Eskay, R. L., and Porter, J. C. (1976). Prostaglandin-induced release of anterior pituitary hormones: structure activity relationships. Endocrinology 98:1135.

354. Harms, P. G., Ojeda, S. R., and McCann, S. M. (1976). Failure of monoaminergic and cholinergic receptor blockers to prevent prostaglandin E_2-induced LH release. Endocrinology 98:318.

355. Ojeda, S. R., Jameson, H. E., and McCann, S. M. Hypothalamic areas involved in prostaglandin (PG) induced gonadotropin release. I. Effect of PGE_2 and $PGF_{2\alpha}$ implants on luteinizing hormone release. Endocrinology 100:1585.

356. Behrman, H. R., Orczyk, G. P., and Greep, R. O. (1972). Effect of synthetic gonadotropin-releasing hormone (GH-RH) on ovulation blockade by aspirin and indomethacin. Prostaglandins 1:245.

357. Ojeda, S. R., Harms, P. G., and McCann, S. M. (1975). Effect of inhibitors of prostaglandin synthesis on gonadotropin release in the rat. Endocrinology 97:893.

358. Brown, M., and Hedge, G. A. (1974). *In vivo* effects of prostaglandins on TRH-induced TSH secretion. Endocrinology 95:1392.

359. Ito, H., Momse, G., Katayama, T., Takagishi, H., Ho, L., Nakajima, H., and Takei, Y. (1971). Effect of prostaglandin on the secretion of human growth hormone. J. Clin. Endocrinol. 32:857.

360. MacLeod, R. M., and Lehmeyer, J. E. (1970). Release of pituitary growth hormone by prostaglandins and dibutyryl adenosine $3',5'$ monophosphate in the absence of protein synthesis. Proc. Natl. Acad. Sci. 67:1172.

361. Ojeda, S. R., Jameson, H. E., and McCann, S. M. Prostaglandin E_2 (PGE_2) induced growth hormone (GH) release: effect of intrahypothalamic and intrapituitary implants. Prostaglandins, in press.

362. Ojeda, S. R., Harms, P. G., and McCann, S. M. (1974). Central effect of prostaglandin E_1 (PGE_1) on prolactin release. Endocrinology 96:613.

363. Ojeda, S. R., Harms, P. G., and McCann, S. M. (1974). Possible role of cyclic AMP and prostaglandin E_1 in the dopaminergic control of prolactin release. Endocrinology 95:1694.

364. Louis, T. M., Stellflug, J. N., Tucker, H. A., and Hofs, H. P. (1974). Plasma prolactin, growth hormone, luteinizing hormone and glucocorticoids after prostaglandin $F_{2\alpha}$ in heifers. Proc. Soc. Exp. Biol. 147:128.

365. Yue, D. K., Smith, I. D., Turtle, J. R., and Shearman, R. P. (1974). Effect of $PGE_{2\alpha}$ on the secretion of human prolactin. Prostaglandins 8:387.

366. Sundberg, D. K., Fawcett, C. P., Illner, P., and McCann, S. M. (1975). The effects of various prostaglandins and a prostaglandin synthetase inhibitor on rat anterior cyclic AMP levels and on hormone release *in vitro*. Proc. Soc. Exp. Biol. Med. 148:53.

367. Moss, R. L., and McCann, S. M. (1983). Induction of mating behavior in rats by luteinizing hormone-releasing hormone. Science 181:177.

368. Pfaff, D. W. (1973). Luteinizing hormone-releasing factor potentiates lordosis behavior in hypophysectomized ovariectomized female rat. Science 182:1148.
369. Moss, R. L., and Foreman, M. M. (1976). Potentiation of lordosis by intrahypothalamic infusion of synthetic luteinizing hormone-releasing hormone. Neuroendocrinology 20:176.
370. Plotnikoff, N. P., and Kastin, A. J. (1976). Neuropharmacology of hypothalamic releasing factors. Biochem. Pharmacol. 25:363.
371. Prange, A. J., Wilson, I. C., Breese, G. R., and Lipton, M. A. (1975). Behavioral effects of hypothalamic releasing hormones in animals and men. Prog. Brain Res. 42:1.
372. Prange, A., Breese, G., Cott, J., Martin, B., Cooper, B., Wilson, I., and Plotnikoff, N. (1974). Thyrotropin releasing hormone: antagonism of pentobarbital in rodents. Life Sci. 14:447.
373. Brown, M., and Vale, W. (1975). Central nervous system effects of hypothalamic peptides. Endocrinology 96:1333.
374. Plotnikoff, N., Prange, A., Bruze, G., Anders, M., and Wilson, I. (1972). Thyrotropin releasing hormone: enhancement of Dopa activity by a hypothalamic hormone. Science 178:417.
375. Havlicek, V., Rezek, M., and Friesen, H. (1976). Somatostatin and thyrotropin releasing hormone: central effect on sleep and motor system. Pharmacol. Biochem. Behav. 4:455.
376. Cohn, M. L., Cohn, M., and Taylor, F. H. (1975). Thyrotropin releasing factor (TRF) regulation of rotation in the non-lesioned rat. Brain Res. 96:134.
377. Metcalff, G. (1974). TRH: a possible mediator of thermoregulation. Nature 252:310.
378. Kastin, A., Schalch, D., Ehrensing, R., and Anderson, M. (1972). Improvement in mental depression with decreased thyrotropin response after administration of thyrotropin-releasing hormone. Lancet 2:740.
379. Mountjoy, C., Wheeler, M., Hall, R., Price, J., Hunter, P., and Dewar, J. (1974). A double-blind crossover sequential trial of oral thyrotrophin-releasing hormone in depression. Lancet 1:958.
380. Cohn, M. L., and Cohn, M. (1975). "Barrel rotation" induced by somatostatin in the nonlesioned rat. Brain Res. 96:138.
381. Plotnikoff, N. P., Kastin, A. J., Anderson, M. S., and Schally, A. V. (1971). Dopa potentiation by hypothalamic factor, MSH release-inhibiting hormone (MIF). Life Sci. 10:1279.
382. Plotnikoff, N., Kastin, A. J., Anderson, M. S., and Schally, A. V. (1972). Oxotremorine antagonism by a hypothalamic hormone, melanocyte hormone release-inhibiting factor (MIF). Proc. Soc. Exp. Biol. Med. 140:811.
383. Hill-Samli, M., and MacLeod, R. M. (1974). Interaction of thyrotropin-releasing hormone and dopamine on the release of prolactin from the rat anterior pituitary in vitro. Endocrinology 95:1189.
384. Moss, R. L., (1976). Unit responses in the preoptic and arcuate neurons related to anterior pituitary function. In L. Martini and W. F. Ganong (eds.), Frontiers in Neuroendocrinology, pp. 95–128. Raven Press, New York.
385. Schally, A. V., Arimura, A., Takahara, J., Redding, T. W., and Dupont, A. (1974). Inhibition of prolactin release in vitro and in vivo by catecholamines. Fed. Proc. 33:237.

386. Schally, A. V., Dupont, A., Arimura, A., Takahara, J., Redding, T. W., Clements, J., and Shaar, C. (1976). Purification of a catecholamine-rich fraction with prolactin release-inhibiting factor (PIF) activity from porcine hypothalami. Acta Endocrinol. 82:1.

387. Schally, A. V., Redding, T. W., Linthicum, G. L., and Dupont, A. (1976). Inhibition of prolactin release *in vivo* and *in vitro* by natural hypothalamic and synthetic gamma aminobutyric acid. Program of the 58th Meeting of the Endocrine Society, No. 310 (Abstr.).

388. Greibrokk, T., Currie, B. L., Johansson, K. N. G., Hansen, J. J., Folkers, K., and Bowers, C. Y. (1974). Purification of a PIF and the revealing of hormone D-GHIG which inhibits the release of GH. Biochem. Biophys. Res. Commun. 59:704.

389. Greibrokk, T., Hansen, J., Knudsen, R., Lau, Y. K., Folkers, K., and Bowers, C. Y. (1975). On the isolation of a PIF. Biochem. Biophys. Res. Commun. 67:338.

390. Dular, R., Labella, F., Vivian, S., and Eddie, L. (1974). Purification of prolactin releasing and inhibiting factors from beef. Endocrinology 94:563.

391. Kokobu, T., Sawano, S., Shiraki, M., Yamasaki, M., and Ishizuka, Y. (1975). Extraction and partial purification of PRF in bovine hypothalamus. Endocrinol. Jap. 22:213.

392. Pearlmutter, A. F., Rapino, E., and Saffran, M. (1975). The ACTH-releasing hormone of the hypothalamus requires a co-factor. Endocrinology 97:1336.

393. Gilham, B., Jones, M. T., Hillhouse, E. W., and Burden, J. L. (1975). Preliminary observations on the nature of CRH from the rat hypothalamus *in vitro*. J. Endocrinol. 65:12P.

394. Jones, M. T., Hillhouse, E., and Burden, J. (1976). Secretion of CRH *in vitro*. *In* L. Martini and W. F. Ganong (eds.), Frontiers in Neuroendocrinology, pp. 195–226. Raven Press, New York.

395. Pearlmutter, A. F., Rapino, E., and Saffran, M. (1974). A semiautomated *in vitro* assay for CRF: activities of peptides related to oxytocin and vasopressin. Neuroendocrinology 15:106.

396. Villareal, J. A., Vale, W., Brown, M., Butcher, M., Brazeau, P., Rivier, C., and Burgus, R. (1976). Immunoreactive GH *in vitro*. Biochim. Biophys. Res. Commun. 70:551.

397. Takahara, J., Arimura, A., and Schally, A. V. (1974). Assessment of GH releasing hormone activity in Sephadex separated fractions of porcine hypothalamic extracts by hypophyseal portal vessel. Acta Endocrinol. 78:428.

398. Wilson, M. C., Steiner, A. L., Dhariwal, A. P. S., and Peake, G. T. (1975). Purified ovine GHRF: effects on GH secretion and pituitary cyclic nucleotide accumulation. Neuroendocrinology 15:313.

399. Wilbur, D. L., Worthington, W. C., and Markwald, R. R. (1975). An ultrastructural and radioimmunoassay study of interior pituitary somatotrophs following pituitary portal vessel infusion of growth hormone releasing factor. Neuroendocrinology 19:12.

400. Ishikawa, H., Nagayama, T., Kato, C., and Takahashi, M. (1976). The effects of GH-RH and thyrosine on the synthesis and release of GH in a clonal strain of rat pituitary cells. Biochem. Biophys. Res. Commun. 70:241.

401. Haar, W., Fermandjian, S., Vicar, J., Blaha, K., and Fromageot, P. (1975). ^{13}C-NMR study of (85% ^{13}C-enriched proline) TRH: [13]C-^{13}C vicinal coupling constants and conformation of the proline residue. Proc. Natl. Acad. Sci. U. S. A. 72:4948.

402. Belloco, A. M., Boilot, J. C., Dupont, E., and Dubien, M. (1973). Conformational analysis of the hypothalamic hormone TRF with Raman spectroscopy. C. R. Acad. Sci. (Paris) 276:423.

403. Burgess, A. W., Momany, F. A., and Scheraga, H. A. (1973). Conformational analysis of TRF. Proc. Natl. Acad. Sci. U. S. A. 70:1456.

404. Imae, T., Fasman, G. D., Hinkle, P. M., and Tashjian, A. H. (1975). Intrinsic tryptophan fluorescence of membranes of GH3 pituitary cells: quenching by TRH. Biochem. Biophys. Res. Commun. 62:923.

405. Barnea, A., Ben-Jonathan, N., Colston, C., Johnston, J. M., and Porter, J. C. (1975). Differential subcellular compartmentalization of TRH and LRH in hypothalamic tissue. Proc. Natl. Acad. Sci. U. S. A. 72:3153.

406. Prasad, C., and Peterkofsky, A. (1976). Demonstration of pyroglutamyl peptidase and amylase activities toward TRH in hamster hypothalamus extracts. J. Biol. Chem. 251:3229.

407. Griffitts, E. C., Hooper, K. C., Jeffcoate, S. L., and White, N. (1975). Peptidases in the rat hypothalamus inactivating TRH. Acta Endocrinol. 79:209.

408. Hinkle, P. M., and Tashjian, A. H. (1975). TRH regulates the number of its own receptors in the GH_3 strain of pituitary cells in culture. Biochemistry 14:384.

409. Hinkle, P. M., and Tashjian, A. H. (1975). Degradation of TRH by the GH_3 strain of pituitary cells in culture. Endocrinology 97:324.

410. Lybeck, H., Leppaluoto, J., Virkkunen, P., Schafer, D., Carlsson, L., and Mulder, J. (1973). TRH induced increase in circulating I[131] reduced by cyclopentyl carbonyl histidyl pyrolidine. Neuroendocrinology 12:366.

411. Sivertsson, H., Castensson, S., Anderson, K., Bjorkman, S., and Bowers, C. Y. (1975). Thyrotropin and prolactin inhibitory studies by compounds related to the thyrotropin releasing hormone. Biochem. Biophys. Res. Commun. 66:1401.

412. Mitnick, M. A., and Reichlin, S. (1972). Enzymatic synthesis of TRH by hypothalamic synthetase. Endocrinology 91:1145.

413. Dixon, J. E., and Acres, S. G. (1975). The inability to demonstrate the non-ribosomal biosynthesis of TRH in hypothalamic tissue. Fed. Proc. 34:658.

414. Bauer, K., and Lipmann, F. (1976). Attempts towards biosynthesis of TRH and studies on its breakdown in hypothalamic tissue preparations. Endocrinology 99:230.

415. McKelvey, J. F. (1974). Biosynthesis of TRH by organ cultures of mammalian hypothalamus. Brain Res. 65:489.

416. McKelvey, J. F., Sheridan, M., Joseph, S., Phelps, C. H., and Perrie, S. (1975). Biosynthesis of TRH in organ cultures of the guinea-pig median eminence. Endocrinology 97:908.

417. Rivier, J., Brown, M., and Vale, W. (1975). D-Trp[8]-somatostatin: an analog of somatostatin more potent than the native molecule. Biochem. Biophys. Res. Commun. 65:746.

418. Marks, N., and Stern, F. (1975). Inactivation of somatostatin and its analogs by crude and partially purified rat brain extracts. FEBS Lett. 55:220.

419. Brazeau, P., Vale, W., Rivier, J., and Guillemin, R. (1974). Acylated des Ala[1], Gly[2]-somatostatin analogs: prolonged inhibition of GH secretion. Biochem. Biophys. Res. Commun. 60:1202.
420. Ferland, L., Labrie, F., Coy, D. H., Arimura, A., and Schally, A. V. (1976). Inhibition by six somatostatin analogs of plasma GH levels stimulated by thianylal and morphine in the rat. Mol. Cell Endocrinol. 4:79.
421. Efendic, S., Luft, R., and Sivertsson, H. (1975). Relative effects of somatostatin and two somatostatin analogues on the release of insulin, glucagon and GH. FEBS Lett. 58:302.
422. Brown, M., Rivier, J., Vale, W., and Guillemin, R. (1975). Variability of the duration of inhibition of GH release by N^α-acylated des (Ala[1] Gly[2])-H_2 somatostatin analogs. Biochem. Biophys. Res. Commun. 65:752.
423. Brazeau, P., and Martin, J. B. (1976). *In vivo* activities of somatostatin and its analogs: prolongation with protamine-zinc. *In* F. Labrie, J. Meites, and G. Pelletier (eds.), Current Topics in Molecular Endocrinology. Vol. III, pp. 379–386. Plenum Press, New York.
424. Immer, H., Abraham, N. A., Nelson, V., Sestany, K., Gotz, M., Brazeau, P., and Martin, J. B. (1976). Analogs of somatostatin. *In* F. Labrie, J. Meites, and G. Pelletier (eds.), Current Topics in Molecular Endocrinology, Vol. III, pp. 373–378. Plenum Press, New York.
425. Wessels, P. L., Feeney, J., Gregory, H., and Gormley, J. J. (1973). High resolution nuclear magnetic resonance studies of the conformation of luteinizing hormone releasing hormone (LH-RH) and its component peptides. J. Chem. Soc. (Perkin I) 2:1691.
426. Deslauriens, R., Levy, G. C., McGregor, W. H., Garantakis, D., and Smith, Z. C. P. (1975). Conformational flexibility of LHRH in aqueous solution: a carbon 13 spin lattice relaxation time study. Biochemistry 14:4335.
427. Mabney, S., and Klotz, I. M. (1976). Conformation of gonadotropin releasing hormone. Biochemistry 15:234.
428. Marks, N., and Stern, F. (1974). Enzymatic mechanisms for the inactivation of LRH. Biochem. Biophys. Res. Commun. 61:1458.
429. Koch, Y., Baram, T., Chobsieng, P., and Fordkin, P. (1974). Enzymatic degradation of LRH by hypothalamic tissue. Biochem. Biophys. Res. Commun. 61:95.
430. Griffiths, E. C., Hooper, K. C., Jeffcote, S. L., and Holland, D. T. (1974). The presence of peptidases in the rat hypothalamus inactivating LRH. Acta Endocrinol. 77:435.
431. Kuhl, H., and Taubert, H. D. (1975). Short loop feedback mechanism of LH: LH stimulates hypothalamic L-cystine arylamidase to inactivate LHRH in the rat hypothalamus. Acta Endocrinol. 78:649.
432. Fawcett, C. P., Beezley, A. E., and Wheaton, J. L. (1975). Chromatographic evidence for the existence of another species of LRF. Endocrinology 96:1311.
433. Sandow, J., Enzmann, F., Arimura, A., Redding, T. W., and Schally, A. V. (1975). Purification and characterization of two porcine hypothalamic fractions with LH releasing activity: evidence for a single LH and FSH releasing hormone. Acta Endocrinol. 80:209.
434. Millar, R., Aenhelt, C., Rossier, G., and Hendricks, S. (1975). Evidence for the existence of a higher molecular weight precursor of LRH. IRCS Rev. Med. Sci. 3:603.
435. Barnea, A., and Porter, J. C. (1975). Demonstration of a macromolecule

cross reacting with antibodies to LHRH and its tissue distribution. Biochem. Biophys. Res. Commun. 67:1346.

436. Burgus, R., Amoss, M., Brazeau, P., Brown, M., Ling, N., Rivier, C., Rivier, J., Vale, W., and Villareal, J. (1970). Isolation and characterization of hypothalamic peptide hormones. *In* F. Labrie, J. Meites, and G. Pelletier (eds.), Current Topics in Molecular Endocrinology, Vol. III, pp. 355–372. Plenum Press, New York.

437. Johansson, K. N. G., Currie, B. L., Folkers, K., and Bowers, C. Y. (1973). On the chemical existence and partial purification of the hypothalamic FSH releasing hormone. Biochem. Biophys. Res. Commun. 50:14.

438. Schally, A. V., Arimura, A., Redding, T. W., Debeljuk, L., Carter, W., Dupont, A., and Vilchez-Martinez, J. A. (1976). Re-examination of porcine and bovine hypothalamic fractions for additional LH and FSH releasing activities. Endocrinology 98:380.

439. Labrie, F., Pelletier, G., Borgeat, P., Drouin, J., Ferland, L., and Belanger, A. (1976). Mode of action of hypothalamic regulatory hormones in the adenohypophysis. *In* L. Martini and W. F. Ganong (eds.), Frontiers in Neuroendocrinology, pp. 63–93. Raven Press, New York.

440. Peake, G. T., Steiner, A. L., And Daughaday, W. H. (1972). Guanosine $3'5'$ cyclic monophosphate is a potent pituitary growth hormone secretagogue. Endocrinology 90:212.

441. Nakano, H., and Fawcett, C. P. The application of enzymatically and mechanically dispersed anterior pituitary cells to studies on the control of gonadotropin release. V. International Congress of Endocrinology Abstr. 751. Hamburg, 1976.

442. Edwardson, J. A., and Gilbert, D. (1975). Sensitivity of the self-potentiating effect of LHRH to cycloheximide. Nature 255:71.

443. Vilchez-Martinez, J. A., Arimura, A., and Schally, A. (1976). Effect of actinomycin D on the pituitary response to LRH. Acta Endocrinol. 81:73.

444. Pickering, A. J. M. C., and Fink, G. (1976). Priming effect of LRH: *in vitro* and *in vivo* evidence consistent with its dependence upon protein and RNA synthesis. J. Endocrinol. 69:373.

445. DeKoning, J., Van Dieten, J. A. M. J., and Van Rees, G. P. (1976). LRH dependent synthesis of protein necessary for LH release from rat pituitary glands *in vitro*. Mol. Cell. Endocrinol. 5:151.

446. DeKoning, J., Van Dieten, J. A. M. J., and Van Rees, G. P. (1976). Inhibitory and augmentative effects of estradiol on LRH induced release by anterior pituitary glands from intact female rats *in vitro*. Mol. Cell. Endocrinol. 5:321.

447. Spona, J. (1975). Sex steroids influence LRH-receptor interactions. Endocrinol. Exp. 9:167.

448. Park, K. R., Saxena, B. B., and Gandy, H. M. (1976). Specific binding of LHRH to the anterior pituitary gland during the oestrus cycle in the rat. Acta Endocrinol. 82:62.

449. Liu, T. C., Jackson, G. L., and Gorski, J. (1975). Effect of synthetic gonadotropin-releasing hormone on incorporation of radioactive glucosamine and amino acids into LH and total protein by rat pituitaries *in vitro*. Endocrinology 98:151.

450. Corbin, A., and Beattie, C. W. (1975). Inhibition of the preovulatory proestrus gonadotropin surge ovulation and pregnancy with a peptide analog of LRH. Endocrine Res. Commun. 2:1.

451. de la Cruz, A., Coy, D. H., Vilchez-Martinez, J. A., Arimura, A., and Schally, A. V. (1976). Blockade of ovulation in rats by inhibitory analogs of LHRH. Science 191:195.

452. Wan, Y.-P., Humphries, J., Fisher, G., Folkers, K., and Bowers, C. Y. (1976). Inhibitors of LHRH based upon modifications in the 2, 3 and 6 positions. J. Med. Chem. 19:199.

453. Reichlin, S., Saperstein, R., Jackson, I. M. D., Boyd, A. E., and Patel, Y. (1976). Hypothalamic hormones. Annu. Rev. Physiol. 38:389.

454. Labrie, F., Meites, J., and Pelletier, G. (eds.) (1976). Hypothalamus and endocrine function. Current Topics in Molecular Endocrinology, Vol. 3, Plenum Press, New York.

455. Martini, L., and Ganong, W. F. (eds.). (1976). Frontiers in Neuroendocrinology, Vol. 4. Raven Press, New York.

International Review of Physiology
Endocrine Physiology II, Volume 16
Edited by S. M. McCann
Copyright 1977   University Park Press   Baltimore

3
The Hypothalamic-Pituitary-Adrenocortical System

A. BRODISH and J. R. LYMANGROVER

Bowman Gray School of Medicine,
Wake Forest University, Winston-Salem, North Carolina,
and Tulane University School of Medicine,
New Orleans, Louisiana

Much of the recent work in endocrinology has been directed at the analytical characterization of the component parts of the endocrine system. The remarkable progress that has been made in the biochemical elucidation of individual endocrine organs has been made primarily by the analytical approach. As a result of the recent progress in studies of the individual components of the endocrine system, it is now important to attempt to understand the overall organization of the system. The broad integrative significance of the entire endocrine machinery within the organism as a whole must now be understood.

The analytical approach has provided an understanding of the components of the endocrine system. The integrative or synthetic approach must now explain how the system functions as a whole. Of these two approaches in biology, the analytical approach has been overwhelmingly the predominant one during the recent period of exponential progress. The integrative understanding of the field now represents a new challenge for the immediate future. Claude Bernard, who provided much of the conceptual foundation for the modern integrative approach, was among the first to recognize clearly that these two strategies are not antithetical but rather are complementary to each other. The integrative study of coordination between the parts obviously presupposes prior analytical characterization of the individual parts. The two approaches then logically go hand and hand; analysis first, then synthesis. The task in biology is not complete, however, after even the most definitive physiochemical analysis of elemental body processes. Sooner or later there must be the task of reassembling the many unit parts into an organized and coordinated system that functions meaningfully in the complex whole organism. In other words, what is needed is the striking of a proper balance between the two approaches. As Claude Bernard said in 1865, "we really must learn then that if we break up a living organism by isolating its different parts, it is only for the sake of ease in experimental analysis and by no means in order to conceive them separately. Indeed when we wish to ascribe to a physiological quality its value and true significance we must always refer to this whole and draw our final conclusion only in relation to its effect in the whole" (1).

CENTRAL NERVOUS SYSTEM
ACTIVATION OF CORTICOTROPIN-RELEASING FACTOR

It is generally accepted that many aspects of adrenocorticotropic hormone (ACTH) release are modulated by the central nervous system (CNS). Such regulation is mediated by a corticotropin-releasing factor (CRF). The site of production of such a factor within the central nervous system and its chemical nature still remain to be elucidated. It is believed that corticotropin-releasing factor production occurs within neurosecretory cells which, in addition to having secretory properties, share with other nerve cells the property of synaptic activation by neurotransmitter substances. It is presumed that some of these neurotransmitters are similar to those whose function has been described in the peripheral nervous system. Chemical and fluorescence techniques have demonstrated the presence of acetylcholine, norepinephrine, serotonin, and dopamine within the central nervous system. Regional and circadian variation of levels of these substances within areas of the hypothalamic-limbic system have also been demonstrated. These are areas which have been shown through lesion and stimulation experiments to have a marked effect on ACTH secretion (2) as well as to be sites of corticosteroid concentration (3). It is likely that these transmitter substances, by acting on the neurosecretory cells involved in the production of CRF, could affect its release or inhibition in response to the varied stimuli which are known to influence ACTH levels. There is no evidence that such neurotransmitter substances may change ACTH release by a direct action on the pituitary gland (4).

Investigations concerned with the role of neurotransmitter substances in the regulation of CRF release have used diverse approaches. These have included the assessment of the effects of various transmitters on pituitary-adrenal function of systemic, intra-, and extrahypothalamic or intraventricular administration of substances or drugs which may block transmitter action or synthesis. Similarly, the effects of lesions or chemical substances which destroy specific neurotransmitter pathways have also been studied. Investigations have at times led to contradictory results. To explore some of the methodological problems that have led to such inconsistencies, Krieger (5) has described some of the problems of methodology that may influence the results in assessing neurotransmitter regulation of ACTH release.

1. The role of the state of consciousness and stress. In evaluating the effects of neurotransmitter agents on basal ACTH or cortisol levels, the use of unrestrained, unstressed conscious animals is desirable. There is evidence that a given chemical or electrical stimulus may have opposite effects on pituitary-adrenal function if the stimulus is given at a time of high or low plasma corticosterone levels. There is also evidence that anesthesia may modify the effect of a given neurotransmitter substance.

2. Site of drug administration. In studies of intracerebral versus intraventricular drug administration, a difference in pituitary-adrenal responsiveness might be expected if a transmitter substance or blocking agent is injected intraventricu-

larly rather than into a specific area of the central nervous system. Thus, implantation of a given neurotransmitter may lead to inhibition or stimulation of pituitary-adrenal function, depending upon the central nervous system area into which it is implanted. On the other hand, intraventricular administration may lead to widespread transport of the administered substance to both stimulatory and inhibitory areas. The exact response would be dependent upon the relative proximity to the ventricular system of such areas. In studies of systemic versus intracerebral drug administration, systemic administration of drugs which modify central neurotransmitter synthesis, metabolism, or action would also be expected to affect equally all intracerebral loci at which the neurotransmitter might exert a stimulatory or inhibitory effect. Systemic administration of drugs which modify neurotransmitter synthesis, metabolism, or action would be expected to affect peripheral as well as central neurotransmitters. It might then be unclear as to whether hormonal changes observed were secondary to direct effects of these drugs on central neurotransmitters or were indirect ones secondary to changes in central neurotransmitters brought about by peripheral changes in blood pressure, intravascular volume, etc.

3. Assay of neurotransmitter content. There is regional variation of specific neurotransmitters. Therefore, studies in which only whole brain levels of such transmitters are determined might mask more specific changes in the loci actually involved in CRF regulation. Since there is circadian variation in neurotransmitter content, studies should specify the time of day at which this is determined. In addition, it is important to measure several neurotransmitters simultaneously. Drugs may affect more than one transmitter at a time. Unless concentrations of several transmitter substances are measured, it would be inaccurate to ascribe any observed effects to changes in just the one transmitter that is being studied. The effects may be specific for a particular transmitter or general for a number of different transmitters. Finally, there is evidence that it is the ratio between two neurotransmitter substances, rather than the actual levels of a given neurotransmitter, that is important in effecting CRF release. This is further reason for measuring levels of several neurotransmitters when studying the effect of a given pharmacological agent.

4. Time of drug administration. In addition to the importance of measuring levels of transmitter substances at a constant time of day because of circadian variation, this is also an important parameter in evaluating the neurotransmitter effect. For example, it has been noted that direct application of norepinephrine during the dark period suppresses feeding behavior, whereas increased feeding is noted following such application during the light period. It is to be expected that other parameters, including hormonal ones, will vary accordingly.

5. Concomitant rather than causal changes. Certain experimental interpretations have assumed cause and effect in the interrelationship of two variables, whereas such a relationship may merely reflect concomitant changes in these variables in response to another factor. For example, the fall in brain norepinephrine levels, which occurs in some stress situations concomitant with elevation of cortico-

steroid levels, has been interpreted as indicating adrenergic inhibition of pituitary-adrenal function. Not only can such parameters be changing independently of each other in response to the stress, but it has been demonstrated that in such stress situations norepinephrine turnover is increased.

6. Site of stimulation as possible site of CRF production. In studies involving direct intracerebral implantation of neurotransmitter, it is important to note that the observation of a hormonal effect of neurotransmitter at a given site does not necessarily imply that that site is directly involved in CRF synthesis. Instead, the site may be a link in a multisynaptic pathway leading to the final common pathway for CRF release.

7. Dose of substance employed. The dose of neurotransmitter employed should be within the physiological range for the tissue being studied. It is axiomatic in neurophysiology that, whereas a physiological dose of acetylcholine leads to transient membrane depolarization, a higher dose causes prolonged depolarization. In the case of the biogenic amines, in addition to these considerations, effects on blood vessel tone and consequent pituitary blood flow of supraphysiological amounts also have to be considered.

8. Parameters of ACTH release studied. As a result of lesion and transection experiments, it is well established that different parameters of ACTH release (i.e., circadian periodicity, stress-evoked release, basal levels, and feedback responsiveness) are differently affected by specific lesions. Therefore, it would also be possible to observe an effect of a given neurotransmitter on one aspect of ACTH release without it affecting any of the others.

9. Miscellaneous factors. Finally, factors of age, sex, species, end-point of pituitary-adrenal function observed, and interval after application of stimulus until pituitary-adrenal function is studied should also be controlled.

NATURE OF HYPOTHALAMIC CORTICOTROPIN-RELEASING FACTOR

What is the nature of the hypothalamic hormone that stimulates ACTH release, and are there other physiological regulators of ACTH from hypothalamic or pituitary sources?

Although CRF was the first hypothalamic-releasing factor to be demonstrated in hypothalamic tissue (6), it remains the least well characterized of the releasing hormones. This lack of understanding of the nature of CRF might be attributed to the difficulty in effectively assaying this substance in hypothalamic tissue, not to mention the difficulties in measuring ACTH itself. Other problems have surfaced in the purification of CRF. It has been reported that CRF activity is lost as purification proceeds, until little or no activity remains (7). Thus, much of the knowledge concerning CRF structure and function is of necessity obtained through indirect methods.

Some clues concerning the nature of CRF have been obtained by studying the action of substances with known structure which can stimulate ACTH secretion in a manner similar to that described for hypothalamic extract

(HSME). Some of the compounds which have been studied are the prostaglandins, vasopressin, and associated compounds. Hedge and Hanson (8) have
presented data which demonstrated that prostaglandins did not directly stimulate ACTH release from the anterior pituitary but apparently acted through the
release of CRF from the hypothalamus. Coudert and Faiman (9) also failed to
demonstrate a direct action of PGF_2 on the anterior pituitary of adult human
subjects. Thus, although hypothalamic tissue contains significant amounts of
prostaglandins (10, 11), there is no direct evidence that CRF activity is due to a
prostaglandin-like substance.

Previous studies showed that CRF was present in the posterior lobe and
possibly influenced posterior pituitary function. Some investigators had proposed
that vasopressin itself was the physiological CRF (12–14). Guillemin et al. (15)
isolated a neurohypophysial CRF termed β-CRF. Schally and Bowers (16)
subsequently proposed a structure for β-CRF of posterior pituitary origin. The
proposed structure consisted of a polypeptide of 13 amino acids which shares a
common sequence with lysine vasopressin for 10 of the amino acids. Previously,
Schally and colleagues (17) postulated that there were several CRF-like substances from the posterior pituitary: vasopressin itself, α-melanocyte-stimulating
hormone, and β-CRF. However, there is considerable evidence that some other
substance from the hypothalamus can release ACTH from the anterior pituitary
(6, 15, 18, 19).

CRF of hypothalamic origin may or may not be identical with or related to
neurohypophysial CRF, but the similarities between the CRF activity of vasopressin and hypothalamic CRF have stimulated additional studies to determine
whether a vasopressin-like compound may be a physiological CRF. Data reported by Andersson et al. (20) indicate that the ability of vasopressin to release
ACTH and cortisol does not depend upon its antidiuretic or pressor activity.
Analogs of vasopressin, which exerted significant pressor and maximal antidiuretic action in human subjects, did not change cortisol levels, whereas 1–10
ng of lysine vasopressin, given intravenously to similar subjects, did cause
significant steroid release.

If vasopressin or related substances are indeed physiologically significant in
the control of ACTH release, or if HSME-CRF is structurally similar to vasopressin, then these substances must be found to be active at physiological levels.
Saffran et al. (21) have shown that the synthetic hexapeptide that corresponds
to the ring of the vasopressin molecule exhibited corticotropin-releasing activity
of incubated rat pituitary quarters in a dose range of 3–30 ng/ml, whereas
greater doses were without effect. These findings were subsequently confirmed
and reported by Hiroshige (22). Both investigators have encountered difficulties
in consistently demonstrating this activity because of an apparent instability of
the peptide. Confirmation of this effect, in an in vivo preparation, has not been
forthcoming.

The CRF-like activity of vasopressin has also been observed in rat anterior
pituitary cell preparations (23 and 24). In contrast with the findings of Arimura

et al. (25) and Chan et al. (26), who have reported similarities in dose-response relationships of HSME extracts and vasopressin preparations in several in vivo and in vitro assay systems, the in vitro cell suspension procedures of Portanova and Sayers demonstrated unique dose-response relationships, permitting distinction between these substances.

Additional recent evidence from Miller et al. (27) indicates that vasopressin or other CRF-like substances from the posterior pituitary or both are not necessarily involved in the control of ACTH release from the anterior pituitary. They found that the axis functions quite normally in the absence of the posterior pituitary gland. Thus, it appears that vasopressin or vasopressin-like compounds may stimulate ACTH release, but it is probably not the normal physiological regulator responsible for stress-induced release of ACTH.

If SME-CRF is not identical with prostaglandins or vasopressin of posterior pituitary origin, what then is the nature of this substance? Chan et al. (26) reviewed some of the chemical properties of CRF of SME origin. Not a great deal of additional information has subsequently been reported. Observations by Chan et al. indicated that there may be two CRFs in the hypothalamic tissue. Acetone precipitation, thin layer chromatography, and gel filtration produced two areas of activity. The fact that thioglycolate produced only partial inactivation suggests that one of the factors contains sulfide bonds, whereas the second does not (26).

The proposal of two components of hypothalamic CRF activity has been recently substantiated by Pearlmutter et al. (28). In general, their data show that there are high and low molecular weight fractions from rat and bovine hypothalamic stalk median eminence tissues which exhibit CRF activity when they are assayed in vitro. The separation of the two fractions, using a Sephadex gel column, resulted in the loss of a large amount of the CRF activity. The larger molecular weight fraction alone had considerable activity, whereas the smaller weight fractions had only minimal activity. The recombination of these two fractions restored the full ACTH-releasing activity. Such findings can do much to explain previous reports of loss of activity with purification and inconsistencies in the characteristics of CRF activity reported from different laboratories. There is now hope that the purification necessary for further chemical analysis can proceed and that an elucidation of the chemical identity of CRF may be forthcoming.

An interesting report by La Bella et al. (29) indicates that when bovine hypothalamic extract was sufficiently purified, a highly active CRF fraction was produced in which the activity was due to the presence of divalent metals. The most abundant metal was copper, which was active at concentrations less than 1 μg/ml in an in vitro releasing factor assay which used bovine pituitary tissue. Zinc and nickel were also present, but were usually less potent than copper ion. These investigators found that these metal ions not only released ACTH but also thyroid-stimulating hormone (TSH), luteinizing hormone (LH), and growth hormone (GH) and inhibited prolactin PRL release at comparable ionic concentrations. Whether these ions play a physiological role in the control of pituitary hormone release remains to be established. However, it is important to recall these observations when one is interpreting data based on different extraction and purification procedures for releasing factors from hypothalamic extracts. Depending upon the extraction procedures, these ions could easily contribute to releasing factor activity when assayed in a biological system.

Bertolini et al. (30) have reported that a fraction of porcine and rat hypothalamic extract, containing a hexapeptide with the proposed amino acid sequence Glu-His-Phe-Arg-Trp-Gly, behaves like CRF when injected, since it causes an increase in corticosteroid activity in the blood of dexamethasone- and pentobarbitone-blocked rats and is inactive in hypophysectomized rats. Additional experiments showed that the labeled amino acid incorporation into this fraction was enhanced by bilateral adrenalectomy, hypophysectomy, and stress. This peptide shares some of the amino acid sequence with ACTH, β-lipotropin (β-LPH), and MSH peptides. These experimental results may indicate that this compound is the organic hypothalamic-releasing factor found in SME extracts, but unfortunately the report suffers from a lack of procedural detail and we must await independent confirmation.

CORTICOTROPIN-RELEASING FACTOR
ACTIVATION OF PITUITARY GLAND

What are the cellular mechanisms by which ACTH secretion is controlled? Douglas and Poisner (31) proposed that pituitary hormones are released by a mechanism somewhat analogous to the excitation-contraction coupling mechanism demonstrated for muscle, which they termed "stimulus-secretion coupling." Generally, as applied to anterior pituitary hormones, this proposal states that hypothalamic hormones activate the pituitary cells by interacting with the pituitary cell membrane, resulting in a change in cell membrane permeability to a specific ion. With this permeability alteration, there would be an influx of ions (e.g., Ca^{2+}) into the cell which would then activate the secretory process for the preformed pituitary hormone. Subsequently, much data have accumulated that suggest such a mechanism in the secretory process for a number of hormones.

In general, the data from many laboratories indicate that a specific ionic environment is necessary for hypothalamic hormones to alter pituitary hormone secretion. Several investigators have shown that hypothalamic-releasing factors obtained from crude hypothalamic tissue of several species require the presence of Ca^{2+}. Additionally, alterations in the external K^+ ion concentration, in the direction which would result in a depolarization of the membrane potential and further changes in permeability, stimulate the release of a number of pituitary hormones.

York et al. (32) have studied the effects of crude hypothalamic extracts on the membrane potential and resistance of rat pituitary tissue in vivo. Although they demonstrated only minimal changes in membrane potentials, there were significant changes in membrane resistance in the population of cells that they studied. Unfortunately, these studies were complicated because they used the entire population of pituitary cells and crude hypothalamic extract, which probably contained both inhibiting and stimulating factors. More definitive experiments must include homogeneous populations of pituitary cells with purified releasing factors. Subsequent experiments by Martin et al. (33) show that depolarization per se is not the cause of ACTH release. Their data indicate that the population of pituitary cells which they investigated could be slightly depolarized in Ca^{2+}-free medium, a condition known to inhibit pituitary hormone release. These data are consistent with the hypothesis of Douglas which would have predicted that in the absence of Ca^{2+} no stimulus-secretion coupling could occur.

Not all data are consistent with the Douglas hypothesis. Although evidence has been presented which shows that there is Ca^{2+} influx into pituitary cells when purified growth hormone-releasing factor (GRH) is introduced (39), similar evidence for ACTH secretion is lacking. In fact, Milligan and Kraicer (34) could not detect any $^{45}Ca^{2+}$ uptake into rat pituitaries after hypothalamic ME extract, db-cAMP, and other compounds which normally provoke ACTH release. The role of Ca^{2+} in ACTH secretion was more intensely examined in a more recent study by these authors (35). These experiments confirmed the finding that there is a minimal requirement of Ca^{2+} for ACTH release, and in addition that different secretagogues require different amounts of Ca^{2+} in the tissue in order to cause hormone release.

Portanova and Sayers (36) have confirmed the requirements of Ca^{2+} for HSME-induced release of ACTH from isolated rat anterior pituitary cells, but they also showed that incubation of these cells with Ca^{2+}-free medium plus EDTA (a Ca^{2+} chelator) resulted in an elevation of basal ACTH release. The importance of the ionic environment on either side of the pituitary cell membrane in the maintenance of pituitary cellular activity was further demonstrated by Fleischer and associates (37). They implicated the Na/K membrane pumps in the mechanisms of the release of these hormones and proposed that the Na/K pumps mediate the Ca^{2+} influx which modulates ACTH release from pituitary cells.

Eto et al. (38) confirmed some of the observations of Milligan et al. (39) that no detectable Ca^{2+} uptake could be demonstrated in rat anterior pituitary cells when they were incubated with hypothalamic extract, lysine vasopressin, thyrotropin-releasing hormone (TRH), db-cAMP, or theophylline, all known secretagogues for pituitary hormones. However, they did show that the Na/K pump inhibitor, ouabain, and elevated potassium levels (which could also hinder the Na/K pump) caused significant uptake of labeled Ca^{2+} into pituitary tissue which could presumably release ACTH. These authors also showed that verapamil, a Ca^{2+} flux inhibitor, blocked both Ca^{2+} influx and ACTH release caused by ouabain or elevated potassium, whereas this compound did not affect ACTH released by HSME, vasopressin, db-cAMP, or theophylline.

With these and other reports in mind, it seems reasonable to conclude that 1) Ca^{2+} is important in the secretory process for ACTH; 2) there are several mechanisms for regulating this secretory process (some may involve Ca^{2+} influx, whereas others may not); 3) Ca^{2+} influx per se does not precede the release of ACTH that is elicited by hypothalamic-releasing factors; 4) one must reject the Douglas stimulus-secretion coupling hypothesis for anterior pituitary cortico-trophs or amend it to include a possible translocation of Ca^{2+} or other ions which are either attached to the internal surface of the cell membrane or are in different intracellular pools; and 5) one must also consider the possibility that another ion besides Ca^{2+} may be a stimulus-secretion coupler in the case of the corticotroph.

Although the exact mechanisms are not absolutely clear, there is some available information concerning the events which follow the initial stimulation of the corticotroph. It appears that the stimulated secretion of ACTH from whole anterior pituitary tissue or single cell preparations is an energy-dependent process. Chan et al. (26) observed that vasopressin-induced release of ACTH in vitro required glucose and oxygen. More recently, Portanova (40), using a preparation of rat anterior pituitary cells, showed that a number of metabolic inhibitors blocked the HSME or vasopressin-induced release of ACTH. Where the energy is required has not been conclusively demonstrated.

One possible sequence of events which may lead to ACTH release from anterior pituitary cells seems to be mediated by the adenylate cyclase-cyclic AMP system. Hypothalamic extracts stimulate anterior pituitary tissue in vitro, with concomitant increases in adenylate cyclase activity (41, 42), as well as in cAMP itself (43). Furthermore, Fleischer et al. (44) have shown that cAMP or db-cAMP can cause the release of ACTH in a manner resembling that mediated by HSME. It has been proposed by many investigators that cAMP action in endocrine tissue involves the stimulation of a protein kinase. Such a protein kinase has been isolated from anterior pituitary tissue (45, 46), and the enzyme has been shown to increase in rat anterior pituitary tissues in response to hypothalamic extract (47). Pelletier et al. (48) reported that after incubation with 3.7 mM monobutyryl cAMP (mb-cAMP) for 30 min there was a significant release of ACTH from the rat anterior pituitary tissue but no significant change in the granulation of the corticotrophs. However, after 3 hr of incubation with mb-cAMP, there were significant ultrastructural changes such as hypertrophy of the Golgi apparatus and marked increases in the number of smooth vesicles in the Golgi area of the corticotrophs. Furthermore, the investigators were unable to find any evidence of exocytosis in the corticotroph cells—possibly indicating a relatively slow turnover in the stored ACTH. The newly synthesized ACTH may be preferentially released, rather than the stored form which is found in the granules. Thus, although it is clear that cAMP is involved in the control of ACTH secretion, it is uncertain whether it is a necessary second messenger or whether there are alternate pathways that mediate ACTH release.

Finally, HSME-stimulated ACTH release from the anterior pituitary probably involves an increase in protein synthesis. However, there are a number of reports that indicate that the acute release of preformed ACTH does not require de novo protein synthesis, whereas subsequent actions of CRF may require protein synthesis.

PITUITARY ADRENOCORTICOTROPIC HORMONE

Although it is generally accepted that ACTH is synthesized and secreted in the pars distalis of the pituitary gland, a number of questions remain to be answered concerning which cell type produces the hormone and whether or not the anterior pituitary is the only site of ACTH synthesis and release. Many of the recent investigations in this area have employed the use of immunohistochemical techniques permitting relatively specific localizations of the hormone on a particular cell type in specific regions of the pituitary gland.

Baker and Drummond (49) employed a peroxidase-labeled antibody technique to localize cells in the rat hypophysis which contain peptides with amino acid sequences common to ACTH and MSH. Small stellate cells were found throughout the pars distalis which accept anticorticotropin β^{1-24} and β^{17-39} (nomenclature recommended by Li (in ref. 49, p. 396) for molecules other than natural ACTH with corticotropic activity). In addition to these cells in the pars distalis, there were cells in the pars intermedia which stained to a lesser extent with antiserum for β^{1-24} $ACTH^{17-39}$. The corticotrophs of the anterior pituitary hypertrophied 1–3 weeks after adrenalectomy and regressed after cortisol administration for 19 days, whereas changes in the cells of the pars intermedia were minimal. MSH was found predominantly in the intermedia and minimally in the pars distalis. Using somewhat similar techniques, Kraicer et al. (50) found a greater concentration of ACTH (β^{17-39}) in the pars intermedia than in the pars distalis and only minimal amounts in the pars nervosa of intact adult rats. An interesting finding by these investigators was that the levels of immunoreactive ACTH in the pars intermedia were not significantly altered 30 days after adrenalectomy or after daily cortisol administration, whereas highly significant changes were observed in the cells of the pars distalis. Microscopically, these ACTH positive-staining cells were distributed throughout the anterior gland but showed a tendency to distribute centrally. The cells were stellate with long projections between other cell types and appeared to end in bulbous enlargements abutting on sinusoidal walls. The granules of these cells were fine and tended to be concentrated in the peripheral cytoplasm.

Additional evidence that immunologically active ACTH-like substances, and possibly biologically active ACTH, are elevated in anterior hypophysectomized rats has been presented by Greer et al. (51). Significant peripheral levels of immunoreactive ACTH (with the use of an antibody which cross-reacts with MSH and ACTH) and corticosteroids were found in ether-stressed and tourniquet-stressed adult rats with the anterior pituitary removed but with intact intermediate and posterior lobes. Using a more specific antibody (specific for α-ACTH$^{1-24}$), these investigators found little or no stress-induced alteration in ACTH and peripheral plasma corticosteroid levels in the anterior hypophysecto-mized group, but found elevated levels in the neural hypophysectomized groups. However, there was a depression in the stress-induced plasma steroid level in neural hypophysectomized rats compared to intact rats, possibly indicating the existence of a factor from the neural lobe which directly influences the adrenal gland.

Since the corticotropic activity of the neurointermediate lobe of the pitui-tary was first described by Mialhe-Voloss (52) and Rochefort et al. (53), a number of confirmatory reports of such activity have appeared, although the physiological role of such activity has not been defined. The more recent studies with the use of immunohistochemical techniques have shed some light on the localization of ACTH activity outside of the anterior pituitary but have com-pounded the question of what the physiological significance of these immuno-reactive ACTH-like compounds is, since some antibodies which may not be specific for ACTH have been employed. Since MSH and ACTH share a common amino acid sequence and MSH is found in high concentrations outside of the pars distalis, it is not surprising that these data are occasionally difficult to interpret. Furthermore, as Stoeckel et al. (54) have suggested, the localization of ACTH in the intermediate or neural lobe cells does not necessarily mean that this polypeptide is synthesized in these cells, but it may possibly be extracted from the circulation or adjoining tissues.

From the available literature, it seems likely that ACTH can be found, and may even be synthesized, in areas of the pituitary outside of the pars distalis, but it has not been shown that this hormone participates in the physiological normal, stress-induced release of corticosteroids.

There are many reports of extrapituitary ACTH synthesis from tumor tissue, and these substances may indeed play an important role in the clinical symptom-ology of patients with such pathological tissue.

Saffran et al. (55) have shown that biologically active ACTH can be found in the ventral hypothalamus of intact rats and that the amino acid composition of this corticotropin activity is similar to that of pituitary ACTH. Again, there is no indication whether this material is synthesized in or simply extracted by the hypothalamic tissue. It is conceivable that such ACTH activity might play a role in the short loop negative feedback proposed for ACTH on CRF release.

There still remains some controversy concerning the cell types in the anterior pituitary that secrete ACTH. Much of the data is based upon electron micro-graphic studies from animals that have been adrenalectomized. These studies rely on the earlier findings of Fortier and de Groot (56), who showed that the anterior pituitary content of ACTH rose dramatically within 24 hr after adrenal-ectomy. Prior to this study, Farquhar (57) found that there were ungranulated follicular cells in the pituitary gland that increased in size after adrenalectomy and might, therefore, be the source of ACTH. Some of the more recent studies from Moriarty and Halmi's laboratory (58) with the use of a combination of electron microscopy and a procedure involving unlabeled antibody—peroxidase—antiperoxidase complex have identified in the rat anterior pituitary stellate-shaped cells with a maximal diameter of 300 nm arranged around the periphery. The granules behaved as one would have predicted from Fortier and de Groot's findings, decreasing immediately after adrenalectomy and increasing 21 days later. The approximate size of the granules and their distribution around the periphery of the cytoplasm are in agreement with the findings of Nakane (59). Cameron and Foster (60) made similar observations with the use of metyrapone in rabbits to enhance the storage of ACTH in a specific cell type. This corticotroph was a polygonal-shaped cell with secretory granules approximately 150 nm in diameter.

There appears to be some discrepancy concerning the size of granule found in the corticotrophs (sizes ranging from 100—300 nm). Recently, Ishikawa et al. (61) and Yoshimura et al. (62) have isolated granules from rat anterior pituitary acidophils and found that a significant amount of biologically active ACTH resided in granules 100—200 nm in diameter and that no activity could be detected in the fraction containing granules 300—450 nm in diameter.

The characterization of the anterior pituitary corticotroph as an acidophil, basophil, or chromophobe does not appear to be resolved with any reasonable degree of certainty (62, 63). However, many of the more recent papers, which used immunohistochemical techniques in conjunction with the classical staining procedures, seem to indicate that the corticotrophs are indeed acidophilic.

In summary, many of the recent reports seem to indicate that there is a characteristic cell type in the anterior pituitary of adult rats, rabbits, and humans which can be distinguished as an acidophil of fine-to-medium granularity which may vary in shape, but appears to be somewhat stellate, with protruding cytoplasmic processes between neighboring cells, and shows definitive alterations after adrenalectomy and metyrapone and cortisol treatment (58, 60—64).

Previous reports have shown a close correlation between plasma β-MSH levels over a wide range of normal and pathological conditions. Donald and Toth found that immunoreactive β-MSH and ACTH usually showed good correlation. However, in this study, as well as in a previous study by Kastin et al. (67), it was reported that there are a number of instances in which MSH and ACTH do not show such good correlation.

Other reports not only show a close correlation between plasma levels of MSH and ACTH, but also indicate that both of these hormones may come from the same pituitary cell. Phifer et al. (68, 69) suggested that their "$\beta(r)$" cell from human pituitary glands was not only an ACTH-producing cell but was also immunostained with their porcine MSH antiserum. Thus, not only may there be similar stimuli for MSH and ACTH release from the pituitary, but they may, in fact, come from the same cells. However, it is hard to reconcile this proposal with the findings of those investigators who have shown a lack of correlation of plasma levels of these two hormones. It is possible that one stimulus could release both MSH and ACTH from the same cell, but, due to differences in threshold, latency of action, or half-life of pituitary hormone, the plasma levels may not always appear to be well correlated.

ADRENOCORTICOTROPIC HORMONE STRUCTURE AND FUNCTION

A question that remains unresolved is whether biologically active ACTH from sources other than the anterior pituitary (and in forms other than the commonly found ACTH$^{1-39}$ molecule) exists and plays a role in the physiological control of the adrenal cortex.

Yalow and Berson (70) described a component of human plasma and pituitary preparations that showed immunological and biological ACTH activity but was of greater molecular weight than ACTH$^{1-39}$. More recently (71), these investigators described this molecule to be chemically distinct but immunologically indistinguishable from ACTH$^{1-39}$. Apparently, it is almost as large as albumin and, upon addition of trypsin, this molecule is broken down to the smaller portions resembling ACTH$^{1-39}$. The data suggested that "big ACTH" is composed of ACTH$^{1-39}$ covalently linked at the amino terminus to a lysine or arginine residue of a more acidic peptide. Of interest was the finding that plasma samples from some patients contained only big ACTH, with little or no ACTH$^{1-39}$. Krieger (72) also reported on a patient that apparently produced only big ACTH. In this patient, the immunoreactive ACTH was elevated, but the bioassay indicated low levels of ACTH; however, if the plasma was trypsinized, then ACTH with biological activity could be demonstrated. Gewirtz et al. (73) confirmed and extended these earlier observations. Originally, the ACTH had 4% of the biological activity of ACTH$^{1-39}$, but after trypsin digestion for 10 s there was a highly significant increase in the biological ACTH activity. The ability to produce biologically active (and immunoreactive) ACTH of a lower molecular weight than the original big ACTH leads these authors to suggest that big ACTH may in fact be a precursor molecule for the ACTH$^{1-39}$.

Large molecular weight fractions, containing ACTH-like activity, have been described from other sources and several other species of animals. Other investigators (74–76) have isolated a biologically active peptide from the pars intermedia of rat and pig pituitaries (and from some human tumors) which is indistinguishable from the 18–39 amino acid or COOH-terminal portion of the ACTH molecule and have termed it "corticotropin-like intermediate lobe peptide" (CLIP). They propose that CLIP and α-MSH are derived from ACTH by cleavage into these two fragments. Furthermore, they speculate that not only might CLIP be a hormone in its own right but it may in fact be a precursor of other biologically active peptides. Although there have been a number of reports to indicate that there might be ACTH-like activity in the human placenta, only recently has there been direct evidence that the placenta or amniotic cells actually produce a substance with such activity. These investigators (77, 78) suggest the term "human chorionic corticotropin" (HCC) to describe this activity, but give little evidence of its chemical nature. Its physiological role, if any, remains to be elucidated. An indication of its possible clinical importance is suggested by Genazzani et al. (79), who have shown that this HCC activity is found in the plasma of pregnant women and cross-reacts in the ACTH immuno-assay, making it difficult to interpret data for pituitary ACTH secretory activity during pregnancy.

The production of ACTH from other extra pituitary sources has been suggested by a number of investigators over many years. The evidence for such ACTH synthetic activity, except from tumor tissue, has been largely indirect. One possible source of ACTH activity is hypothalamic tissue. Pearlmutter et al. (80) showed that there are significant levels of ACTH activity in extracted hypothalamic tissue of rats. The possibility exists that ACTH is produced by hypothalamic or other CNS tissue. Similarly, several investigators have shown ACTH activity in the cerebrospinal fluid (CSF) of a number of species, including man (81, 82). They have shown that there is no equilibration of immunoreactive ACTH activity across the human and cat blood-brain-CSF barrier, suggesting that the activity which is found in the CSF is not coming from the peripheral circulation but is presumably arising within the CNS itself. Additional roles for "ACTH" molecules of different sizes, or amino acid composition, have been proposed. Data from a number of laboratories have suggested that the types of corticosteroids that are secreted at any given time, in a specific series, depend upon the nature of the ACTH molecule secreted. Prolonged administration of porcine ACTH altered the type of corticosteroid which was secreted by rabbits by decreasing corticosterone and increasing cortisol secretion (83, 84). Drummond and Fevold (85) prepared ACTH-containing fractions from rabbit and steer pituitaries and assayed equal quantities of activity in an in vitro preparation of rat adrenal tissue. When these preparations were administered to rabbits over a 2-day period, porcine ACTH stimulated 10 times the cortisol production compared to rabbit ACTH, whereas bovine ACTH stimulated cortisol production to the same degree as did porcine ACTH. Thus, one type of ACTH can stimulate the 17-α-hydroxylation to a much lesser extent than another. More recently, Coslovsky and Yalow (86) demonstrated an intermediate size ACTH compound in the pituitaries of rabbits, rats, and mice. These species have as their principal glucocorticoid, corticosterone, whereas other species, which produce predominantly the ACTH$^{1-39}$ (such as man, monkey, sheep, dog, cat, and guinea pig), produce mainly cortisol. Bovine pituitaries contain an intermediate ACTH as well as ACTH$^{1-39}$ and produce both cortisol and corticosterone in approximately equal quantities.

There is substantial experimental evidence that has served to clarify the physiological functions of portions of the ACTH molecule. Starting from the NH$_2$-terminal part of the amino acid sequence, there is considerable evidence that the active site of the ACTH molecule resides in the first 14 amino acids (87), more specifically, amino acids 5–10 (88). Even with doses as high as 1 mg in an isolated cell suspension assay, Seelig and Sayers (88) could detect no corticosterone-stimulating action for the ACTH amino acids 11–24. This fraction, however, did act as a competitor and thus may represent the binding site configuration that determines the affinity of the ACTH molecule for the adrenal cell. The tryptophan at the ninth position appears to be involved in the excitation of the receptor, according to the data of Seelig et al. (89). Furthermore, the positive charge on amino acid 11 is also required for binding to the membrane receptor (90). The data of Blade and Li (91) also indicated that the peptide sequence 11–14 not only acts as a bridge between the active site and the binding site but contributes to the actual potency of the molecule.

The amino acid sequence 15–18 was intensively investigated by Nakamura (87), using isolated rat adrenal cells. From these studies, it was concluded that the Lys-Lys-Arg-Arg in position 15–18 increase the affinity of the ACTH molecule.

What then is the functional significance of the remaining 15 amino acids of the ACTH molecule (i.e., amino acids 25–39)? Hajós et al. (92), in an in vivo assay which used various segments of the amino acid sequence of ACTH, suggest that synthetic $ACTH^{1-24}$ is less potent than human $ACTH^{1-28}$, which in turn is less potent than human $ACTH^{1-39}$. Graf et al. (93) have shown that the deamidation of the porcine ACTH molecule, which they suggest affects only the asparagine at position 25 in the sequence, resulted in a 50% decrease of its biological activity, as measured in a rat in vivo bioassay. Bennett et al. (94) demonstrated that the longer chained $ACTH^{1-39}$ molecule is less susceptible to proteolytic attack than $ACTH^{1-24}$. The COOH-terminal part of the molecule apparently protects the molecule from proteolytic degradation.

A number of other analogs of ACTH have been synthesized and studied. For example, Kumar et al. (95) have shown that Trp (Dnps)^9 $ACTH^{5-24}$ can block the corticosteroid and AMP production elicited by $ACTH^{1-24}$ in isolated adrenal cortical cells. Hoffman et al. (96) also have shown that the tryptophan residue of the ACTH molecule on position 9 is essential for the activation of the adrenal cell. They showed that substitution of the tryptophan by a phenylalanine or N^2-methyltryptophan resulted in a compound which had a high affinity for the ACTH receptor but failed to activate the adenylate cyclase on the adrenal cell membrane. Thus, simply binding to the receptor site is not a sufficient stimulus for the expression of the hormone action.

ASSAYS FOR ADRENOCORTICOTROPIC HORMONE AND CORTICOTROPIN-RELEASING FACTOR

Impact of Radioimmunoassays

Prior to the development of radioimmunoassay by Berson and Yalow, investigation into pituitary-adrenal physiology was hampered by the lack of suitable methods for measuring most of the hormones of the hypothalamic-pituitary-adrenal system. Only cortisol and its metabolites could be measured easily and reliably. Methods for other hypothalamic-pituitary-adrenal hormones were either nonexistent or too impractical for extensive use. The situation improved greatly with the advent of radioimmunoassay into the field in 1964 when Berson and Yalow and their co-workers published their first paper on a plasma ACTH radioimmunoassay (97).

Even though these radioimmunoassays have been used for only a very short time, they have contributed much new and important information that has led to a better understanding of pituitary-adrenal physiology (98). One of the most important contributions the radioimmunoassay has made has been in the area of circadian rhythm. New information on how cortisol and ACTH are secreted have led to important revisions in old, established concepts about hypothalamic-pituitary-adrenal circadian rhythm.

Prior to radioimmunoassays for plasma ACTH and cortisol, large volumes of blood were required, and measurements were carried out at infrequent intervals of 4–6 hr. These infrequent assays were interpreted to mean that cortisol and ACTH blood levels change slowly but continuously in a smooth diurnal pattern that peaked out in the early morning and reached a minimal level around midnight.

With the increased sensitivity of the radioimmunoassay, much smaller volumes of blood were required, and samples could be collected as frequently as every 10 min throughout the day. These frequent assays revealed that past concepts were wrong. The adrenal secretes cortisol intermittently in short bursts lasting only a few minutes (99, 100).

The largest number of secretory episodes occurs most frequently during the 6–8 hr of sleep, whereas the fewest secretory episodes occur in the period 2–4 hr prior to the onset of sleep. Plasma ACTH levels are usually parallel to cortisol levels except that ACTH precedes cortisol by a few minutes, as expected (101). This type of secretion has been designated "episodic secretion" to distinguish it from the usual concept of diurnal variation. It is now known that several hormones other than hypothalamic-pituitary-adrenal hormones are secreted episodically. It has been suggested that a control center or biological clock in the hypothalamus or higher brain centers initiates or terminates this cortisol secretion by stimulating or suppressing the secretion of CRF by the hypothalamus, followed by pituitary ACTH release. The critical question is what tells the CNS control center when to initiate this process, presumably because the body needs more cortisol, and what tells it when to stop to avoid overproduction? For years it was felt that blood cortisol levels served this function. However, the following observations, from episodic secretion studies and other sources, have led to serious doubts that blood cortisol levels are directly involved.

1. Plasma cortisol levels may fall to zero levels for several hours without stimulating an ACTH response (100).
2. ACTH secretion may occur at a time when cortisol levels are in the high normal range (100).
3. An essentially normal circadian rhythm for plasma ACTH at higher than normal levels persists in adrenal insufficiency in spite of undetectable cortisol levels (102, 103).

4. Following adrenalectomy in rats, there is a considerable time lag between the fall in corticosterone and the rise in ACTH (104).

If episodic secretion is independent of blood cortisol concentration, it is conceivable that cortisol concentration in the central nervous system control center itself might regulate its activity. The observations that hypothalamic-pituitary-adrenal activity can be inhibited by implanting corticosteroids in the hypothalamus, and that radioactive corticosteroids localize in the hypothalamus and higher brain centers following systemic administration, lend some support to this theory (105).

The possibility that blood cortisol concentration might influence the CNS control center has not been completely ruled out. If the maximal cortisol levels (i.e., peak values for each secretory episode throughout the day) are plotted against time, one obtains a fairly smooth curve with a maximum during the early morning hours and a minimum at midnight, a curve somewhat reminiscent of those drawn to illustrate cortisol diurnal variation prior to the discovery of episodic secretion. This curve appears to represent the cortisol level that terminates ACTH secretion at any given time. Since this threshold level is continuously changing in a smooth gradient, this theory has been called the "variable set-point theory."

A similar plot of the minimal cortisol levels for each secretory episode appears to represent the threshold level at which ACTH secretion is initiated. It appears to operate only during the early morning hours; throughout the rest of the day other factors must initiate ACTH secretion.

If blood cortisol levels are maintained at a level over 7.5 μg/100 ml. throughout the day by means of a constant intravenous infusion, ACTH secretion is completely abolished in normal subjects (106). If plasma cortisol levels are maintained at lower levels, ACTH is secreted in the usual pattern, but in smaller amounts. These findings suggest that there is a threshold blood cortisol level that turns ACTH secretion off. It can be argued equally effectively that it is not the level of cortisol in the blood but the level in the CNS control center that is responsible. It has been observed, in episodic secretion studies, that blood cortisol levels frequently rise to levels much higher than 7.5 μg/100 ml before ACTH secretion is terminated. This observation suggests that the level of cortisol in the control center must build up to a critical level before ACTH secretion is shut off and that blood levels may not accurately reflect the levels in the control center.

There are objections to the "variable set-point theory."

1. In most normal subjects, the cortisol threshold curves for inhibition and stimulation are fairly continuous and smooth, but the basic pattern is interrupted sporadically by large bursts of secretion for no apparent reason.
2. In some normal subjects, the secretory episodes seem to occur erratically throughout the day with no basic underlying pattern.

3. In a very short period of time, the levels of cortisol associated with both ACTH suppression and stimulation may fluctuate widely.

To explain these objections, it has been suggested that a variable set-point operates to establish a base line pattern of secretion, but that this base line pattern can be overridden by the hypothalamus and higher brain centers in response to a variety of stimuli.

Since most of the ectopic secretory episodes occur during times when the patient is awake and active, it may be that stimuli such as exercise, psychic and physical stress, or eating override the basic rhythm of secretion (107, 108).

Whatever physiological mechanisms control the activity of the hypothalamic-pituitary-adrenal system, they must be sensitive to the amount of cortisol produced per unit of time in order to maintain the normal state. It would appear that blood cortisol concentrations are not normally directly involved. That concentrations of cortisol in the CNS control center might be the key controlling mechanism appears to be an attractive theory at the present time.

Radioimmunoassay for Adrenocorticotropic Hormone

Radioimmunoassay has only been used for a relatively short time to study the hypothalamic-pituitary-adrenal system, but the findings have already contributed immeasurably toward a better understanding of the physiology of this system. In some instances, classical concepts have been confirmed and extended. Other findings have led to revisions of old concepts and the formulation of new ones. These physiological studies have produced new and better laboratory tests for pituitary-adrenal function that are simple and reliable enough to be used not only in clinical research, but also in the routine practice of medicine. Even greater contributions from radioimmunoassay can be expected in the future.

One of the most difficult problems which is raised by radioimmunoassay of ACTH is that of suitable antibodies for ACTH assays in human plasma. The first difficulty is related to the low antigenicity of the ACTH molecule because of its low molecular weight (4,542), the small species differences in the amino acid sequence of the ACTH molecules, the lack of a disulfide bridge for molecular stability, the rapid destruction of the molecule in vivo, and induced hypercortisolism in animals since corticoids inhibit the production of antibodies. Secondly, it is necessary to obtain an antibody directed to the NH_2-terminal portion of the molecule (1–24). This biologically active portion is common to all mammals.

Finally, the antibody must have a great affinity for ACTH since the molar concentration of ACTH in human plasma is about 10 times less than that of the glycoprotein hormones. Proeschel et al. (109) developed a method for the rapid screening of ACTH antibodies. They compared different immunization methods according to the type of antigen and its preparation. They also compared the rhythm of injections, as well as the amount of ACTH injected. With the use of

267 guinea pigs, these investigators found that among different methods the injection of some with 30 I.U. of human ACTH resulted in 7 antibodies that were suitable for specific and sensitive radioimmunoassay of ACTH in human plasma without necessity of previous extraction. These antibodies reacted with the 17–24 portion of the ACTH molecule. When they studied patients with varying adrenal-pituitary-axis disorders, they found that the radioimmunoassay compared favorably with those results reported by other investigators using bioassay techniques.

Vaitukaitis et al. (110) described methodology that could be used to generate sensitive antisera to weakly antigenic molecules such as ACTH. Using these methods, Rose and Newsome (111) examined the feasibility of producing sensitive antisera to several hormones such as ACTH, angiotensin, and 11-desoxy-corticosterone (DOC), which are normally found in peripheral plasma in extremely low concentrations. They reported success in producing antisera to two small peptides, ACTH and angiotensin II, and one steroid (DOC) with the use of a small number of animals. These antisera were produced within 4 months of the initial immunization. From their data, it appears that multiple injections of antigen over a long period of time are not necessary for the production of highly sensitive antisera to small polypeptides. This was in contrast to the authors' previous experience with ACTH when more than 18 months were required for the production of suitable antisera (112) and to the experience of others such as Orth et al. (113) where over 200 animals were immunized before a satisfactory antiserum was produced.

Plasma ACTH in humans has been determined by both bioassay and radioimmunoassay. Although radioimmunoassay has been shown to be as specific as the bioassay in measuring ACTH, there is a fundamental difference in principle between bioassay, which measures the steroidogenic potency of ACTH residing in the first 18 amino acids of the molecule, and the radioimmunoassay, which measures immunochemical reactivity of ACTH. The steroidogenic and immunochemical activities are not necessarily identical. Both agreement and discrepancy between the two could occur and, in fact, have been demonstrated by studies involving intact ACTH and its fragments and by comparisons of both parameters in rats.

Additional studies have been carried out by Matsuyama et al. (114) to demonstrate comparative biological and immunological levels of human plasma ACTH in the same sample. These investigators found that the immunologically determined amounts of ACTH were almost always equal to or greater than those determined by biological assays. These results suggested to these authors that, although the biologically active ACTH is measured by the immunological assay, some of the ACTH measured immunologically lacks biological activity. Matsuyama et al. (114) concluded that individual immunological determinations were almost always higher than biological determination, possibly due to the presence of ACTH fragments which retain immunological specificity but lack biological potency.

In a further study, Matsuyama et al. (115) studied the disappearance rates of exogenous and endogenous ACTH from rat plasma measured by bioassay and radioimmunoassay. They found that when α-ACTH (Li) was given intravenously to hypophysectomized rats, it disappeared with a half-time of 2.9 min by bioassay and 4.1 min by radioimmunoassay. Endogenous ACTH in stressed 14-day adrenalectomized rats had a half-time of 1.7 min by bioassay and 3.6 min by radioimmunoassay. Intact stressed rats showed a similar decrease in ACTH as measured by radioimmunoassay with a half-life of 4.1 min. These results suggested to these authors that ACTH fragments, which are biologically inert but immunologically active, arise in circulating plasma during the metabolism of ACTH. The antibody used in these studies is probably reactive to the COOH-terminal portion of ACTH since it does not cross-react with α-ACTH$^{1-24}$. Therefore, as the molecule is degraded, COOH-terminal fragments remaining in the circulation could still react immunologically and become additive to the intact biologically active ACTH measured by the radioimmunoassay. This could partly explain the discrepancy under certain conditions between bioassay and radioimmunoassay results. It is, therefore, possible that ACTH fragments that are biologically active appear in rat plasma under conditions of increased ACTH output. The biological and immunological half-lives of both exogenous and endogenous ACTH in man and in the pig, however, are much longer than in rats, possibly due to differences in metabolism between small and large mammals.

It is well known that steroid hormones, as well as hormones of the thyroid gland, are bound specifically to plasma proteins. More recently, a binding protein for neurohypophysial hormones, neurophysin, has been demonstrated in blood by means of radioimmunoassay. On the other hand, the binding of other polypeptide hormones to plasma proteins has not been convincingly shown. While working on a radioimmunoassay for ACTH, Fehm et al. (116) found increasing evidence for the existence of a plasma factor with ACTH-binding activity. Since this factor may disturb the radioimmunological system and because of its suspected biological validity, they tried to elucidate its nature. These investigators found that there is a factor present in plasma, at varying activity, which prevents adsorption of ACTH to silicates. Column chromatography of ^{125}I-ACTH on Sephadex G-200, after incubation of plasma, revealed a large molecular weight fraction of ACTH. From these results, Voight et al. (117) concluded that ACTH is bound to a plasma factor with large molecular weight and that this binding factor and the silicates compete for ACTH. Although the physiological significance of the binding phenomenon remains obscure, it may well explain the difficulties of radioimmunological measurement of ACTH in untreated plasma.

Since its original application to the measurement of plasma insulin, radioimmunoassay has been used for the assay of many polypeptide hormones. In addition to the specificity and great sensitivity obtainable by the use of carefully selected antisera to hormones, this method readily allows precise measurement of hormone concentrations on a large number of specimens. Disadvantages have been that the basis for the specificity is immunological rather than biological and that relatively long incubation periods are usually required to achieve maximal sensitivity.

Analogous competitive protein-binding assays have been developed in which other materials such as thyroxin-binding globulin are used in place of specific antibodies, but again the structural features of the ligand that determine the degree of binding are not identical with those needed for biological activity.

Polypeptide hormones, including ACTH, appear to act by binding to specific receptors which are on the outer surface of cells. In most cases, the receptor-hormone complex, in some undetermined way, activates adenyl cyclase, an enzyme bound to the plasma membrane that markedly accelerates the conversion of adenosine triphosphate to cyclic adenosine monophosphate. The latter appears to be the intracellular mediator of ACTH activity.

Fate of Circulating Adrenocorticotropic Hormone

Both endogenous and exogenous ACTH are rapidly removed from the circulation with half-lives varying from approximately 1–30 min, depending upon the assay used and the experimental conditions.

ACTH appears to be removed faster when measured by bioassay than when measured by radioimmunoassay. If an antiserum directed toward the NH_2-terminal portion of the ACTH molecule is used, the removal rate is usually slower than when a COOH-terminal antiserum is used (118). Since biological activity resides in the NH_2-terminal portion of the ACTH molecule, these findings have been interpreted to indicate that circulating ACTH undergoes rapid proteolysis to form peptides that have lost biological activity but retain their immunological activity. Where in the body this metabolism occurs is unknown.

There are other observations in support of this notion. When ACTH is measured by both radioimmunoassay and bioassay on identical plasma samples, the value obtained by radioimmunoassay is usually higher. When the patient or the experimental animal is stimulated to produce more ACTH, the difference between radioimmunoassay increases strikingly (119, 120). The latter observation suggests that, under conditions of stress, biologically inactive but immunologically active peptide precursors to ACTH may be released into or accumulate in the circulation.

Radioreceptor Assay for Adrenocorticotropic Hormone

Lefkowitz and Roth (121) have developed a radioreceptor assay of adrenocorticotropic hormone as a new approach to the assay of polypeptide hormones in plasma. They have prepared monoiodo ^{125}I-ACTH of very high specific radioactivity and adrenal extracts that contain both the ACTH receptors and the ACTH-sensitive adenylate cyclase. With these as reagents, they have developed a rapid, sensitive assay for ACTH based upon competition of ^{125}I-labeled and unlabeled ACTH for binding sites on specific ACTH receptors.

Reactivity in this system appears to be based upon the biological properties of ACTH. Of the ACTH derivatives tested, only those which retain biological activity occupy the receptors. The authors claim that the assay permits easy measurement of ACTH in unextracted plasma in a few hours. This method, which in principle is widely applicable to other hormones, has the advantages of immunoassay and also affords greater speed and specificity that is biological, rather than immunological. The authors claim that the successful application of ACTH receptors to assay of ACTH in plasma represents the first time that target tissue receptors have been used for the measurement of a polypeptide hormone.

A substantial advantage of the radioreceptor assay is its specificity for biologically active ACTH. Reactivity in the system is proportional to biological activity. This system provides not only a direct method for studying the interaction of hormones with their target tissues but also a general approach to the assay of biologically active substances in body fluids.

Wolfsen et al. (122) modified the method of Lefkowitz et al. (121) by using normal adrenal glands as the source of the ACTH receptor rather than the adrenal tumor tissue used by Lefkowitz et al. By using the competitive binding assay employing the cortical receptor from normal adrenal glands, it was possible to reproducibly quantify ACTH in less than 250 μl of unextracted plasma from normal subjects. The major advantage of using normal adrenal glands, rather than the tissue culture of mouse adrenal tumor used by Lefkowitz et al., is the widespread availability of the normal tissue. An additional advantage of this assay, with the use of high affinity receptor, is the rapid equilibration and, therefore, short incubation time which minimized the problems of incubation damage and adsorption to glass and plastic surfaces.

As shown by Lefkowitz et al. (121) and Hofmann et al. (123), the receptor assay measures the portion of the ACTH molecule which must bind to initiate biological activity. The correlation of ACTH values in normal and pathological states of pituitary-adrenal function supports the validity of the assay.

In Vivo Bioassay Modifications

Nicholson and Van Loon (124) have reported some innovations in the biological assay of ACTH. The three practical innovations include modification of the fluorometric assay of corticosterone, earlier collection of blood, and preliminary treatment of the 24–48 hr hypophysectomized rats with ACTH.

These changes have increased the sensitivity of the Guillemin et al. assay (125) while still retaining its simplicity. First, the use of the fluorescence assay of Mattingly (126), which employs ethanolic rather than aqueous sulfuric acid as the fluorescence reagent, has improved the corticosterone method by lowering plasma background fluorescence and increasing the intensity of corticosterone fluorescence. Secondly, the collection of blood for corticosterone determination at 10 min, rather than at a later time, increases the sensitivity of the method by measuring near-peak responses to small doses of ACTH. Thirdly, the use of

ACTH to sensitize the 24- or 48-hr hypophysectomized rat has relieved the investigator of the necessity of performing this operation in his own laboratory. With these improvements, the simple method of Guillemin has been made as sensitive as the more tedious method of Lipscomb and Nelson (127). The limit of useful sensitivity with each method is about 0.03 mu (300 pg of ACTH). This has been accomplished without losing any desirable features of the Lipscomb-Nelson method, such as precision. The present method, using commercially available hypophysectomized rats, places the assay of ACTH within easy reach of anyone who can perform the simple fluorometric assay for corticosterone.

Oxidation-Reduction Cytochemical Adrenocorticotropic Hormone Assay

Most biological assays for ACTH cannot measure normal circulating levels without the use of prohibitively large volumes of plasma. Because of its sensitivity, the oxidation-reduction cytochemical assay for corticotropin was developed by Chayen et al. in 1972 (128). The oxidation-reduction assay is able to determine normal and subnormal ACTH concentrations in plasma using very small μl samples. ACTH depletes reducing groups in the guinea pig adrenal cortex maintained in organ culture. This depletion can be quantitatively determined by scanning and integrating microdensitometry of sections of the zona reticularis after appropriate staining. An inverse correlation has been demonstrated between the intensity of the stain and the logarithmic concentration of ACTH over the range of 0.0027–2.7 pg/ml (129, 130). The general procedure, after recent modifications (131), is as follows. Segments of the adrenal glands of a guinea pig are first maintained in vitro at $37°C$ for 5 hr with Trowell T-8 medium. The gas phase is 95% oxygen. At the end of this 5-hr period, the culture medium is removed and replaced by fresh T-8 ascorbate medium at pH 7.6, containing 0.0005 pg/ml of the standard ACTH (3rd International Working Standard). After 4-min exposure to this priming concentration of ACTH (the effect of which cannot be detected by the cytochemical bioassay method), the segments are chilled to $-70°C$ and stored at $-70°C$. Sections are then cut at 20 μm in a cryostat fitted with an automatic cutting device to insure regular thickness of the sections. The sections are flash dried onto warm glass slides and kept at room temperature for 1 hr before being used. They are then clipped in pairs, back to back, and immersed in the relevant compartment of the assay trough (each containing its particular concentration of ACTH or plasma) for 1 min. The sections are then immediately immersed in a second trough containing the ferricyanide reaction medium for 5 min. The reaction medium is replaced with freshly prepared reaction medium in which the sections are immersed for another 5 min. This procedure is repeated to give a total reaction time of 15 min. The sections are then rinsed in tap water and left to dry, after which they are cleared in xylene and mounted under a cover slip. Once mounted under a cover slip, the sections must be kept in the dark to avoid fading. The amount of color produced by the reduction of ferricyanide to produce a blue fine precipitate of ferric ferricyanide in the zona reticularis is measured by its absorption at

640 nm. For this purpose, a scanning and integrating microdensitometer is used. The relative absorption per field recorded by this instrument is converted to the absolute value. The amount of blue stain in the zona reticularis was found to vary linearly and inversely with the logarithmic concentration of ACTH applied to the sections over the range of 0.05—5 pg/ml. The sensitivity was improved to that of the segment assay (0.0005 pg/ml) when the segments of the gland were primed with 0.0005 pg/ml of ACTH for 4 min prior to chilling. The results show that it is possible to assay ACTH in human plasma by the effect this hormone has on sections of guinea pig adrenal glands, provided that the sections are suitably prepared and protected during exposure to the hormone. This method is extremely sensitive (132) and, as the authors state, it would not be unreasonable to expect one worker to be able to do 20 assays in 2 days. The oxidation-reduction assay has been validated and seems to be the most sensitive assay for ACTH currently available (133).

Isolation of Cells of Anterior Pituitary and Adrenal Cortex

Previous studies of the action and secretion of hormones had been derived largely from studies in the whole animal, tissue slices, and tissue homogenates, and more recently by the use of isolated cells. Isolated cells of the endocrine glands or of the target tissues of the hormones represent a new approach since these preparations retain the advantages of the intact cell, yet eliminate problems of penetration of diffusion barriers inherent in the tissue slice. Most of the cell separation techniques originate with the studies of Rodbell (134), who developed a simple and highly reproducible technique for the isolation of adipocytes. Collagenase, combined with gentle agitation, frees the cells of the epididymal fat pad of the rat. The isolated cells synthesize and release fatty acids, processes which are exquisitely sensitive to the addition of insulin, epinephrine, and other hormones to the incubation medium. The metabolic activities of the isolated adipocytes and the regulation of these activities by insulin and other hormones appear to be a close representation of the events as they occur in the intact animal.

For the dispersion of adrenal cells, several methods have been developed. Kloppenborg et al. (135) and Haning et al. (136) used collagenase, whereas Halkerston and Feinstein (137) employed a combination of five different enzymes. Swallow and Sayers (138) and Sayers et al. (139) reported on a method which used trypsin as a dispersing enzyme. Swallow and Sayers have modified and refined the trypsin technique so that the preparation of isolated cells of the rat adrenal responded with increased production of corticosterone to the addition of less than 1 pg of ACTH.

The trypsin technique has also been used successfully by Portanova et al. (140) in the isolation of cells of the rat anterior pituitary. The isolated pituitary cells maintained a high concentration of ACTH when incubated under appropriate conditions. The use of trypsin has an advantage in that it can subsequently be inhibited with trypsin inhibitor. Isolated adrenal cells elaborate corticosteroids in response to physiological concentrations of ACTH and also offer the advantage that many aliquots from a homogenous suspension can be used to compare samples over a range of dilutions.

Barofsky et al. (141) have systematically compared various dissociation procedures, with the use of collagenase, hyaluronidase, and trypsin in varying amounts and in varying combinations. These authors have systematically evaluated the enzymatic and mechanical requirements for the dissociation of rat adrenal tissue and have interpreted the results in terms of known characteristics of the tissue used.

One of the difficulties encountered in the isolation of adrenal cells is the cell damage caused by over-trypsinization and mechanical rupture. Rodbell (142) found that the rupture of isolated fat cells in a medium free from serum albumin can be prevented by the addition of bovine serum albumin (BSA). Kono (143) observed in his experiments on the preparation of fat cell suspensions that approximately one-half of the cells in a medium free from serum albumin are ruptured within 30 min, regardless of the presence or absence of trypsin. He also demonstrated that this rupture of isolated fat cells is prevented by the addition of BSA to the medium. Although the mechanism of the BSA effect is still unknown, Nakamura and Tanaka (144) applied BSA to the dispersion of adrenal tissue. They described a simple and reproducible method for the preparation of isolated adrenal cells which involves the combined use of trypsin and bovine serum albumin to prevent cell damage during the digestion period. Not only did the BSA prevent cell rupture occurring in a protein-free medium, but it also aided in the buffering during the proteolytic action of trypsin. These investigators obtained a linear relationship between the corticosterone production and the log concentration of ACTH over a range of 60–500 mU/ml.

In contrast to the "in vitro" method of Saffran and Schally (145), based on the incubation of rat adrenal quarters, which gave a dose-response relationship ranging from 10–400 mU per flask of ACTH, the present method, with the use of isolated adrenal cells, showed a sensitivity that was about 1,000 times greater than that of Saffran and Schally's adrenal slice method. Lowry et al. (146) reported on a method for isolating intact cells from the adrenal glands of a small number of rats (4–6) so that a large number of incubations could be carried out with each batch of cells. They found an increased potency of corticotropin (1–24 tetracosapeptide) when compared with the full corticotropin 1–39 sequence. The response of isolated adrenal cells to cAMP has been reported by Sayers et al. (147) and by Kitabchi and Sharma (148). In the latter publication, the dog dose-response curve to cyclic AMP was much steeper than that obtained with corticotropin, whereas, in the former, parallel dose-response curves were reported. Lowry et al. obtained results that were similar to those of Kitabchi and Sharma in which the increase in steepness was so great that, on a linear plot, the response to cAMP was markedly sigmoid, whereas the response to corticotropin at low concentrations was suggestive of simple drug-receptor interaction. The authors suggested that, if cAMP is the mediator of corticotropin activation, it is surprising that the shapes of the dose-response curves would be so different. However, the difference cannot be taken as conclusive evidence against mediation by cAMP since other explanations might account for the anomaly, for example, lack of linearity in the cell penetration characteristics of AMP at the very high extracellular concentrations required for steroidogenesis.

Sayers and Beall (149) reported that, after hypophysectomy, isolated adrenal cortex cells became hypersensitive to ACTH. Cells from the adrenals of hypophysectomized rats required less ACTH to induce one-half maximal rate of $3':5'$-AMP production than did the cells from intact rats. A corresponding increase in sensitivity was also demonstrated in the steroidogenic response to ACTH, up to 2 days after hypophysectomy, before drastic reductions in steroidogenic capacity developed. Although the total steroidogenic capacity is decreased 2 days after hypophysectomy, the steroidogenic sensitivity to administered ACTH is enhanced.

Fehm et al. (150) confirmed the findings of Sayers et al. (139) and Giordano and Sayers (151) of a factor in plasma that inhibits ACTH-mediated corticosterone production of isolated adrenal cells. Fehm and co-workers excluded degradation as a likely cause and found that the inhibitory factor differed from one plasma to another, making valid measurements almost impossible. However, because the inhibitory factor, in contrast to ACTH, is not adsorbed to ultrafine precipitated silica (QUSO), QUSO extraction of ACTH from plasma successfully circumvents the problem. Liotta and Krieger (152) used silicic acid adsorption of plasma, with a subsequent acid wash and aqueous acetone desorption, to remove the substances which had interfered with steroidogenic response of dispersed adrenal cells when unextracted plasma was employed. Approximately 75% of the ACTH in the plasma was extracted, and 2 pg of ACTH could be consistently detected. When compared to the Lipscomb-Nelson bioassay (127), this method offers advantages of sensitivity (2 pg/ml rather than 100 pg/ml) and the ability to assay a greater number of samples per day (approximately 25). The cytochemical oxidation-reduction assay (128–132) is still more sensitive (50 fg/ml) and does not require extracted plasma, but it suffers from the disadvantage that only a few samples can be processed because of the effort necessary to carry out the procedures. Furthermore, with the oxidation-reduction method, it is not adrenal steroidogenesis, but loss of reducing potency in the adrenal cortex, that is measured, so that it is comparable to, but more sensitive than, the ascorbic acid depletion technique of Sayers et al (153).

The availability of the more sensitive assays for ACTH has enabled investigators to assess more precisely the inter-relationships of the central nervous system and pituitary-adrenal axis. Thus, Krieger and Allen (154) measured plasma ACTH and cortisol concentrations at 5-min intervals over a 3-4 hr sampling period in normal subjects and in hypersecreting patients with Cushing's disease. Although, in general, there was good correlation between plasma ACTH immunoassay and plasma ACTH bioassay, they found episodes during which a lack of correlation existed between ACTH levels and plasma cortisol levels in both normal subjects and in patients with Cushing's disease. Episodes of lack of correlation could not be attributed to biological inactivation of ACTH, but instead were thought to be due to an abnormality of ACTH regulatory mechanisms. Studies by Buckingham and Hodges (155) suggest that the synthesis and basal release of ACTH are directly controlled by the concentration of corticosteroids in the blood, but the corticosteroids exert only a delayed effect in modulating the stress-induced release of ACTH. Finally, severe and chronic depletion of catecholamines in the rat forebrain did not appear to interfere with pituitary-adrenal function as far as basal diurnal periodicity and responsiveness of the system to stressful or feedback stimuli were concerned (156).

Procedures have been developed for the continuous flow incubation of isolated adrenal cells, thereby combining the advantages of isolated cell suspension and the superfusion system (157, 158). The superfusion system allows dynamic studies into the functioning of the adrenal gland. Previous superfusion studies employing whole or sectioned glands have not overcome the limitations associated with studying kinetic cellular function with the use of blocks of tissue, in which the permeability of the tissue mass itself may influence the characteristics of the response. Cells internally located in blocks of tissue may suffer from restricted access to medium components. Employing superfusion of isolated cells allows for the investigation of the dynamic control systems operating in the cells. Lowry and McMartin (159) perfused isolated adrenal cells in a small column of Bio-Gel polyacrylamide as an inert supporting matrix and studied the dynamics of the steroidogenic response to ACTH, ACTH-analogs, and cAMP. They found a difference in the time course of response to ACTH and cAMP which suggested that there may be a second mediator to ACTH in addition to cAMP. Furthermore, the extremely rapid response to cAMP suggested the possibility that initiation of protein synthesis may not be necessary for steroidogenesis.

Assays for Corticotropin-releasing Factor

At the present time, corticotropin-releasing activity is detected and quantitatively determined by means of bioassay. In vivo or in vitro methods have been used which essentially measure the amount of ACTH released into the peripheral circulation or into the medium, respectively, after administration of extracts containing CRF (160).

The ideal in vivo CRF assay requires a physiological preparation in which the response to stress has been abolished without altering the functional integrity of the anterior pituitary. Although no single in vivo CRF assay is available which fulfills these criteria, several attempts have been made to approximate these requirements. Stereotaxic lesions (161) have been employed, adrenocortical suppression (162) has been used, and central depressants (163) have been administered for the purposes of assaying CRF. Each of these preparations has its merits and limitations in regard to ease of preparation, specificity, sensitivity, and successful utilization.

Hedge et al. (164) developed an assay for CRF by stereotaxically injecting material directly into the pituitary gland in pharmacologically blocked rats (dexamethasone, nembutal, and morphine sulfate). Because of the difficulty in localizing intrapituitary injections by stereotaxic methods, Hiroshige et al. (165) developed a direct intrapituitary microinjection technique in which tissue extracts are administered in 0.5-μl volumes into the adenohypophysis which is exposed parapharyngeally in a pharmacologically blocked (dexamethasone, chlorpromazine, nembutal) rat. These investigators have successfully demonstrated quantitative physiological changes in hypothalamic CRF with this technique (166, 167). Witorsch and Brodish (168) have systematically analyzed the conditions that must be met in order to use the lesioned rat reliably for the assay of CRF in tissue extracts. Most efforts to improve assays for CRF have been designed to enhance sensitivity without appreciable change in specificity and without the means to examine the dose-related responsiveness of a particular extract preparation. Lymangrover and Brodish (169) described a procedure for the multiple use of a lesioned assay preparation that makes it possible for an investigator to evaluate the animal's sensitivity to a standard CRF preparation, its blockade effectiveness or specificity, and its dose-related responsiveness (slope) after administration of two different doses of an unknown CRF preparation.

Sayers and his colleagues have employed dispersed pituitary cells for CRF assays and for elucidating CRF effects on pituitary cells. Employing suspensions of trypsin-dispersed anterior pituitary cells, Portanova et al. (170) showed that extracts of hypothalamic median eminence (HME) added to these cells produced increased release of ACTH into the medium in a log-dose relationship to the amount of extract. Energy dependence (171) was demonstrated, and vasopressin and other neurohypophysial-like peptides stimulated ACTH release in a manner suggesting that they are partial agonists of corticotropin secretion (172). Portanova and Sayers (173, 174) have developed the isolated pituitary cell suspension into a sensitive assay for CRF. Lowry (175) has recently developed the technique of cell column perfusion so that isolated cells, packed in an inert matrix and continuously perfused with incubation medium, can then be allowed to recover from the trauma of isolation before any stimulation is started, thereby leading to lower background levels and greater sensitivity. A 4-min pulse of SME extract, followed by a 4-min wash, was sufficient to obtain adequate stimulation and relaxation profiles when fractions of the effluent were collected and assayed for ACTH (175). Mulder and Smelik (176) applied Lowry's column perfusion system (175) in order to study the dynamics of ACTH release from isolated cells. Short pulses of CRF-containing extract caused bursts of ACTH release from the cells; these bursts were diminished by prior inclusion of corticosterone in the superfusion medium. Similarly, prior treatment of the pituitary donor animals with corticoids in vivo also had a profound effect on ACTH release in vitro (176).

A further modification of the dispersed cell technique for CRF assay is the use of monolayer cultures of pituitary cells. Fleischer and Rawls (177) prepared pituitary cell monolayer cultures to quantitatively determine ACTH synthesis, storage, and release and to measure the effect of the glucocorticoids, dexamethasone, and corticosterone on these parameters. They showed that new synthesis of ACTH does occur in monolayer pituitary cell culture and that ACTH secretion can decrease without apparent change in ACTH synthesis. Thus, ACTH synthesis and secretion can be dissociated. Other investigators (178) have used the cloned mouse pituitary tumor cell line as a model system to study the effects of glucocorticoids on ACTH production. Their results suggest that the response of these neoplastic cells resembles that of normal pituitary cells and support the localization of negative feedback inhibition of ACTH secretion, at least in part, at the level of the pituitary.

Availability of pituitary cells which synthesize and secrete hormones in culture provides a system that allows long-term studies of hormone regulation and synthesis which cannot be carried through with some of the other in vitro models, which are hampered by limited viability. With the use of monolayer cultures, it is possible to view the cells during the experiments and to correlate the biochemical with the morphological findings. Although the inhibition of ACTH secretion by glucocorticoids has been demonstrated in cultures of rat pituitary cells (177) and mouse pituitary tumor cells (178), effects of stimulating agents were not studied. Thus, Lang et al. (179) used cyclic AMP and theophylline as a stimulus for ACTH release in rat pituitary monolayer cultures. Both substances promoted the secretion of ACTH in a dose-dependent fashion, and the authors further demonstrated clearly the synthesis of new hormone by incorporation of labeled amino acids into the hormone during culture. They used a sensitive immunoprecipitation assay for the measurement of ACTH synthesis. The assay was specific for this hormone, since it was shown that the presence of excess authentic ACTH reduced radioactivity in the immunoprecipitate to background levels. These results present direct evidence for the ability of rat anterior pituitary cells growing in culture to synthesize ACTH and may allow for the study of the metabolism of ACTH molecules after their synthesis by employing pulse-chase experiments.

Takebe et al. (180) developed a reliable and relatively simple technique for CRF assay with the use of cultured rat anterior pituitary cells based on the method of Vale et al. (181) and Tang and Spies (182). The authors believe that the combined use of pooled cultured anterior pituitary cells and ACTH measurement by radioimmunoassay provides a convenient method for CRF assay which gives more accuracy and sensitivity than most of those previously described, while possessing the general advantages of in vitro assays. Graded doses of rat hypothalamic extract (HE) were added to dishes containing dispersed, pooled rat adenohypophysial cells cultured for several days. ACTH secretion into the medium gave a linear log-dose response curve over a 100-fold range between 0.01 mg and 1 mg of NIH-HE (0.0125–1.25 rat hypothalamus). Forty percent of the maximal ACTH secretion in response to a given dose of HE occurred within 3 min. No decrease in intracellular ACTH occurred at any time or with any dose of HE, indicating that secretion was always balanced by production. The same cultured cells could be used in repetitive assays performed on the same or different days (180). Yasuda et al. (183) applied their technique to study the basal and CRF-induced ACTH secretion and intracellular ACTH content in cultured adenohypophysial cells derived from adrenalectomized, dexamethasone treated, or intact rats. They found that even after 4 days of culture pituitary cells preserved characteristic supra- or infranormal secretion of ACTH induced by in vivo adrenalectomy or dexamethasone administration, respectively.

IN VITRO HYPOTHALAMIC INCUBATION

The effect of incubating the hypothalamus of the rat in vitro with various putative neurotransmitters was studied by Hillhouse et al. (184). The rat hypothalamus in vitro showed a considerable degree of metabolic activity, released corticotropin-releasing hormone in response to neurotransmitters, and also synthesized the releasing hormone CRH during in vitro incubation. Three hypothalami were incubated in 1 ml of medium and exposed to the test substance for 10 min, followed by a 20-min period of rest before being challenged with the test substance for a further 10 min. Samples were pooled, and CRH activity in the medium was assayed in 48-hr median eminence-lesioned rats; the corticosterone production of excised adrenals in vitro was used as the end-point of the assay. Acetylcholine (1–5 pg) caused a dose-dependent release of CRH which was antagonized by hexamethonium (1–10 ng) and partially antagonized by atropine. Neither norepinephrine, dopamine, nor histamine had any effect on the basal secretion of CRH. Norepinephrine (10 ng) was able to inhibit the release of CRH in response to acetylcholine (3 pg), and this action of norepinephrine was reduced by phentolamine, an α-adrenergic blocking agent. Serotonin (5-hydroxytryptamine, 100 pg–10 ng/ml) also caused a dose-dependent release of CRH. The stimulatory action of serotonin was prevented by the presence of norepinephrine in the incubating medium. The response to serotonin was also inhibited by hexamethonium and atropine, which would indicate that it is acting via a cholinergic pathway. The model that these studies propose concerning the role of neurotransmitters in the regulation of CRH is that acetycholine and serotonin are excitatory, the serotonin acting via a cholinergic interneuron; acetylcholine acts at the dendritic level of the CRH neuron via a nicotinic receptor mechanism. Both GABA and norepinephrine are neuroinhibitory, with GABA inhibiting at the axonal level and norepinephrine at the dendritic level via an α-adrenergic receptor mechanism.

Edwardson et al. (185) carried out studies to determine whether electrical and potassium stimulation would cause the release of neurosecretory substances and amino acids from hypothalamic synaptosomes prepared from sheep. Synaptosomes were prepared and suspended in Krebs phosphate medium containing glucose for 20-min periods of incubation, with and without electrical stimulation of the suspension or addition of potassium to the medium. Unstimulated suspensions of synaptosomes from the same preparation served as controls. The suspensions were centrifuged after incubation, and CRF activity in the super-natants was measured with the use of mice in which the release of endogenous CRF was blocked by pretreatment with chlorpromazine and sodium pentobarbi-tone. The results of these studies suggest that nerve endings isolated from sheep hypothalamus contain CRF, prolactin-inhibiting-factor (PIF), and perhaps all of the hypophysiotropic factors which control the secretion of hormones by the anterior pituitary gland. Stimulation released greater amounts of CRF, and the possibility of de novo synthesis is suggested by the relatively high levels of CRF that are present even after the lengthy period of preparation.

MECHANISM OF ADRENOCORTICOTROPIC HORMONE ACTION ON ADRENAL STEROIDOGENESIS

The initial sequence of cellular events which have been proposed to be involved in the regulation by ACTH of adrenocortical cellular activity is usually described as follows. ACTH is bound to a specific receptor site on the adrenal cell membrane. During this time the ACTH molecule is inactivated, but in turn activates various membrane-bound enzyme systems, for example, adenylate cyclase. Through the action of this enzyme, cAMP is formed from ATP. Cyclic AMP reacts with an intracellular receptor-protein kinase complex to activate the kinase enzyme which is then involved in the activation of a number of meta-bolic- and growth-controlling systems within the cell. In general, this sequence of events seems logical and largely explains most of the data which are now available. However, like most models of a biological system, there are several aspects of the system that are not explained by this sequence. There is compell-ing evidence to indicate that there may be alternative second messengers in addition to cAMP. One must also be concerned with the mechanism by which ACTH activates the adenylate cyclase enzyme. Currently there is insufficient evidence to indicate the exact relationship between these two molecules, al-though it is proposed that the binding site closely approximates, or may be in contact with, the enzyme complex. This hypothesis of the mechanism of action of ACTH on adrenal cells also fails to take into account the role various ions play in the regulation of adrenal cortical cell function. The roles of Ca^{2+}, Mg^{2+}, Na^+, K^+, or Cl^- are largely ignored in many reviews of the mechanism of action of ACTH; yet it is recognized that they are essential for hormone action and that alterations of these ionic concentrations within the cell can greatly influence enzymatic activities. Thus, a second messenger could logically involve the move-ment of ions across cell membranes to initiate intracellular processes.

In this section, the initial events in the process of ACTH stimulation of adrenal cortical cells are discussed. Some of the more recent data suggest that cAMP or other nucleotides may not be the only second messenger for ACTH action. Additional information has also become available concerning some of the biochemical steps after cAMP formation. Finally, some of the data which describe the role of ions in these processes and try to establish how they might influence ACTH action on the adrenal are considered.

First, there is a need to establish that ACTH is bound to the external surface of the cell membrane and that it need not actually enter the cell to exert its effect intracellularly. It is fairly well established that ACTH is bound to a specific membrane receptor, but it has largely been assumed that ACTH does not actually enter the cell. To our knowledge, there has been no convincing evidence to show that ACTH is actually present inside an adrenal cell. Several reports have shown that ACTH can stimulate steroidogenic activity of adrenal cortical cells without being able to actually enter the cell. In general, it was found that combinations of ACTH with large impermeable substances are compatible with retention of its potent steroidogenic activity, thereby suggesting that ACTH does not require entry into the cell to exert its effect.

It appears that ACTH need not enter the cell to exert its action on steroidogenesis; presumably this may also be the case for its tropic action. ACTH must then activate an adrenal cortical site on the outside of the adrenal membrane—a specific membrane receptor. There is considerable evidence for a specific binding site for ACTH on the adrenal cortical membrane based upon in vitro and in vivo studies. The binding of ACTH to these receptor sites has been related to the activation of adenylate cyclase enzyme. There are some indications, however, that there exists a heterogeneity of adrenal receptors for ACTH on the adrenal cell membrane. Data from several laboratories have suggested that there may be two populations of receptors for ACTH on the adrenal cortical cell membrane; one of the receptors for ACTH has a high affinity but relatively low capacity, whereas another has a relatively low affinity but 10 times the capacity (i.e., 10 times the number of sites per cell). Thus, a "spare receptor" is postulated for ACTH in these cells.

Once the ACTH has become attached to the adrenal cortical cell membrane, there must be some change in the membrane or structures associated with it to transmit information to the inside of the cell. Virtually nothing is known about the changes that occur at the membrane level which permit the information contained in the ACTH-receptor complex to activate intracellular processes. One possibility is that ACTH might cause a change in membrane permeability by altering membrane electrophysiological properties, much as neurotransmitters do on postsynaptic junctions, but this still does not elucidate the nature of the membrane changes. One approach to this problem has been to observe the effects of removal of sialic acid from the cell membrane by treating adrenal cortical cells with neuraminidase; sialic acid has been implicated in various cellular functions related to the cell membrane. Haksar et al. (186) have studied the effect of this membrane constituent on the relationship between ACTH stimulation and cAMP formation in isolated rat adrenal cortical cells and indicate that sialic acid of the membrane may be involved in the transmission of the information imparted to the cell by the ACTH molecule from the membrane-receptor complex to the intracellular activities regulated by the hormone.

CYCLIC AMP AND STEROIDOGENESIS

There is considerable evidence that one of the second messengers for the steroidogenic action of ACTH on adrenal cortical cells is by means of changes in cAMP levels. Haynes (187) was the first to show that ACTH increased cAMP concentrations in bovine adrenal cortex slices and that cAMP could mimic the steroidogenic action of ACTH in vitro. Since that time, many investigators have shown that cyclic AMP accumulation in adrenal tissue or incubation medium or both usually preceded the steroidogenic activity brought on after stimulation with ACTH. These and other reports have consistently shown a close correlation between ACTH-induced steroidogenic activity and cAMP. However, other evidence suggests that the cAMP second messenger is not the only substance that can stimulate steroidogenesis. Besides other cyclic nucleotides (such as GMP), there is the possibility that moieties such as inorganic ions or possibly even a prostaglandin could act as an intracellular mediator.

Many criteria must be met before one can conclude that cAMP is a second messenger for ACTH-induced steroidogenesis in the adrenal cortex. One particularly important criterion is that cAMP must be temporally related to steroidogenesis so that it appears in the cell prior to steroid synthesis and possibly before release. A second important criterion is whether steroidogenic activity can occur in the absence of detectable changes in the level of cAMP in the tissue. The first of the two criteria seems to be reasonably well resolved. The experiments related to the second now provide evidence that cAMP is not the unique second messenger in the adrenal cortex.

First, what are the early factors that are involved in the sequence of events leading to steroid formation in the adrenal cortex? Many in vivo and in vitro experiments have shown that the time lag between ACTH introduction to the tissue and steroid hormone release from the tissue takes approximately 3 min. If the response to the administered ACTH is normalized so that time zero is taken as the time when the applied pulse of ACTH reaches 50% of the final concentration, then there is an even quicker response to the peptide hormone.

Using various in vitro preparations of rat adrenal tissue, a number of investigators have reported significant increments in cAMP concentration in the tissue with 1—2 min after stimulation with ACTH. Similar findings have been reported by many other investigators. Richardson and Schulster (188) demonstrated that a similar temporal relationship exists for the cAMP-dependent protein kinase activity and ACTH-induced steroidogenesis.

Thus, the question of the necessary temporal sequence for ACTH, cAMP, and corticosteroid release has now been resolved satisfactorily: cAMP levels do rise prior to steroidogenesis. At least in this respect, cAMP does meet the criterion for a second messenger.

It is becoming increasingly clear that there are instances in which cAMP may not act as a second messenger for ACTH steroidogenic activity. There are a number of situations in which steroidogenesis can be stimulated, seemingly without involvement of cAMP. Kumar et al. (95) examined the steroidogenic- and cAMP-producing activities of two analogs of ACTH by using an isolated rat adrenal cortical cell preparation. In both cases, doses of peptides which could produce corticosteroid at a rate of 10% of the maximum did not produce detectable increments in cAMP. Greater doses of the peptides stimulated production of both cAMP and steroids. Nakamura et al. (189) observed similar results with the use of other analogs of ACTH. In their isolated cell incubations, they too could not detect cAMP increments with a dose of ACTH analog that produced a significant corticosteroid response, even after 1 hr of incubation. They could detect cAMP levels as low as 0.4 pmol and up to 50 pmol. Beall and Sayers (190) reported that ACTH, at a dose of 25 and 50 μU, in an incubation vial containing about 300,000 isolated rat adrenal cells, incubated for 60 min, produced steroid levels of from 50 to 75% of maximum, without significant elevations in cAMP. Only with a dose of 100 μU of ACTH (4 $\times$ the minimal dose for corticosteroid) were there significant increase in cAMP levels.

Similar to the reports of Kumar et al. (95) and Nakamura et al. (189), other investigators examined the activity of an analog of ACTH in which an o-nitrophenylsulfonyl group was attached to the indole group of the single tryptophan residue of the native peptide. Moyle et al. (191), using isolated rat adrenal cortical cells, showed that these cells responded to ACTH and this analog over a wide range of concentrations in terms of steroidogenic activity, but that the analog was much less active and, in combination with ACTH, was actually inhibitory. Of great interest was the finding that with very high doses of the analog it was possible to stimulate steroidogenesis up to maximal levels, but that it was not possible to raise cAMP levels with any dose of this analog much above the control levels. In some cases, both intracellular as well as total cAMP levels were measured at 5-, 8-, 15–16-min intervals after ACTH or the analog was introduced. Using an isolated rat adrenal cortical cell incubation procedure, Sharma and co-workers (192) and Shirma et al. (193) presented data which indicate that one cyclic nucleotide (GMP) may be involved in the mediation of ACTH activity at low levels of stimulation, whereas cAMP may act as the messenger signal for steroid output at higher doses of ACTH.

Peytremann et al. (194) observed the release of corticosterone and cAMP into the peripheral plasma of adult rats, and again the finding was that cAMP was first detected at a dose which produced a maximal level of corticosterone. Results from isolated calf adrenal cortical cells were reported by the same laboratory, and the conclusions were similar even when the incubation of the cells was stopped after 3 min of stimulation by ACTH (195). In fact, the literature includes many similar examples. These data indicate that, at least at the lower doses, cAMP may not play a role in the steroidogenic response. The obvious rebuttal is that there are changes in cAMP levels at all steroidogenic doses of ACTH, but that the increments in cAMP are too small and/or the cAMP is too labile at these levels to be detected.

There are other indications that cAMP may not be essential to mediate the ACTH steroidogenic response. Among these are the findings of Richardson and Schulster (188, 196), who showed that at low doses of ACTH there was a submaximal steroidogenic response, but without evidence of stimulation of cAMP-dependent protein kinase activity in isolated rat adrenal cortical cells. However, from the same laboratory there was a further observation that suggests that there may be an inability to detect sufficiently small cAMP increments. In the report by Mackie and Schulster (197), 1.0 mM theophylline (a phosphodiesterase inhibitor) was found to enhance the steroidogenic effect of ACTH but did not potentiate the effect on cAMP and protein synthesis in isolated rat adrenal cells. If theophylline enhanced the steroidogenic activity of ACTH in this system, why then were they not able to detect increased cAMP levels? Assuming that theophylline is acting through phosphodiesterase, then one possible explanation is that, indeed, they were unable to measure the physiologically significant levels of cAMP which were presumably responsible for the increased steroid production by the gland.

More convincing data arguing against cAMP as the necessary intermediate for steroidogenesis come from the studies of Rubin and co-workers (198–200). Using isolated cat adrenal glands perfused in situ with Locke's solution, they demonstrated that it was possible to dissociate cAMP content and steroid output and content of the adrenal tissue. The administration of ACTH elicited a significant increment in tissue cAMP content as well as in steroid output and content. However, if the tissue was perfused with a Ca^{2+}-free Locke's solution, then there was a highly significant increase in cAMP without significant steroid output or change in steroid content. The use of a K^+-free solution, again, resulted in an increase in cAMP content without increase in steroid secretion, but an increase in steroid concentration in the tissue was observed. Thus, not only was there a dissociation between steroid secretion from the tissue and the tissue cAMP concentration (which in the case of Ca^{2+}-free medium was 10 X that observed with a dose of ACTH), but there was also a dissociation between adrenal steroid content and steroid output, indicating that, in the case of the K^+-free medium, cAMP might have been involved in the synthesis of the steroid but not in the regulation of the secretory process. Therefore, an increase in cAMP alone is not necessarily sufficient to initiate the release of the corticosteroids; additional factors must also be involved. In a subsequent report from this same laboratory, experiments were described with the use of $[^3H]$ acetate as a precursor, which showed that the pattern of incorporation of the radioactive label into intermediates following K^+-deprivation was different from that observed after ACTH. More recent experiments by Tait et al. (201) demonstrated that K^+ concentrations above normal resulted in significant release of cortico-steroids from rat adrenal cortical tissue, but that at very high levels of K^+ (13 mM) there was a drop in steroid output despite continued high level of cAMP release from the tissue. They attributed most of this steroidogenic activity to the glomerulosa of the adrenal.

There is considerable evidence that one of the rate-limiting steps for the steroidogenic action of ACTH, or its mediator cAMP, is the conversion of cholesterol to (20S)-20-hydroxycholesterol. Sharma (202, 203) has shown that ACTH stimulated the synthesis of corticosterone from (20S)-20-hydroxy-cholesterol and that cycloheximide did not show inhibitory effects at this step. cAMP or db-cAMP did not stimulate activity of this rate-limiting step in isolated rat adrenal cortical cells. These findings led Sharma to propose that ACTH stimulates the synthesis or corticosterone by two different mechanisms. One mechanism involves cAMP mediation and is cycloheximide-sensitive; the second mechanism is independent of cAMP or cGMP and involves the rate-limiting steps of (20S)-20-hydroxycholesterol conversion to the corticosteroid.

TROPIC ACTION OF CYCLIC AMP
AND ADRENOCORTICOTROPIC HORMONE

There is considerable evidence that cAMP is at least one of the primary mediators of ACTH-induced steroidogenic action on the adrenal cortical zona fasciculata cells. However, there has been little definitive evidence to indicate that ACTH mediates its growth-promoting influence on this tissue through the same second messenger. Ney (204) has shown that cAMP can partially maintain the adrenal weight of hypophysectomized rats. However, Marton et al. (205) and Nussdorfer and Mazzocchi (206) showed that theophylline, a phosphodiesterase inhibitor, increased the ACTH corticosteroid response but did not influence its tropic action. More recently, Roos (207) has studied the effects of ACTH and cAMP on the steroidogenesis and growth of human adrenal cortical cells in monolayer culture over a 12-day period. He found that ACTH, but not cAMP, stimulated both steroidogenesis and growth of these cells.

The possibility that cAMP may be able to mimic some of the actions of ACTH on the growth of adrenal cells but is not an essential second messenger is also suggested by morphological studies on the ultrastructure of the cells. Nussdorfer and Mazzocchi (208) found that there were essentially no differences between groups in the morphology of adrenal cells from hypophysectomized rats given ACTH or cAMP. On the other hand, Milner (209) has shown that cAMP could elicit some but not all of the changes in the morphology of adrenal cortical cells in culture that were treated with ACTH. A possible explanation for the apparent contradiction in results reported by Nussdorfer's and Milner's laboratories may be the fact that entirely different systems were employed to test for the action of these compounds. Nussdorfer used an in vivo system, whereas Milner worked with an in vitro system. This difference is particularly important in light of the report of Kahri (210) and others who have shown that corticosterone can cause ultrastructural changes in tissue cultures of fetal rat adrenal cells. For example, high doses of corticosteroids inhibited ACTH-induced differentiation of the cortical cells. Since Milner used a static system, it is possible that some of the effects she observed were due to the release of corticosteroids into the incubation medium.

O'Hare and Neville (211) examined the effects of cAMP and ACTH on enzyme systems of rat adrenal cortical cells in monolayer culture. They found that both ACTH and cAMP, or db-cAMP, present for 4–5 days, could restore many of the adrenal enzyme systems involved in steroidogenesis to their original pattern of activity, similar to that found in the intact animal. Both ACTH and db-cAMP were shown to increase the ornithine decarboxylase enzyme activity in the adrenal cortex 4 hr after administration to hypophysectomized rats (212). Fuhrman and Gill (213) showed that 14 hr after administration both ACTH and cAMP produced significant increases in nuclear RNA polymerase in guinea pig adrenals.

As in the case of the steroidogenic action of ACTH, the tropic action of this hormone could, but may not necessarily, involve cAMP as a second messenger. It is important to recall the report of Richman et al. (212), who showed that the changes in cAMP in adrenal tissue, after ACTH stimulation, more closely followed the patterns of the steroid output than the long-term, tropic actions of this hormone. However, it is possible that the initial burst of cAMP activity may set into motion the long-term mechanisms involved in growth and development of this tissue. As with the steroidogenic action of ACTH, cAMP can mimic many of the actions of ACTH, but this in itself does not prove it is the second messenger.

There is increasing evidence that cyclic nucleotides other than cAMP may be involved in the tropic action of ACTH on adrenal cortical tissue. Nussdorfer and Mazzocchi (214) gave various cyclic nucleotides to hypophysectomized rats 5–10 days after surgery. After killing of the experimental animals, various morphological parameters were examined in the adrenal fasciculata cells. cAMP and, to a lesser extent, cGMP both reversed some of the effects of hypophysectomy, whereas cUMP-TMP-IMP or cCMP caused no significant changes. There were a number of qualitative as well as quantitative differences between the tropic action of cAMP and cGMP. Cyclic GMP did not induce structural changes in the adrenal mitochondria nor enhance uridine incorporation into adrenal mitochondria. Thus, unlike cAMP, cGMP may stimulate the adrenal cells primarily by altering nuclear RNA synthesis. These investigators showed that the combined regime of cAMP and cGMP completely restored many of the morphological characteristics that neither compound alone could bring about.

ROLE OF IONS IN ADRENOCORTICOTROPIC HORMONE ACTION

What roles do various ions play in the mechanism of action of ACTH? It has been pointed out that zinc ion plays a role in the binding of ACTH to the surface of the cell membrane (215). Another ion which has been implicated in adrenal cortical cellular activity is Ca^{2+}. That Ca^{2+} was required for steroidogenic action of ACTH on the adrenal cortex was first demonstrated by Birmingham et al. (216). Subsequent reports from these and other laboratories have clearly shown that Ca^{2+} is essential for ACTH-induced steroid release from adrenal cortical tissue.

A number of reports indicate that Ca^{2+} may be involved in the binding of ACTH to its membrane receptor site. More recently, Haksar and Peron (217) have reported that, at low doses of ACTH, EDTA caused some inhibition in binding to rat adrenal cells in suspension. However, at higher hormone concentrations this inhibition was not as evident. Therefore, inhibition of binding may not explain completely the failure of ACTH to initiate corticosterone synthesis in the presence of the Ca^{2+} chelator (EDTA).

The next point to be established was whether there was net transport of Ca^{2+} across the membrane of adrenal cortical cells when they were stimulated by ACTH. Leier and Jungman's data (218) indicate that there was net uptake of Ca^{2+} into adrenal cortical cells upon stimulation with ACTH, db-cAMP or theophylline. In vivo administration of ACTH to rats resulted in significant elevation of steroids and accumulation of labeled Ca^{2+} in the adrenal cells 90 min after the injection. When large doses of ACTH were applied to adrenal cortical cells in vitro, there was significant Ca^{2+} uptake within 3 min preceding the release of corticosterone. Additionally, there appeared to be a decreased Ca^{2+} uptake of the stimulated adrenal of hypophysectomized rats compared to normal rats. Of great interest is the finding that not only ACTH, but also db-cAMP, stimulated net accumulation of Ca^{2+} ion and that elipten, an inhibitor of cholesterol side chain cleavage, blocked the action of ACTH on Ca^{2+} accumulation in this tissue. Finally, these studies showed that Ca^{2+} uptake and steroidogenesis were abolished by treatment of the rats with cycloheximide, but not with actinomycin, indicating the need in both cases for de novo protein syntheses, but not for RNA synthesis. It must be remembered that movement of Ca^{2+} across the external limiting membrane is not the only means of changing internal Ca^{2+} concentrations within a given intracellular pool. There can also be a readjustment of Ca^{2+} within intracellular pools which might alter enzymatic machinery within the cells. Jaanus and Rubin (219) showed that the addition of ACTH to the isolated perfused cat adrenal cortex resulted in a small but significant increase in radiocalcium space and content, although the total Ca^{2+} content was not altered. These findings, and others, led these investigators to suggest that translation of Ca^{2+} occurs during stimulation of the adrenal cortex by ACTH and that the source is probably not the extracellular fluid but rather the Ca^{2+} that may be shifted by ACTH from a rapidly exchanging cellular pool to a more slowly exchanging cellular pool. In a more recent publication, Rubin et al. (220) presented data to suggest that Ca^{2+} inhibited cyclase activity. They proposed that cyclase activity is kept at low levels by the presence of calcium and that ACTH activates cyclase by displacing the Ca^{2+} fraction.

Translocation of this fraction to the interior of the cell, such as the endoplasmic reticulum or mitochondria, may be responsible for initiating steroid release.

What is the relationship of Ca^{2+} to cAMP activity? Does it stimulate cAMP or does it act at a later stage, beyond cAMP formation? There is evidence that Ca^{2+} works both before and after cAMP formation.

Some of the earlier reports indicated that activation of adenyl cyclase by ACTH required Ca^{2+}. However, other investigators have shown that a Ca^{2+}-free solution actually augmented adrenal cyclase activity. Recalling the reports of Haksar and Peron, as well as Lefkowitz: calcium in some circumstances may actually inhibit the binding of ACTH to its receptor sites, which might explain the decrease in adenylate cyclase activity reported by Carchman et al. (221). However, as Sayers et al. (222) point out, there is no convincing experimental evidence or theory that compels one to draw the conclusion that depression of binding is equated with a decrease in biological activity. Some of the discrepancies about the role of calcium in initiating or participating in some of the initial events of ACTH stimulation of adrenal cortical cells may be related to dose dependency, as shown by Haksar and Peron (217). In general, these investigators conclude that, at low concentrations of Ca^{2+}, this ion is necessary for ACTH enhancement of steroidogenesis in rat adrenal cell suspensions. However, the calcium requirement was decreased when higher concentrations of ACTH were employed. Additionally, they showed that there was no comparable change in the db-cAMP requirement for Ca^{2+} at the higher dose of the ion and, at all levels of db-cAMP tested, the Ca^{2+} requirement was about the same. These studies suggested that the events prior to the formation of cAMP were more dependent upon Ca^{2+} than upon the events which followed.

The dual role of Ca^{2+} in ACTH action on the adrenal cortical cell was also demonstrated by Bowyer and Kitabchi (223). At physiological concentrations, ACTH-stimulated steroidogenesis was proportional to Ca^{2+} concentration in a preparation of isolated rat adrenal cells. Much greater concentrations of ACTH were needed in the "absence" of Ca^{2+}. Maximal corticosteroid formation, in response to db-cAMP, was also dependent upon Ca^{2+} in the incubation medium. They also concluded that Ca^{2+} may act both before and after the elaboration of cAMP. Using a preparation of dispersed bovine adrenal cortical cells enriched with plasma membranes, Finn et al. (224) showed that the addition of Ca^{2+} (as little as 50 μM) caused inhibition of cAMP formation, and, at the same time, they also showed that the chelating agent EGTA inhibited ACTH-activated adenylate cyclase. Thus, in the same preparation, the presence or absence of Ca^{2+} can have the same effect. It is probable that some Ca^{2+} is necessary for cyclase activation, but where this Ca^{2+} exerts its effect and in what form it is active still remain to be elucidated. Obviously, this system is very responsive to changes in Ca^{2+} concentration within the cell. The fact that Ca^{2+} influenced ACTH-stimulated steroid output, but not cyclic AMP-induced steroid output, in mouse adrenal tumor cells indicates that Ca^{2+} is active (at least in this preparation) prior to cAMP formation. Finally, Birmingham and Bartova (225) have shown that an in vitro preparation of intact gland required Ca^{2+} for both the steroidogenic and glycolytic response to ACTH stimulation. In contrast, db-cAMP-stimulated steroidogenic and glycolytic response proceeded in calcium-free medium, suggesting that exogenous Ca^{2+} enhanced ACTH-stimulated synthesis of cAMP or prevented its destruction.

What sites beyond cyclic AMP might require Ca^{2+} for the steroidogenic action of ACTH? Farese (226) has reported data that suggest that Ca^{2+} may have direct effects on protein synthesis. It has also been demonstrated that Ca^{2+} is involved in the process of mitochondrial swelling, enhancement of pregnenolone synthesis, and the stimulation of 11-β-hydroxylation. Pfeiffer and Tchen (227) have shown that the reduction of extramitochondrial NADP by malic enzyme in intact mitochondria isolated from the bovine adrenal cortex was dependent upon the Ca^{2+} concentration. Although there are still many unresolved questions, it seems fairly certain that Ca^{2+} is involved in processes at a number of sites in the adrenal cortical cell.

Not only has Ca^{2+} been shown to influence the cellular action of ACTH on adrenal cortical cells, but other ions have been implicated to have an effect on this system. A high concentration of Mg^{2+} (20 mM) in the external medium was shown to partially inhibit ACTH-induced steroidogenic action (228), a finding that has been confirmed by Matthews and Saffran (229). Strontium can replace extracellular Ca^{2+}, thereby permitting normal responsiveness to ACTH in rabbit (229), rat (230), and cat (228) adrenal cortical cells. Lanthanum (La) has been shown to block membrane calcium fluxes (231) and at low concentrations of La in superfused rabbit adrenal cortical tissue the ACTH-evoked steroid output was almost completely blocked (229), further demonstration of calcium involvement in ACTH stimulation of adrenal tissue. Choline could replace Na^+ as an extracellular ion, and the steroidogenic action of ACTH would remain intact (229); however, LiCl could not replace NaCl. Using adrenal tissue homogenates (with, apparently, broken cell fragments), Halmi et al. (232) showed that there was a rise in basal adenylate cyclase activity with increasing concentrations of Mg^{2+} in the medium, whereas Li^+ (25 mM and 100 mM) depressed basal enzyme activity. It is not quite clear just how these data fit our overall view of the mechanism of ACTH action on the adrenal, but they indicate that ions other than Ca^{2+} may be important in ACTH-mediated action on the adenylate cyclase enzyme.

Jaanus et al. (233) used cat adrenal glands, perfused in situ, to investigate the effects of K^+ ions on corticosteroid secretion. Their data seemed to indicate that an increase in cAMP formation, as a result of removing K^+ from the superfusing medium, was associated with an increase in synthesis of steroid. Differences were observed in the steroidogenic response of these adrenals to ACTH and to K^+ removal, suggesting a different mechanism of action.

A number of investigators have initiated studies on the relationships between the electrophysiological properties and the function of adrenal cortical cells. It is reasoned that alterations in such characteristics as membrane resistance and potential may reflect alterations in membrane permeability to ions. Permeability alterations to specific ions could produce changes in intracellular concentrations of these ions which may result in alterations in adrenal cortical cellular activity. Thus, the use of the tools of the electrophysiologist can possibly provide insight into the cellular events which immediately follow hormonal stimulation.

EXTRAHYPOTHALAMIC REGULATION OF ADRENOCORTICOTROPIC HORMONE-TISSUE-CORTICOTROPIN-RELEASING FACTOR

The pituitary-adrenal system may be activated by hypothalamic median eminence CRF (ME-CRF) and also by extrahypothalamic mechanisms, one of which Brodish (234) has termed "tissue-CRF." Tissue-CRF has been distinguished from CRF of median eminence origin on the basis of its physical-chemical properties, its extreme potency, its prolonged action on the pituitary-adrenal system, and its existence even after the entire hypothalamus had been removed.

Recent reports by Lymangrover and Brodish (235, 236) clearly demonstrate a humoral factor in the peripheral blood of stressed rats which can activate the pituitary-adrenal axis, resulting in a massive and prolonged secretion of corticosterone. Because the substance appeared in animals with extensive ventral hypothalamic lesions that were also hypophysectomized 5 hr earlier, it seems unlikely that this potent pituitary-adrenal activation was evoked by ME-CRF or ACTH.

Nonhypothalamic CRF (tissue-CRF) seems to stimulate the pituitary-adrenal system in a sufficiently unique manner to suggest that it is not identical with hypothalamic ME-CRF. The term tissue-CRF is suggested to characterize the nonhypothalamic humoral substance that can directly stimulate the secretion of ACTH. There are a number of reasons why such terminology is suggested. This substance is probably not of hypothalamic origin; therefore, it is not unreasonable to assume that it is released from a more peripheral site in response to stress. The studies of Brodish and other investigators suggest that the types of stress that presumably activate an extrahypothalamic mechanism are extensive surgery (237), caval constriction (237–239), laparotomy, and prolonged cold exposure (240) and high altitude (241); all seem to possess, as a common factor, tissue anoxia or tissue destruction or both. Gordon (242) and Guillemin et al. (244) had earlier speculated that there may be substances present in all tissues which could directly activate the pituitary adrenal axis. Reports have also appeared to show that substances extracted from a variety of peripheral tissues can directly stimulate the pituitary-adrenal axis (168, 243, 244). It is postulated that intense and prolonged stress, which results in tissue change, may evoke the release of tissue-CRF to supplement the rapid ME-CRF mechanism and thereby produce a prolonged and massive output of adrenal cortical steroids in time of need.

What is the possible physiological role of tissue-CRF? Transient secretion of ACTH, presumably by hypothalamic activation, may be an appropriate response to acute stress. The subsequent feedback suppression of the hypothalamic-pituitary system by the secreted hormones may be a means of preventing overstimulation and excessive secretion of the system.

In cases of severe trauma associated with extensive tissue damage, hypothalamic-pituitary suppression by the secreted hormones may be premature and inappropriate. Therefore, a mechanism may exist whereby the affected tissues themselves may sustain adrenocortical activation by releasing tissue-CRF as a signal to the pituitary for continued need. Tissue-CRF release would represent a valuable mechanism for damaged tissues to sustain the signals for the hormones or metabolites that are needed. When the tissue damage has been repaired or stabilized, then tissue-CRF release would cease.

One can further speculate that the mechanism of suppression by corticosterone on tissue-CRF secretion is similar to the membrane stabilization theory proposed by Weissman and Thomas (245). If tissue-CRF is a common factor which is found in all tissues and is released as a result of tissue destruction, then the suppression could be mediated through corticosterone acting at the cell membrane and lysosome level to stabilize the cellular lysosomes and prevent the release of enzymes that could disrupt the cell and release tissue-CRF. Further clarification must await purification of tissue-CRF and studies of its secretory process.

The significance of this new finding is that it suggests that tissue-CRF is under physiological regulation and thus may play a role in an animal's ability to adapt to its environment. What previously appeared to be a possible artifact of the lesioned animal preparation now appears to be related to a possible fundamental mechanism for the control of ACTH secretion. Normally, a transient response to stress is observed which if sufficient may be terminated by neural adaptive mechanisms that prevent over-stimulation and over-secretion of the pituitary-adrenal system. During continued stress of relatively high intensity, the needs of the organism may not be met by the hypothalamic mechanism and another system (tissue-CRF) may be brought into play to sustain pituitary adrenal secretions. Obviously, these studies require confirmation because of their significance in our comprehension of pituitary-adrenal regulation. The conclusion is inescapable that CRFs are produced at sites other than the central nervous system.

REFERENCES

1. Bernard, C. (1957). Introduction to the Study of Experimental Medicine, pp. 89. Dover Publications, Inc., New York.
2. Mangili, G., Motta, M., and Martini, L. (1967). Control of adrenocorticotropic hormone secretion. *In* Martini, L. and Ganong, W.F. (eds.), Neuroendocrinology, Vol. I, p. 297. Academic Press, New York.
3. McEwen, B. S., Weiss, J. M., and Schwartz, L. S. (1970). Retention of corticosterone by cell nuclei from brain regions of adrenalectomized rats. Brain Res. 17:471.

4. Guillemin, R., and Rosenberg, B. (1955). Humoral hypothalamic control of anterior pituitary. Endocrinology 57:599.
5. Krieger, D. T. (1973). *In* D. T. Krieger (ed.), Neurotransmitter Regulation of ACTH Release, Peptide Hormone Assay and Action. Intercontinental Medical Book Corporation, New York.
6. Saffran, M., and Schally, A. V. (1955). The release of corticotrophin by anterior pituitary tissue *in vitro*. Can. J. Biochem. 33:408.
7. Chan, L. T., Schall, S. M., and Saffran, M. (1970). The rat median eminence as a source of CRF. *In* Meites, J. (ed.), Hypophysiotropic Hormones of the Hypothalamus, p. 253. Williams & Wilkins, Co., Baltimore.
8. Hedge, G. A., and Hanson, S. D. (1972). The effects of prostaglandins on ACTH secretion. Endocrinology 91:925.
9. Coudert, S. P., and Faiman, C. (1973). Effect of prostaglandin F on anterior pituitary function in man. Prostaglandins 3(1):89.
10. Holmes, S. W., and Horton, E. W. (1967). The nature and distribution of prostaglandins in the central nervous system of the dog. J. Physiol. (Lond.) 191:134P.
11. Hinman, J. W. (1967). The prostaglandins. Bioscience 17:779.
12. Sobel, H., Levy, R. S., Marmorston, J., Schapiro, S., and Rosenfeld, S. (1955). Increased excretion of urinary corticoids by guinea pigs following administration of Pitressin. Proc. Soc. Exp. Bio. Med. 89:10.
13. Martini, L., and Morpurgo, C. (1955). Neurohumoral control of the release of ACTH. Nature 175:1127.
14. McCann, S. M. (1957). The ACTH-releasing activity of extracts of the posterior lobe of the pituitary *in vivo*. Endocrinology 60:664.
15. Guillemin, R., Hearn, W. R., Cheek, W. R., and Householder, D. F. (1957). Control of ACTH release: further studies with *in vitro* methods. Endocrinology 60:488.
16. Schally, A. V., and Bowers, C. Y. (1964). Corticotropin-releasing factor and other hypothalamic peptides. Metabolism 13:1190.
17. Schally, A. V., Anderson, R. N., Lipscomb, H. S., Long, J. M., and Guillemin, R. (1960). Evidence for the existence of two corticotropin-releasing factors. Nature 188:1192.
18. McDonald, R. K., Wagner, E. N., Weise, V. K. (1957). Relationship between endogenous ADH hormone activity and ACTH release in man. Proc. Soc. Exp. Biol. Med. 96:652.
19. Royce, P. D., and Sayers, G. (1958). Corticotropin releasing activity of a pepsin labile factor in the hypothalamus. Proc. Soc. Exp. Biol. Med. 98:677.
20. Andersson, K. E., Arner, B., Hedner, P., and Mulder, J. L. (1972). Effects of lysine-vasopressin and synthetic analogues on release of ACTH. Acta Endocrinol. 69:640.
21. Saffran, M., Pearlmutter, A. F., Rapino, E., and Upton, G. V. (1972). Pressinoic Acid: A peptide with corticotrophin-releasing activity. Biochem. Biophys. Res. Commun. 49(3):748.
22. Hiroshige, T. (1973). Attempts to physiologically validate the circadian rhythm of corticotropin-releasing activity in the rat hypothalamus. Fourth International Meeting of the International Society for Neurochemistry, Tokyo, Japan, p. 147, Abstr. No. R-6-6.
23. Portanova, R., and Sayers, G. (1973). An *in vitro* assay for CRF using suspensions of isolated pituitary cells. Neuroendocrinology 12:236.

24. Portanova, R., and Sayers, G. (1973). Isolated pituitary cells: CRF-like activity of neurohypophysial and related peptides. Proc. Exp. Biol. Med. 143:661.
25. Arimura, A., Schally, A. V., and Bowers, C. Y. (1969). Corticotropin-releasing activity of lysine vasopressin analogues. Endocrinology 84:579.
26. Chan, L. J., deWied, D., and Saffran, M. (1969). Comparison of assays for CRF. Endocrinology 84:967.
27. Miller, R. E., Yueh-Chien, H., Wiley, M., and Hewitt, R. (1974). Anterior hypophyseal function in the posterior-hypophysectomized rat: normal regulation of the adrenal system. Neuroendocrinology 14:233.
28. Pearlmutter, A. F., Rapino, E., and Saffran, M. (1975). The ACTH-releasing hormone of the hypothalamus requires a co-factor. Endocrinology 97:1336.
29. LaBella, F., Dular, R., Vivian, S., and Queen, G. (1973). Pituitary hormone releasing or inhibiting activity of metal ions present in hypothalamic extracts. Biochem. Biophys. Res. Commun. 52(3):786.
30. Bertolini, A., Gentile, G., Greggia, A., Sternieri, E., and Ferrari, W. (1971). Possible role of hypothalamic CRF in the induction of sexual excitation in adult male rats. Riv. Farmacol. Ter. 11:243.
31. Douglas, W. W., and Poisner, A. M. (1964). Stimulus-secretion coupling in a neurosecretory organ: the role of calcium in the release of vasopressin from the neurohypophysis. J. Physiol. (Lond.) 172:1.
32. York, D. H., Baker, F. L., and Kraicer, J. (1973). Electrical changes induced in rat adenohypophysial cells, *in vivo,* with hypothalamic extract. Neuroendocrinology 11:212.
33. Martin, D., York, D. H., and Kraicer, J. (1973). Alterations in transmembrane potential of adenohypophysial cells in elevated potassium and calcium free media. Endocrinology 92:1084.
34. Milligan, J. V., and Kraicer, J. (1971). Ca^{++} uptake during *in vitro* release of hormones from the rat adenohypophysis. Endocrinology 89:766.
35. Milligan, J. V., and Kraicer, J. (1974). Physical characteristics of the Ca^{++} compartments associated with *in vitro* ACTH release. Endocrinology 94:435.
36. Portanova, R., and Sayers, G. (1973). An *in vitro* assay for corticotropin releasing factor(s) using suspensions of isolated pituitary cells. Neuroendocrinology 12:236.
37. Fleischer, N., Zimmerman, G., Schindler, W., and Hutchins, M. (1972). Stimulation of ACTH and GH release by ouabain: relationship to calcium. Endocrinology 91:1436.
38. Eto, S., Wood, J. M., Hutchins, M., and Fleischer, N. (1974). Pituitary $^{45}Ca^{++}$ uptake and release of ACTH, GH and TSH: effect of verapamil. Am. J. Physiol. 226:1315.
39. Milligan, J. V., Kraicer, J., Fawcett, C. P., and Illner, P. (1972). Purified GH-RF increase of Ca^{++} uptake into pituitary cells. Can. J. Physiol. Pharmacol. 50:613.
40. Portanova, R. (1972). Release of ACTH from isolated pituitary cells: an energy dependent process. Proc. Soc. Exp. Biol. Med. 140:825.
41. Zor, U., Kaneko, T., and Schneider, H. P. G. (1969). Stimulation of anterior pituitary adenylcyclase activity and adenosine 35-cyclic phosphate by hypothalamic extract and prostaglandin E. Proc. Natl. Acad. Sci. U. S. A. 63:918.

42. Steiner, A. L., Peake, G. T., and Utiger, R. D. (1970). Hypothalamic stimulation of growth hormone and thyrotropin *in vitro* and pituitary 3,5-adenosine cyclic monophosphate. Endocrinology 86:1354.
43. Zor, U., Kaneko, T., and Schneider, H. P. G. (1970). Further studies of stimulation of anterior pituitary C-3,5-AMP formation by hypothalamic extract and prostaglandin. J. Biol. Chem. 245:2883.
44. Fleischer, N., Donald, R. A., and Butcher, R. W. (1969). Involvement of adenosine 3,5-monophosphate in release of ACTH. Am. J. Physiol. 217:1287.
45. Kuo, J. F., and Greengard, P. (1969). Cyclic nucleotide dependent protein kinases. IV. Widespread occurrence of CAMP dependent protein kinase in various tissues and phyla of the animal kingdom. Proc. Natl. Acad. Sci. U. S. A. 64:1349.
46. Labrie, F., Lemaire, S., and Courte, C. (1971). CAMP dependent protein kinase from bovine anterior pituitary gland. I. Properties. J. Biol. Chem. 246:7293.
47. Zor, U., Chayoth, R., Kaneko, T., Schneider, H., McCann, S., and Field, J. B. (1974). Effects of hormone treatment with age on the stimulation of rat anterior pituitary adenylate cyclase and CAMP by hypothalamic extract. Metabolism 23:549.
48. Pelletier, G., Lemay, A., Beraud, G., and Labrie, F. (1972). Ultrastructural changes accompanying the stimulatory effect of N^6-monobutyryl adenosine 3,5-monophosphate on the release of GH, PRL, and ACTH in rat anterior pituitary gland *in vitro*. Endocrinology 91:1355.
49. Baker, B. L., and Drummond, T. (1972). The cellular origins of corticotropin and melanotropin as revealed by immunochemical staining. Am. J. Anat. 134:395.
50. Kraicer, J., Gosbee, J. L., and Bencosme, S. A. (1973). Pars intermedia and pars distalis: Two sites of ACTH production in the rat hypophysis. Neuroendocrinology 11:156.
51 Greer, M. A., Allen, C. F., Panton, P., and Allen, J. P. (1975). Evidence that the pars intermedia and pars nervosa of the pituitary do not secrete functionally significant quantities of ACTH. Endocrinology 96:718.
52. Mialhe-Voloss, C. (1958). Posthypophyse et activite corticotrope. Acta Endocrinol. (Kbh.) 35:1.
53. Rochefort, G. J., Rosenberger, J., and Saffran, M. (1959). Depletion of pituitary corticotrophin by various stresses and by neurohypophysial preparations. J. Physiol. (Lond.) 146:105.
54. Stoeckel, M. E., Dellmann, H. D., Porte, A., Klein, J. J., and Stutinsky, F. (1973). Corticotrophic cells in the rostral zone of the pars intermedia and in the adjacent neurohypophysis of the rat and mouse. Z. Zellforsch. 136:97.
55. Saffran, M., Pearlmutter, A. F., and Rapino, E. (1973). *In vitro* assays of corticotropin-releasing factors. *In* Brodish, A., and Redgate, E. D. (eds.), Brain-Pituitary-Adrenal Interrelationships, p. 47. Karger Publishing, Basel.
56. Fortier, C., and de Groot, J. (1959). Adenohypophysial corticotrophin and plasma free cortico steroids during regeneration of the enucleated rat adrenal gland. Am. J. Physiol. 196:589.
57. Farquhar, M. G. (1957). Corticotrophs of the rat adenohypophysis as revealed by electron microscopy. Anat. Rec. 127:291.
58. Moriarty, G. C., and Halmi, N. S. (1972). Electron microscopic study of the adrenocorticotropin-producing cell with the use of unlabeled anti-

body and the soluble peroxidase-anti-peroxidase complex. J. Histochem. Cytochem. 20:590.

59. Nakane, P. K. (1970). Classification of anterior pituitary cell types with immunoenzyme histochemistry. J. Histochem. Cytochem. 18:9.

60. Cameron, E., and Foster, C. L. (1972). Ultrastructural changes in the adenohypophysis of metyrapone-treated rabbits. J. Endocrinol. 52:343.

61. Ishikawa, H., Ohtsuka, Y., Soyama, F., and Yoshimura, F. (1972). Separation of the two different sizes of storage granules with GH and ACTH activity from the pellets of acidophils isolated from rat anterior pituitaries. Endocrinol. Jap. 19(3):215.

62. Yoshimura, F., Soji, T., Takasaki, Y., and Kiguchi, Y. (1974). Pituitary acidophils with small or medium-sized granules alone in normal and adrenalectomized rats with special reference to possible ACTH secretion. Endocrinol. Jap. 21(4):297.

63. Sipperstein, E. R., and Miller, K. J. (1970). Further cytophysiologic evidence for the identity of the cells that produce adrenocorticotrophic hormone. Endocrinology 86:451.

64. Kurosumi, K., and Kobayashi, Y. (1966). Corticotrophs in the anterior pituitary glands of normal and adrenalectomized rats as revealed by electron microscopy. Endocrinology 78:745.

65. Abe, K., Nicholson, W. E., Liddle, G. W., Orth, D. N., and Island, D. P. (1969) Normal and abnormal regulation of B-MSH in man. J. Clin. Invest. 48:1580.

66. Donald, R. A., and Toth, A. (1973). A comparison of the B-melanocyte-stimulating hormone and corticotropin response to hypoglycemia. J. Clin. Endocrinal. Metab. 36:925.

67. Kastin, A. J., Beach, G. D., Hawley, W. D., Kendall, J. W., Edwards, M. S., and Schally, A. V. (1973). Dissociation of MSH and ACTH release in man. J. Clin. Endocrinol. Metab. 36:770.

68. Phifer, R. F., Spicer, S. S., and Orth, D. M. (1970). Specific demonstration of the human hypophyseal cells which produce adrenocorticotropic hormone. J. Clin. Endocrinol. Metab. 31:346.

69. Phifer, R. F., Orth, D. N., and Spicer, S. S. (1974). Specific demonstration of the human hypophyseal adrenocortico-melanotropic (ACTH/MSH) cell. J. Clin. Endocrinol. Metab. 39:684.

70. Yalow, R. S., and Berson, S. A. (1971). Size heterogeneity of immunoreactive human ACTH in plasma and in extracts of pituitary glands and ACTH-producing thymoma. Biochem. Biophys. Res. Commun. 44:439.

71. Yalow, R. S., and Berson, S. A. (1973). Characteristics of "big-ACTH" in human plasma and pituitary extracts. J. Clin. Endocrinol. Metab. 36(3):415.

72. Krieger, D. T. (1974). Glandular end organ deficiency associated with secretion of biologically inactive pituitary peptides. J. Clin. Endocrinol. Metab. 38:964.

73. Gewirtz, G., Schneider, B., Krieger, D., and Yalow, R. S. (1974). Big ACTH: Conversion to biologically active ACTH by trypsin. J. Clin. Endocrinol. Metab. 38:227.

74. Orth, D. N., Nicholson, W. E., Mitchell, W. M., Island, D. P., Shapiro, M., and Byyny, R. L. (1973). ACTH and MSH production by a single cloned mouse pituitary tumor cell line. Endocrinology 92:385.

75. Lang, R. E., Fehm, H. L., Voigt, K. H., and Pfeiffer, E. F. (1973). Two ACTH species in rat pituitary gland. FEBS Lett. 37(2):197.

76. Scott, A. P., Ratcliffe, J. G., Ress, L. H., Landon, J., Bennett, H. P. J., Lowry, P. J., and McMartin, C. (1973). Pituitary peptide. Nature (New Biol.) 244(133):65.

77. Genazzani, A. R., Rvedi, B., Aubert, M. L., and Felber, J. P. (1972). Pituitary response to hypoglycemia in pituitary disease. Horm. Metab. Res. 4:470.

78. Genazzani, A. R., Fraioli, F., Hurlimann, J., Felber, J. P., and Fioretti, P. (1973). Detection and partial purification of a ACTH-like placental hormone: the human chorionic corticotrophin (HCC). Acta. Endocrinol. (Kbh) 177:240.

79. Genazzani, A. R., Fraioli, F., Hurlimann, J., Fioretti, P., and Felber, J. P. (1975). Immunoreactive ACTH and cortisol plasma levels during pregnancy: detection and partial purification of corticotrophin-like placental hormone: the human chorionic corticotrophin (HCC). Clin. Endocrinol. 4:1.

80. Pearlmutter, A. F., Rapino, E., and Saffran, M. (1974). A semi-automated in vitro assay for CRF: activities of peptides related to oxytocin and vasopressin. Neuroendocrinology 15:106.

81. Kleerekoper, M., Donald, R. A., and Posen, S. (1972). Corticotrophin in cerebrospinal fluid of patients with Nelson's syndrome. Lancet 1:74.

82. Allen, J. P., Kendall, J. W., McGilvra, R., and Vancura, C. (1974). Immunoreactive ACTH in cerebrospinal fluid. J. Clin. Endocrinol. Metab. 38:586.

83. Kass, E. H., Hechter, O., Macchi, I. A., and Mou, T. W. (1954). Changes in patterns of secretion of corticosteroids in rabbits after prolonged treatment with ACTH. Proc. Soc. Exp. Biol. Med. 85:583.

84. Slaga, T. J., and Krum, A. A. (1973). Modification of rabbit steroid biosynthesis by prolonged ACTH administration. Endocrinology 93:517.

85. Drummond, H. B., and Fevold, H. R. (1972). The effect of a rabbit ACTH preparation on adrenal steroid biosynthesis. Biochem. Biophys. Res. Commun. 46:605.

86. Coslovsky, R., and Yalow, R. S. (1974). Influence of the hormonal forms of ACTH on the pattern of corticosteroid secretion. Biochem. Biophys. Res. Commun. 60(4):1351.

87. Nakamura, M. (1972). Studies on the role of basic amino acid residues of ACTH peptide in steroidogenesis by isolated adrenal cells. J. Biochem. 71:1029.

88. Seelig, S., and Sayers, G. (1973). Isolated adrenal cortex cells: ACTH agonists, partial agonists, antagonists, cyclic AMP, and corticosterone production. Arch. Biochem. Biophys. 154:230.

89. Seelig, S., Kumar, S., and Sayers, G. (1972). Isolated adrenal cells: the partial agonists $(Trp(Nps)^9)ACTH^{1-39}$ and $(Trp(Nps)^9)ACTH^{1-24}$ (nitrophenylsulfonyl derivatives of ACTH), Proc. Soc. Exp. Biol. Med. 139:1217.

90. Geiger, R., and Schroder, H. G. (1973). Synthetische analoga des corticotropins. Z. Physiol. Chem. 354:156.

91. Blade, J., and Li, C. H. (1972). The synthesis and steroidogenic activity of (2-N-methylphenyl)alanine. Int. J. Peptide Protein Res. 4:343.

92. Hajós, G. T., Szparny, L., Karpati, E., and Fekete, G. (1972). Studies of the potency of polypeptides with ACTH action by a new method based on continuous measurement of plasma corticosterone. Steroids Lipid Res. 3:225.

93. Graf, L., Hajos, G., Patthy, A., and Cseh, G. (1973). The influence of deamidation on the biological activity of porcine ACTH. Horm. Metab. Res. 5:142.
94. Bennett, H. P. J., Bullock, G., Lowry, P. J., McMartin, C., and Peters, J. (1974). Fate of corticotrophins in an isolated adrenal-cell bioassay and decrease of peptide breakdown by cell purification. Biochem. J. 138: 185.
95. Kumar, S., Seelig, S., and Sayers, G. (1972). Isolated adrenal cortex cells: [Trp (Dmps)^9] ACTH 5-24, an inhibitor of ACTH 1-24-induced cyclic AMP and corticosterone production. Biochem. Biophys. Res. Commun. 49(5):1316.
96. Hoffman, K., Montibelle, J. A., and Finn, F. M. (1974). ACTH antagonists. Proc. Natl. Acad. Sci. 71(1):80.
97. Yalow, R. S., Glick, S. M., Roth, J., and Berson, S. A. (1964). Radioimmunoassay of human plasma ACTH. J. Clin. Endocrinol. Metab. 24:1219.
98. Erlanger, B. F., Borek, F., Beiser, S. M., and Lieberman, S. (1957). Steroid protein conjugates. I. Preparation and characterization of conjugates of bovine serum albumin with testosterone and with cortisone. J. Biol. Chem. 228:713.
99. Hellman, L., Nakada, F., Curti, J., Weitzman, E. D., Kream, J., Roffwarg, H., Ellman, S., Fukushima, D. K., and Gallagher, T. F. (1970). Cortisol is secreted episodically by normal man. J. Clin. Endocrinol. Metab. 30:411.
100. Weitzman, E. D., Fukushima, D., Nogeire, C., Roffwarg, H., Gallagher, T. F., and Hellman, L. (1971). Twenty-four hour pattern of the episodic secretion of cortisol in normal subjects. J. Clin. Endocrinol. Metab. 33:14.
101. Berson, S. A., and Yalow, R. S. (1968). Radioimmunoassay of ACTH in plasma. J. Clin. Invest. 47:2725.
102. Graber, A. L., Givens, J. R., Nicholson, W. E., Island, D. P., and Liddle, G. W. (1965). Persistence of diurnal rhythmicity in plasma ACTH concentrations in cortisol-deficient patients. J. Clin. Endocrinol. Metab. 25:804.
103. Besser, G. M., Cullen, D. R., and Irvine, W. J. (1970). Immunoreactive ACTH levels in adrenocortical insufficiency. Biol. Med. J. 1:374.
104. Smelik, P. G. (1970). Adrenocortical feedback control of pituitary-adrenal activity. Prog. Brain Res. 32:20.
105. Kendall, J. W., Jacobs, J. J., and Kramer, R. M. (1972). Studies on the transport from the cerebrospinal fluid to hypothalamus and pituitary. Brain-Endocrine Interaction: median eminence structure and function, p. 342. International Symposium, Munich, 1971. Karger Publishing Company, Basal.
106. Jubiz, W., Matsukura, S., Meikle, A. W., Harada, G., West, C. D., and Tyler, F. H. (1970). Plasma metyrapone, ACTH, cortisol, and deoxycortisol levels. Arch. Intern. Med. 125:468.
107. Krieger, D. T. (1970). Factors influencing the circadian periodicity of adrenal steroid levels. Trans. N. Y. Acad. Sci. 32:316.
108. Krieger, D. T., Allen, W., Rizzo, F., and Krieger, H. P. (1971). Characterization of the normal temporal pattern of plasma corticosteroid levels. J. Clin. Endocrinol. 32:266.
109. Proeschel, M. F., Courvalin, J. C., Donnadien, M., and Girard, F. (1974). Preparation and evaluation of ACTH antibodies. Acta Endocrinol. 75:461.

110. Vaitukaitis, J., Robbins, J. B., Nieschlag, E., and Ross, G. T. (1971). A method for producing specific antisera with small doses of immunogen. J. Clin. Endocrinol. Metab. 33:988.
111. Rose, J. C., and Newsome, H. H., Jr. (1972). The rapid production of antisera to ACTH, angiotensin II and deoxycorticosterone with sufficient sensitivity for use in radioimmunoassays. J. Clin. Endocrinol. Metab. 35:469.
112. Newsome, H. H., and Rose, J. C. (1971). The response of human adreno-corticotrophic hormone and growth hormone to surgical stress. J. Clin. Endocrinol. Metab. 33:481.
113. Orth, D. N., Island, D. P., Nicholson, W. E., Abe, K., Woodham, J. P. (1968). In R. L. Hayes, R. A. Groswitz, and B. E. P. Murphy (eds.), Radioisotopes in Medicine: In Vitro Studies, p. 251. U.S. Atomic Energy Commission, Oak Ridge.
114. Matsuyama, H., Harada, G., Ruhmann-Wennhold, A. (1972). A comparison between bioassay and radioimmunoassay for plasma ACTH in man. J. Clin. Endocrinol. Metab. 34:713.
115. Matsuyama, H., Ruhmann-Wennhold, A., Johnson, L. R., and Nelson, D. H. (1972). Disappearance rates of exogenous and endogenous ACTH from rat plasma measured by bioassay and radioimmunoassay. Metabolism 21:30.
116. Fehm, H. L., Voigt, K. H., and Pfeiffer, E. F. (1972). Problems and artifacts in ACTH assay. Horm. Metab. Res. 4:477.
117. Voight, K. H., Fehm, H. L., and Pfeiffer, E. F. (1971). Evidence for an "ACTH binding factor" in plasma. Horm. Metab. Res. 3:227.
118. Besser, G. M., Orth, D. N., Nicholson, W. E., Byyny, R. L., Abe, K., and Woodham, J. P. (1971). Dissociation of the disappearance of bioactive and radioimmunoactive ACTH from plasma in man. J. Clin. Endocrinol. Metab. 32:595.
119. Matsuyama, H., Mims, R. B., Ruhmann-Wennhold, A., and Nelson, D. H. (1971). Bioassay and radioimmunoassay of plasma ACTH in adrenalectomized rats. Endocrinology 88:696.
120. Matsuyama, H., Ruhmann-Wennhold, A., and Nelson, D. H. (1971). Radioimmunoassay of plasma ACTH in intact rats. Endocrinology 88:692.
121. Lefkowitz, R. J., and Roth, J. (1970). Radioreceptor assay of adrenocorticotropic hormone: new approach to assay of polypeptide hormones in plasma. Science 170:633.
122. Wolfsen, A. R., McIntyre, H. B., and Odell, W. D. (1972). Adrenocorticotropin measurement by competitive binding receptor assay. J. Clin. Endocrinol. 34:684.
123. Hofmann, K., Wingender, W., and Finn, F. M. (1970). Correlation of adrenocorticotropic activity of ACTH analogs with degree of binding to an adrenal cortical particulate preparation. Proc. Natl. Acad. Sci. U. S. A. 67:829.
124. Nicholson, W. E., and Van Loon, G. R. (1973). Some practical innovations in the biological assay of adrenocorticotropic hormone (ACTH). J. Lab. Clin. Med. 81:803.
125. Guillemin, R., Clayton, G. W., Lipscomb, H. S., and Smith, J. D. (1959). Fluorometric measurement of rat plasma and adrenal corticosterone concentration. J. Lab. Clin. Med. 58:830.
126. Mattingly, D. (1962). A simple fluorometric method for the estimation of free 11-hydroxycorticoids in human plasma. J. Clin. Pathol. 15:374.

127. Lipscomb, H. S., and Nelson, D. H. (1962). A sensitive biological assay for ACTH. Endocrinology 71:13.
128. Chayen, J., Loveridge, N., and Daly, J. R. (1972). A sensitive bioassay for adrenocorticotrophic hormone in human plasma. Clin. Endocrinol. 1: 219.
129. Chayen, J., Loveridge, N., and Daly, J. R. (1971). The measurable effect of low concentrations (pg/ml) of ACTH on reducing groups of adrenal cortex maintained in organ culture. Clin. Sci. 41:2P.
130. Daly, J. R., Loveridge, N., Bitensky, L., and Chayen, J. (1972). Early experience with a highly sensitive bioassay for ACTH. Ann. Clin. Biochem. 9:81.
131. Alaghband-Zadek, J., Daly, J. R., Bitensky, L., and Chayen, J. (1974). The cytochemical section assay for corticotrophin. Clin. Endocrinol. 3:319.
132. Chayen, J., Bitensky, L., Chambers, D. J., Loveridge, N., and Daly, J. R. (1974). Studies on the mechanism of cytochemical bioassays. Clin. Endocrinol. 3:349.
133. Holdaway, I. M., Rees, L. H., Ratcliffe, J. G., Besser, G. M., and Kramer, R. M. (1974). Validation of the redox cytochemical assay for corticotrophin. Clin. Endocrinol. 3:329.
134. Rodbell, M. (1964). Metabolism of isolated fat cells. I. Effects of hormones on glucose metabolism and lipolysis. Biol. Chem. 239:375.
135. Kloppenborg, P. W. C., Island, D. P., Liddle, G. W., Michelakis, A. M., and Nicholson, W. E. (1968). A method of preparing adrenal cell suspensions and its applicability to the "in vitro" study of adrenal metabolism. Endocrinology 82:1053.
136. Haning, R., Tait, S. A. S., and Tait, J. F. (1970). "In vitro" effects of ACTH, angiotensins, serotonin and potassium on steroid output and conversion of corticosterone to aldosterone by isolated adrenal cells. Endocrinology 87:1147.
137. Halkerston, I. D. K., and Feinstein, M. (1968). Preparation of ACTH responsive isolated cells from rat adrenal. Fed. Proc. 27:626.
138. Swallow, R. L., and Sayers, G. (1969). A technic for the preparation of isolated rat adrenal cells. Proc. Soc. Exp. Biol. 131:1.
139. Sayers, G., Swallow, R. L., and Giordano, N. D. (1971). An improved technique for the preparation of isolated rat adrenal cells: a sensitive, accurate and specific method for the assay of ACTH. Endocrinology 88:1063.
140. Portanova, R., Smith, D. K., and Sayers, G. (1970). A trypsin technique for the preparation of isolated rat anterior pituitary cells. Proc. Soc. Exp. Biol. Med. 133:573.
141. Barofsky, A. L., Feinstein, M., and Halkerston, I. D. K. (1973). Enzymatic and mechanical requirements for the dissociation of cortical cells from rat adrenal glands. Exp. Cell. Res. 79:263.
142. Rodbell, M. (1966). The metabolism of isolated fat cells. IV. Regulation of release of protein by lipolytic hormones and insulin. J. Biol. Chem. 241:3909.
143. Kono, T. (1969). Destruction of insulin effector system of adipose tissue cells by proteolytic enzymes. J. Biol. Chem. 244:1772.
144. Nakamura, N., and Tanaka, A. (1971). A simple method for the preparation of ACTH responsive isolated cells from rat adrenals. Endocrinol. Jpn. 18:291.

145. Saffran, M., and Schally, A. V. (1955). *In vitro* bioassay of corticotropin: modification and statistical treatment. Endocrinology 56:523.
146. Lowry, P. J., McMartin, C., and Peters, J. (1973). Properties of a simplified bioassay for adrenocorticotrophic activity using the steroidogenic response of isolated adrenal cells. J. Endocrinol. 59:43.
147. Sayers, G., Ma, R. M., and Giordano, N. D. (1971). Isolated adrenal cells: corticosterone production in response to cyclic adenosine-3′,5′-monophosphate. Proc. Soc. Exp. Biol. Med. 136:619.
148. Kitabchi, A. E., and Sharma, R. K. (1971). Corticosteroidogenesis in isolated adrenal cells of rats. I. Effects of corticotrophins and 3′,5′-cyclic nucleotides on corticosterone production. Endocrinology 88:1109.
149. Sayers, G., and Beall, R. J. (1973). Isolated adrenal cortex cells: hypersensitivity to adrenocorticotropic hormone after hypophysectomy. Science 179:1330.
150. Fehm, H. L., Voigt, K. H., Lang, R., Ozyol, M. B., and Pfeiffer, E. F. (1973). Influence of plasma on ACTH stimulated corticosterone production of isolated adrenal cells. FEBS Lett. 36:109.
151. Giordano, N. D., and Sayers, G. (1971). Isolated adrenal cells: assay of ACTH in rat serum. Proc. Soc. Exp. Biol. Med. 136:623.
152. Liotta, A., and Krieger, D. T. (1975). A sensitive bioassay for the determination of human plasma ACTH levels. J. Clin. Endocrinol. Metab. 40:268.
153. Sayers, M. A., Sayers, G., and Woodbury, L. A. (1948). The assay of adrenocorticotrophic hormone by the adrenal ascorbic acid-depletion method. Endocrinology 42:379.
154. Krieger, D. T., and Allen, W. (1975). Relationship of bioassayable and immunoassayable plasma ACTH and cortisol concentrations in normal subjects and in patients with Cushing's Disease. J. Clin. Endocrinol. Metab. 10:675.
155. Buckingham, J. C., and Hodges, J. R. (1974). Interrelationships of pituitary and plasma corticotrophin and plasma corticosterone in adrenalectomized rats. J. Endocrinol. 63:213.
156. Kaplanski, J., van Delft, A. M. L., Nyakas, C., Stoof, J. C., and Smelik, P. G. (1974). Circadian periodicity and stress responsiveness of the pituitary-adrenal system of rats after central administration of 6-hydroxydopamine. J. Endocrinol. 63:299.
157. Schulster, D. (1973). Regulation of steroidogenesis by ACTH in a superfusion system for isolated adrenal cells. Endocrinology 93:700.
158. Falke, H. E., Degenhart, H. J., Abeln, G. J. A., Visser, H. K. A., and Croughs, R. J. M. (1975). Studies on isolated rat adrenal cells. I. Continuous flow and batch incubations. Acta Endocrinol. 78:110.
159. Lowry, P. J., and McMartin, C. (1974). Measurement of the dynamics of stimulation and inhibition of steroidogenesis in isolated rat adrenal cells by using column perfusion. Biochem. J. 142:287.
160. Brodish, A. (1973). Corticotrophin-releasing factor (CRF). *In* Berson, S. A., and Yalow, R. S. (eds.), Methods in Investigative and Diagnostic Endocrinology, p. 391. North Holland Publishing Company, Amsterdam.
161. Brodish, A. (1963). Diffuse hypothalamic system for the regulation of ACTH secretion. Endocrinology 73:727.
162. Vernikos-Danellis, J. (1964). Estimation of corticotropin-releasing activity of rat hypothalamus and neurohypophysis before and after stress. Endocrinology 75:514.

163. Arimura, A., Saito, T., and Schally, A. V. (1967). Assays for corticotropin-releasing factor (CRF) using rats treated with morphine, chlorpromazine, dexamethasone and nembutal. Endocrinology 81:235.

164. Hedge, G. A., Yates, M. B., Marcus, R., and Yates, F. E. (1966). Site of action of vasopressin in causing corticotropin release. Endocrinology 79:328.

165. Hiroshige, T., Kunita, H., Yoshimura, K., and Itoh, S. (1968). An assay method for corticotropin-releasing activity by intrapituitary microinjection in the rat. Jap. J. Physiol. 18:179.

166. Hiroshige, T., Sato, T., Ohta, R., and Itoh, S. (1969). Increase of corticotropin-releasing activity in the rat hypothalamus following noxious stimuli. Jap. J. Physiol. 19:866.

167. Hiroshige, T., and Sato, T. (1970). Postnatal development of circadian rhythm of corticotropin-releasing activity in the rat hypothalamus. Endocrinol. Jap. 17:1.

168. Witorsch, R. J., and Brodish, A. (1972). Conditions for the reliable use of lesioned rats for the assay of CRF in tissue extracts. Endocrinology 90:552.

169. Lymangrover, J. R., and Brodish, A. (1973). Time-course of response to hypothalamic extract and multiple use of lesioned rats for CRF assay. Neuroendocrinology 12:98.

170. Portanova, R., Smith, D. K., and Sayers, G. (1970). A trypsin technique for the preparation of isolated rat anterior pituitary cells. Proc. Soc. Exp. Biol. Med. 133:573.

171. Portanova, R. (1972). Release of ACTH from isolated pituitary cells: an energy dependent process. Proc. Soc. Exp. Biol. Med. 140:825.

172. Portanova, R., and Sayers, G. (1973). Isolated pituitary cells: CRF-like activity of neurohypophysial and related polypeptides. Proc. Soc. Exp. Biol. Med. 143:661.

173. Portanova, R., and Sayers, G. (1973). An in vitro assay for corticotropin releasing factor(s) using suspensions of isolated pituitary cells. Neuroendocrinology 12:236.

174. Portanova, R., and Sayers, G. (1972). Isolated pituitary cells: assay of CRF. In Brodish, A., and Redgate, E. S. (eds.), Brain-Pituitary-Adrenal Interrelationships, p. 319. Karger Publishing Company, Basel.

175. Lowry, P. J. (1974). A sensitive method for the detection of corticotropin releasing factor using a perfused pituitary cell column. J. Endocrinol. 62:163.

176. Mulder, G. H., and Smelik, P. G. (1975). Release of ACTH by rat anterior pituitary cells in a superfusion system. Acta Endocrinol. (Suppl.) 199:207.

177. Fleischer, N., and Rawls, W. E. (1970). ACTH synthesis and release in pituitary monolayer culture: effect of dexamethasone. Am. J. Physiol. 219:445.

178. Watanabe, H., Nicholson, W. E., and Orth, D. N. (1973). Inhibition of adrenocorticotropic hormone production by glucocorticoids in mouse pituitary tumor cells. Endocrinology 93:411.

179. Lang, R. E., Hilwig, I., Voigt, K. H., Fehm, H. L., and Pfeiffer, E. F. (1975). Growth in monolayer culture of rat pituitary cells which synthesize and release ACTH. Acta Endocrinol. 79:421.

180. Takebe, K., Yasuda, N., and Greer, M. A. (1975). A sensitive and simple in vitro assay for corticotropin-releasing substances utilizing ACTH release from cultured anterior pituitary cells. Endocrinology 97:1248.

181. Vale, W., Grant, G., Amoss, M., Blackwell, R., and Guillemin, R. (1972). Culture of enzymatically dispersed anterior-pituitary cells: functional validation of a method. Endocrinology 91:562.
182. Tang, L. K. L., and Spies, H. G. (1974). Effect of synthetic LH-releasing factor (LRF) on LH secretion in monolayer cultures of the anterior pituitary cells of Cynomolgus monkeys. Endocrinology 94:1016.
183. Yasuda, N., Takebe, K., and Greer, M. A. (1976). Studies on ACTH dynamics in cultured adenohypophyseal cells: effect of adrenalectomy or dexamethasone in vivo. Endocrinology 98:717.
184. Hillhouse, E. W., Burden, J., and Jones, M. T. (1975). The effect of various putative neurotransmitters on the release of corticotropin releasing hormone from the hypothalamus of the rat in vitro. I. The effect of acetylcholine and noradrenaline. Neuroendocrinology 17:1.
185. Edwardson, J. A., Bennett, G. W., and Bradford, H. F. (1972). Release of amino acids and neurosecretory substances after stimulation of nerve-endings (synaptosomes) isolated from the hypothalamus. Nature 240:554.
186. Haksar, A., Maudsley, D. V., Kimmel, G. L., Peron, F. G., Robidoux, W. F., and Gagnon, G. (1974). Adrenocorticotrophin stimulation of cyclic adenosine 3,5-monophosphate formation in isolated rat adrenal cells: the role of membrane sialic acid. Biochim. Biophys. Acta 362:356.
187. Haynes, R. C. (1958). The activation of adrenal phosphorylase by the adrenocorticotropic hormone. J. Biol. Chem. 233:1220.
188. Richardson, M. C., and Schulster, D. (1972). Corticosteroidogenesis in isolated rat adrenal cells: effect of ACTH, c-AMP and 1-24 ACTH diazotized to polyacrylamide. J. Endocrinol. 55:127.
189. Nakamura, M., Ide, M., Okabayashi, T., and Tanaka, A. (1972). Relation between steroidogenesis and 3,5-cyclic-AMP production in isolated adrenal cells. Endocrinol. Jap. 19(5):443.
190. Beall, R. J., and Sayers, G. (1972). Isolated adrenal cells: steroidogenesis and c-AMP accumulation in response to ACTH. Arch. Biochem. Biophys. 148:70.
191. Moyle, W. R., Kong, Y. C., and Ramachandran, J. (1973). Steroidogenesis and cyclic adenosine 3,5-monophosphate accumulation in rat adrenal cells. J. Biol. Chem. 248(7):2409.
192. Sharma, K., Ahmed, N. K., Sutliff, L. S., and Brush, J. S. (1974). Metabolic regulation and steroidogenesis in isolated adrenal cells of the rat: ACTH regulation of cGMP and c-AMP levels and steroidogenesis. FEBS Lett. 45(1):107.
193. Shirma, S., Mitsunaga, M., Kawashima, Y., Taguchi, S., and Nakao, T. (1974). Studies on cyclic nucleotides in the adrenal gland. Biochim. Biophys. Acta 341:56.
194. Peytremann, A., Nicholson, W. E., Hardman, J. G., and Liddle, G. W. (1973). Effect of adrenocorticotropic hormone on extracellular adenosine 3,5-monophosphate in the hypophysectomized rat. Endocrinology 92:1502.
195. Peytremann, A., Nicholson, W. E., Brown, R. D., Liddle, G. W., and Hardman, J. D. (1973). Comparative effects of angiotensin and ACTH on cyclic AMP and steroidogenesis in isolated bovine adrenal cells. J. Clin. Invest. 52(4):835.
196. Richardson, M. D., and Schulster, D. (1972). Corticosteroidogenesis in

isolated rat adrenal cells: effect of ACTH, c-AMP and [1-24] ACTH diazotized to polyacrylamide. J. Endocrinol. 55:127.
197. Mackie, C., and Schulster, D. (1973). Phosphodiesterase activity and the potentiation by theophylline of ACTH stimulated steroidogenesis and adenosine 3,5-monophosphate levels in isolated rat adrenal cells. Biochem. Biophys. Res. Commun. 53(2):545.
198. Jaanus, S. D., Rosenstein, M. J., and Rubin, R. P. (1970). On the mode of action of ACTH on the isolated perfused adrenal gland. J. Physiol. 209:539.
199. Carchman, R. A., Jaanus, S. D., and Rubin, R. P. (1971). The role of adrenocorticotropin and calcium in adenosine cyclie 3,5-phosphate production and steroid release from the isolated, perfused cat adrenal gland. Mol. Pharmacol. 7:491.
200. Rubin, R. P., Carchman, R. A., and Jaanus, S. D. (1972). Role of cyclic 3,5-adenosine monophosphate on corticosteroid synthesis and release from the intact adrenal gland. Biochem. Biophys. Res. Commun. 47(6): 1492.
201. Tait, S. A. S., Tait, J. F., Gould, R. P., Brown, B. L., and Albano, J. D. M. (1974). The preparation and use of purified and unpurified dispersed adrenal cells and a study of the relationship of their c-AMP and steroid output. J. Steroid Biochem. 775(5):787.
202. Sharma, R. K. (1973). Regulation of steroidogenesis by adrenocorticotropic hormone in isolated adrenal cells of rat. J. Biol. Chem. 248(15): 5473.
203. Sharma, R. K. (1974). Metabolic regulation of steroidogenesis in isolated adrenal cells in rat: effect of actinomycin D on cGMP-induced steroidogenesis. Biochem. Biophys. Res. Commun. 59(3):992.
204. Ney, R. L. (1969). Effects of dibutyryl cyclic AMP on adrenal growth and steroidogenic capacity. Endocrinology 84:168.
205. Marton, J., Stark, E., and Mihaly, K. (1972). Effect of imidazole on the adrenal response to ACTH and to stress. Acta Physiol. Acad. Sci. Tomus 42(3):225.
206. Nussdorfer, G. G., and Mazzocchi, G. (1973). Effects of 3,5-cyclic nucleotides on adrenocortical cells of hypophysectomized rats. Lab. Invest. 28(3):332.
207. Roos, B. A. (1974). Effect of ACTH and c-AMP on human adrenocortical growth and function in vitro. Endocrinology 94:685.
208. Nussdorfer, G. C., and Mazzocchi, G. (1972). A stereologic study of the effects of intact and hypophysectomized rats. Lab. Invest. 26(1):45.
209. Milner, A. J. (1973). Morphological differentiation of adrenal cortical cells induced by a 40 minute exposure to corticotrophin. J. Endocrinol. 56:325.
210. Kahri, A. I. (1973). Inhibition of ACTH-induced differentiation of cortical cells and their mitochondria by corticosterone in tissue culture of fetal rat adrenal. Anat. Rec. 176(3)253.
211. O'Hare, M. J., and Neville, A. M. (1973). Steroid metabolism by adult rat adrenocortical cells in monolayer culture. J. Endocrinol. 58:477.
212. Richman, R., Dobbins, C., Voina, S., Underwood, L., Mahaffee, D., Gitelman, H. J., Van Wyk, J., and Ney, R. L. (1973). Regulation of adrenal ornithine decarboxylase by adrenocorticotropic hormone and cyclic AMP. J. Clin. Invest. 52(8):2007.

213. Fuhrman, S. A., and Gill, G. N. (1974). Hormonal control of adrenal RNA polymerase activities. Endocrinology 94:691.
214. Nussdorfer, G. G., and Mazzochi, G. (1973). Further studies on the trophic effect of a c-GMP on rat adrenal cortex. J. Endocrinol. 57:559.
215. Flynn, A., Strain, W. H., and Pories, W. J. (1972). Corticotrophin dependency of zinc ions. Biochem. Biophys. Res. Commun. 46(3):1113.
216. Birmingham, M. D., Elliott, F. H., and Valere, P. H. (1953). The need for the presence of Ca^{++} for the stimulation *in vitro* of rat adrenal glands by ACTH. Endocrinology 53:687.
217. Haksar, A., and Peron, F. G. (1972). Comparison of the Ca^{++} requirement for the steroidogenic effect of ACTH and dibutyryl cyclic AMP in rat adrenal cell suspensions. Biochem. Biophys. Res. Commun. 47:445.
218. Leier, D. J., and Jungman, R. A. (1973). Adrenocorticotropic hormone and dibutyryl adenosine cyclic monophosphate-mediated Ca^{++} uptake by rat adrenal glands. Biochim. Biophys. Acta 329:196.
219. Jaanus, S. D., and Rubin, R. P. (1971). The effect of ACTH on calcium distribution in the perfused cat adrenal gland. J. Physiol. 213:581.
220. Rubin, R. P., Jaanus, S. D., and Carchman, R. A. (1972). Role of calcium and adenosine cyclic 3,5-phosphate in action of adrenocorticotropin. Nature (New Biol.) 240(100):150.
221. Carchman, R. A., Jaanus, S. D., and Rubin, R. P. (1971). The role of adrenocorticotropin and calcium in adenosine cyclic 3,5-phosphate production and steroid release from the isolated, perfused cat adrenal gland. Mol. Pharmacol. 7:491.
222. Sayers, G., Beall, R. J., and Seelig, S. (1972). Isolated adrenal cells: adrenocorticotropic hormone, calcium, steroidogenesis, and cyclic adenosine monophosphate. Science 175:131.
223. Bowyer, F., and Kitabchi, A. E. (1974). Dual role of calcium in steroidogenesis in the isolated adrenal cell of rat. Biochem. Biophys. Res. Commun. 57(1):100.
224. Finn, F. M., Montibeller, J. A., Ushifima, Y., and Hofmann, K. (1975). Adenylate cyclase system of bovine adrenal plasma membranes. J. Biol. Chem. 250(4):1186.
225. Birmingham, M. D., and Bartova, A. (1973). Effects of calcium and theophylline on ACTH and dbCAMP stimulated steroidogenesis and glycolysis by intact mouse adrenal glands *in vitro*. Endocrinology 92:743.
226. Farese, R. V. (1971). On the requirement for calcium during the steroidogenic effect of ACTH. Endocrinology 89:1057.
227. Pfeiffer, D. R., and Tchen, T. T. (1973). The role of Ca^{++} in control of malic enzyme activity in bovine adrenal cortex mitochondria. Biochem. Biophys. Res. Commun. 50(3):807.
228. Jaanus, S. D., Rosenstein, M. J., and Rubin, R. P. (1970). On the mode of action of ACTH on the isolated perfused adrenal gland. J. Physiol. 209:539.
229. Matthews, E. K., and Saffran, M. (1973). Ionic dependence of adrenal steroidogenesis and ACTH-induced changes in the membrane potential of adrenocortical cells. J. Physiol. 234:43.
230. Peron, F. G., and Kortiz, S. B. (1958). On the exogenous requirements for the action of ACTH in vitro on rat adrenal glands. J. Biol. Chem. 233:256.
231. Van Breeman, C., and De Weer, P. (1970). Lanthanum inhibition of Ca^{++} efflux from the squid giant axon. Nature (Lond.) 226:760.

232. Halmi, K. A., Halmi, N. S., and Anderson, D. J. (1974). Effects of ions on ACTH-sensitive adenylate cyclase of rat adrenals. Proc. Soc. Exp. Biol. Med. 147:399.
233. Jaanus, S. D., Carchman, R. A., and Rubin, R. P. (1972). Further studies on the relationship between c-AMP levels and adrenocortical activity. Endocrinology 91:887.
234. Brodish, A. (1973). Hypothalamic and extrahypothalamic corticotrophin-releasing factors in peripheral blood. In Brodish, A., and Redgate, E. S. (eds.), Brain-Pituitary-Adrenal Interrelationships, p. 128. Karger Publishing Company, Basel.
235. Lymangrover, J., and Brodish, A. (1973). Tissue-CRF: an extrahypothalamic corticotrophin releasing factor (CRF) in the peripheral blood of stressed rats. Neuroendocrinology 12:225.
236. Lymangrover, J. R., and Brodish, A. (1973/4). Physiological regulation of tissue-CRF. Neuroendocrinology 13:234.
237. Egdahl, R. H. (1962). Further studies on adrenal cortical function in dogs with isolated pituitaries. Endocrinology 71:926.
238. Egdahl, R. H. (1960). Adrenal cortical and medullary response to trauma in dogs with isolated pituitaries. Endocrinology 66:200.
239. Egdahl, R. H. (1961). Corticosteroid secretion following caval constriction in dogs with isolated pituitaries. Endocrinology 68:226.
240. Brodish, A. (1964). A delayed secretion of ACTH in rats with hypothalamic lesions. Endocrinology 74:28.
241. Lau, C., and Timiras, P. S. (1972). Adrenocortical function in hypothalamic deafferented rats maintained at high altitude. Am. J. Physiol. 222:1040.
242. Gordon, M. L. (1950). An evaluation of afferent nervous impulses in the adrenal cortical response to trauma. Endocrinology 47:347.
243. Guillemin, R., Hearn, W. R., Cheek, W. R., and Householder, D. E. (1957). Control of corticotrophin release: further studies with in vitro methods. Endocrinology 60:488.
244. Witorsch, R., and Brodish, A. (1972). Evidence for acute ACTH release by extrahypothalamic mechanisms. Endocrinology 90:1160.
245. Weissman, G., and Thomas, L. (1964). The effects of corticosteroids upon connective tissue and lysosomes. Recent Progr. Horm. Res. 20:215.

International Review of Physiology
Endocrine Physiology II, Volume 16
Edited by S. M. McCann
Copyright 1977   University Park Press   Baltimore

4
Glucagon Physiology in Health and Disease

R. SHERWIN and P. FELIG

Yale University School of Medicine,
New Haven, Connecticut

In the last 5–10 years, investigative interest has increasingly focused on the role of glucagon in normal physiology and in the pathogenesis of diabetes mellitus. The development of radioimmunoassay procedures for measurement of glucagon, the infusion of crystalline glucagon into intact subjects in physiological amounts, and the availability of an agent (somatostatin) which inhibits glucagon secretion have markedly enhanced our understanding of glucagon physiology. In this chapter, a variety of recent studies is discussed in which the nature of circulating glucagon, the secretion and catabolism of this hormone, its interaction with insulin in glucose and ketone metabolism, and the role of tissue receptors are considered. Much of the discussion focuses on observations in humans, reflecting the investigative interest of the authors.

CIRCULATING GLUCAGON

The study of glucagon physiology in man was greatly advanced by the development of a radioimmunoassay for plasma glucagon by Unger and co-workers (1) which demonstrated minimal cross-reactivity with gut peptides (glucagon-like immunoreactivity). The assay was thought to be relatively specific for glucagon of pancreatic origin. Recent studies with the use of gel filtration techniques, however, have demonstrated that only 40–50% of total glucagon immunoreactivity as measured by most assays for glucagon represents biologically active hormone of pancreatic origin (2, 3). Most of the remaining glucagon immunoreactivity in normal human plasma elutes with the void volume (with plasma proteins) and has an estimated molecular weight of 160,000 (4). This fraction has been termed big plasma glucagon and probably is devoid of biological activity. Two additional fractions with molecular weights of approximately 9,000 and 2,000 have been identified in small amounts in normal plasma. The biological significance of these fractions remains to be determined, although the 9,000 material is thought to possibly represent proglucagon activity (3). In support of this notion is the recent report of a marked elevation in the 9,000 molecular weight species in patients with the glucagonoma syndrome (5). This fraction is also increased in patients with chronic renal failure, presumably because of impaired renal removal processes (3).

Although basal levels of immunoreactive glucagon represent both biologically active and nonactive hormone, alterations in circulating immunoreactivity in response to physiological stimulation (e.g., amino acids) or suppression (e.g., glucose) generally reflect changes in the biologically active form of the hormone. Thus, changes in plasma glucagon in response to physiological stimuli or suppressors as determined by currently available assays of immunoreactivity are probably reflective of changes in pancreatic glucagon.

GLUCAGON SECRETION

The rate of pancreatic glucagon secretion in man is extremely small when compared to the doses of glucagon previously employed to study the metabolic effects of this hormone. Basal secretory rates of glucagon in normal man are not greater than 100–150 μg/day (6). These values are probably an overestimate when one takes into account that portion of glucagon immunoreactivity that is not biologically active (2, 3). Thus, earlier studies employing bolus injections of as little as 0.1 mg of glucagon are clearly pharmocological. On the basis of these observations and the small portal-peripheral gradient for glucagon (as compared to insulin), the molar ratio of pancreatic insulin and glucagon secretion is actually about 8–12:1 (7, 8) rather than 3–4:1, as determined by circulating peripheral hormone levels.

Glucagon secretion does not markedly fluctuate throughout the day in normal subjects receiving mixed meals (9). The plasma glucagon level is fairly constant throughout the day. This contrasts with insulin secretion which shows an increase with ingestion of mixed meals (9). Increases in glucagon secretion in normal man generally result from the ingestion of large, purely protein meals (10, 11). Glucagon secretion is reduced following the consumption of large amounts of carbohydrate (11). Although basal glucagon levels are rarely, if ever, suppressed in circumstances other than pure glucose ingestion, a number of physiological conditions are capable of increasing plasma glucagon concentration. α-Cell hypersecretion is associated with acute hypoglycemia (12), prolonged heavy exercise (13), hypercorticism (14), and stimulation of the ventromedial hypothalamus (15) or the adrenergic nervous system (16). These stimuli are most likely required for emergency glucose needs and not responsible for day to day changes in circulating glucagon. Neither episodic α-cell release nor diurnal fluctuations in glucagon secretion have been reported in normal subjects. In fasting, a circumstance characterized by hyperglucagonemia (6), altered catabolism, rather than hypersecretion, is responsible for the elevated plasma levels (see below).

GLUCAGON CATABOLISM

Recent studies indicate that, in contrast to insulin, the kidney rather than the liver is the principal site of glucagon degradation. Consistent renal extraction of glucagon has been observed in the autotransplanted dog kidney (17). The fractional extraction ratio of glucagon across the kidney in the intact dog and rat is 40–50% (18, 19). Renal clearance of glucagon following administration of physiological doses of this hormone to normal dogs accounts for approximately 50% of total glucagon removal (18). Furthermore, renal artery clamping (20) or ureteral ligation (21) results in a rapid rise in plasma glucagon. In contrast, a decrease in circulating glucagon is observed after successful renal transplantation in man (22). Finally, elevations of glucagon (MW 3,500) observed in chronic renal failure in man are solely a result of decreased hormonal degradation (23) (Figure 1). After the induction of renal failure by 75% nephrectomy in rats, a consistent renal uptake of glucagon is no longer observed, indicating that the reduction in glucagon clearance in uremia is likely to be secondary to alterations in renal removal processes (19). These studies support a prime role for the kidney in glucagon catabolism and indicate that renal function must be taken into account in interpreting plasma glucagon levels in a variety of pathological states. Hyperglucagonemia associated with traumatic shock (24), acute myocardial infarction (25), diabetic ketoacidosis (26), and hyperosmolar coma (27) may thus, in part, be explained by altered renal hemodynamics associated with these conditions.

Regarding the nature of the physiological processes involved in glucagon catabolism by the kidney, it is noteworthy that glucagon removal by the kidney exceeds the filtered load of this hormone (19). Furthermore, urinary excretion of glucagon accounts for less than 1% of total renal glucagon removal (19).

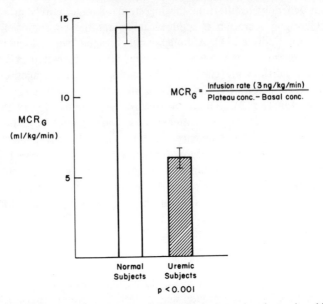

METABOLIC CLEARANCE RATE OF GLUCAGON (MCR$_G$)
IN NORMAL AND UREMIC SUBJECTS

$$MCR_G = \frac{\text{Infusion rate } (3\,ng/kg/min)}{\text{Plateau conc.} - \text{Basal conc.}}$$

MCR$_G$
(ml/kg/min)

15

10

5

Normal   Uremic
Subjects   Subjects
p < 0.001

Figure 1. The metabolic clearance of glucagon in normal and uremic subjects. Hyperglucagonemia in uremia is a consequence of decreased glucagon catabolism rather than hypersecretion. Based on the data of Sherwin et al. (23).

These studies suggest that peritubular uptake of this hormone may account for a significant portion of total renal glucagon clearance. Glucagon degradative enzymes have, in fact, recently been demonstrated in kidney tissue (28).

In contrast to the kidney, the liver is a relatively minor site of glucagon catabolism. The portal-peripheral gradient for glucagon in intact man is only 1.3:1 (as compared to 3:1 for insulin) (7). A consistent extraction of glucagon is not demonstrable in the rat liver (29). Furthermore, in circumstances of decreased liver function such as cirrhosis, the metabolic clearance rate of glucagon remains normal (30).

The key role of altered hormonal catabolism in determining plasma glucagon concentration is underscored by recent studies of glucagon turnover during fasting (6). In prolonged fasting, plasma glucagon levels transiently increase during the 1st week of fasting and then gradually return to base line levels (31). The rise in glucagon observed at 3 days is primarily the result of a 20% reduction in the metabolic clearance rate of glucagon. No significant increase in glucagon delivery is observed at this time (6). As fasting continues for 3–4 weeks, decreased glucagon secretion (40%) accounts for the return of plasma glucagon to base line values despite a further reduction in glucagon turnover (6) (Figure 2). Thus, after prolonged fasting, clearance and secretion have been equally reduced, resulting in normalization of plasma concentration. These studies,

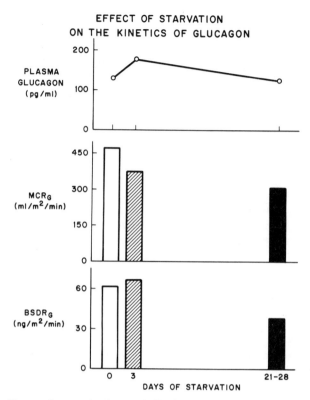

Figure 2. Plasma glucagon levels, metabolic clearance rate (MCR_g), and basal systemic delivery rate ($BSDR_G$) of glucagon during prolonged fasting. The initial rise in plasma glucagon early in fasting is due to a fall in clearance (catabolism) rather than an increase in secretion. The late fall in plasma glucagon is due to a decline in secretion. Based on the data of Fisher et al. (6).

therefore, demonstrate that changes in blood concentration of the hormone cannot be assumed to reflect altered secretion. On the other hand, α-cell hypersecretion is undoubtedly an important contributory factor in certain hyperglucagonemic states. For example, studies in cirrhotic patients with portal-systemic shunting indicate that marked elevations in plasma glucagon result from increased hormonal secretion (30). Interestingly, glucagon secretory rates in this condition are inversely related to the glycemic response to glucagon, suggesting that a feedback system may exist between sensitivity to glucagon and its own secretion (30).

GLUCAGON AND CARBOHYDRATE HOMEOSTASIS IN NORMAL MAN

Studies with the use of doses of glucagon which are 100–1,000 times the normal secretory rate have suggested that glucagon is a potent insulin antagonist in man. Glucagon consistently stimulates glycogenolysis and gluconeogenesis in vitro

(32). In intact man, supraphysiological doses of glucagon (causing plasma levels of 5,000 pg/ml) augment splanchnic output of glucose and cyclic AMP (33). Although the pharmacological effects of glucagon on glucose homeostasis are well established, the significance of these observations to normal physiology has recently been questioned. Studies involving physiological doses of glucagon (3 ng/kg/min) in normal subjects, which result in increments in plasma glucagon comparable to those reported in a variety of hyperglycagonemic states (e.g., diabetic ketoacidosis (26)), produce only small (5–10 mg/100 ml), transient increases in blood glucose levels (34). Blood glucose concentration returns to base line levels within 2–3 hr despite persistent hyperglucagonemia and normal peripheral levels of insulin (34). The transient rise in blood glucose after physiological infusions of glucagon is a consequence of a very evanescent increase in splanchnic glucose production (35, 36). In response to physiological increments in glucagon, splanchnic glucose output rapidly increases by 2–3 fold within 7–15 min, but returns to base line levels within 30 min (Figure 3) (35). This fall in splanchnic glucose output occurs in the face of stable insulin levels

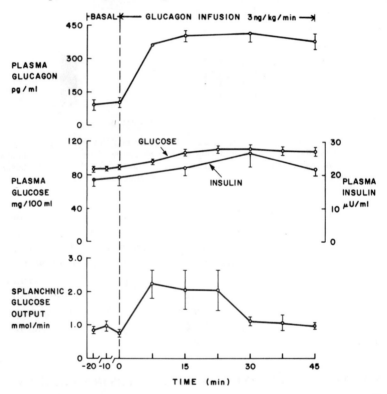

Figure 3. The evanescent effect of physiological hyperglucagonemia on splanchnic glucose output. Despite ongoing hyperglucagonemia, splanchnic glucose output returns to base line levels within 30 min. A similar response is observed in diabetics, indicating that this loss of responsiveness to glucagon is not insulin-dependent. Based on the data of Felig et al. (35).

and is equally demonstrable in diabetic patients (35, 36). The evanescent hepatic response to glucagon is thus not dependent upon increased insulin secretion. The transient nature of the stimulatory response suggests the rapid development of inhibition or reversal of glucagon action in man. Interestingly, this loss of glucagon action is not observed when pharmacological doses (50 ng/kg/min) are infused (33), emphasizing further the need to differentiate physiological from pharmacological effects of glucagon.

In contrast to glucagon, the effects of physiological increments in plasma insulin persist during periods of insulin administration lasting 1 hr or more (37, 38) and continue for 30–45 min after cessation of an insulin infusion (37, 38). These differences in time course of the biological action of physiological perturbations in glucagon and insulin raise serious questions regarding the significance of the insulin to glucagon ratio in determining normal glucose homeostasis.

The bihormonal response (hyperinsulinemia and hypoglucagonemia) to ingestion of large carbohydrate loads has prompted speculation that the combined α- and β-cell response (i.e., the insulin to glucagon ratio), rather than changes in insulin alone, may be required for normal glucose disposal (11, 39). That the rise in insulin is essential for normal glucose disposal is indisputable as attested to by the effects of pancreatectomy, alloxan, and streptozotocin. On the other hand, evidence for the essentiality of glucagon suppression has been entirely indirect. The possibility of a bihormonal influence on oral glucose disposal is consistent with data demonstrating that the liver (the major physiological site of glucagon action), rather than muscle or adipose tissue, is quantitatively the most important site of glucose uptake after carbohydrate feeding (40). However, when the effects of physiological hyperglucagonemia and an altered insulin to glucagon ratio on oral glucose tolerance are evaluated in normal subjects, the concept of bihormonal regulation is not supported. To evaluate the essentiality of glucagon suppression in normal glucose tolerance, glucagon was infused in physiological amounts (3 ng/kg/min) prior to and during oral glucose tolerance testing. Rather than the usual fall in plasma glucagon accompanying carbohydrate feeding, 3–4 fold increments in plasma glucagon were maintained (34). Despite elevations in plasma glucagon comparable to those reported in diabetic ketoacidosis (26), uremia (21, 23), cirrhosis (41), fasting (6, 31), or trauma (24), glucose tolerance was no different from that observed during a control study in which saline solution was infused (Figure 4) (34). Particularly noteworthy was the fact that normal glucose tolerance was maintained in the absence of compensatory hyperinsulinemia (Figure 4) (34). Thus, despite a 5–6-fold fall in the peripheral insulin to glucagon ratio (from 34:1 to 6:1) during the glucagon infusion, no change in glucose tolerance occurred. The argument has been raised that glucose intolerance would not be expected unless the glucagon to insulin ratio had been reduced to levels well below 6:1 (42). However, to achieve such a ratio would require either absolute insulin deficiency or hyperglucagonemia in excess of that observed in most disease states (i.e., pharmacological hyperglucagonemia).

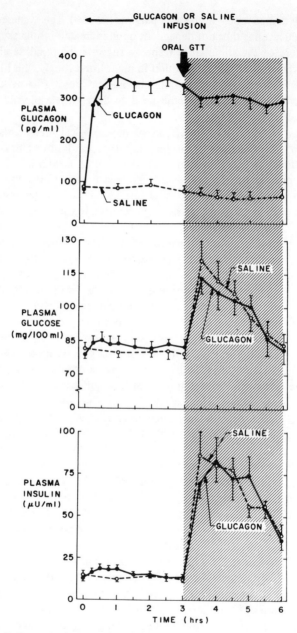

Figure 4. Failure of physiological hyperglucagonemia to alter glucose tolerance in normal subjects. Reproduced from Sherwin et al. (34), with permission of the *New England Journal of Medicine*.

These findings indicate that the fall in plasma glucagon observed after carbohydrate feeding is not essential for the maintenance of normal glucose tolerance. Rather, the primary determinant of normal glucose disposal is the insulin secretory response. Furthermore, these observations suggest that, so long as insulin is available and in the absence of pharmacological elevations or altered sensitivity to glucagon, the insulin to glucagon ratio provides a no more useful index of glucose homeostasis than is available from the absolute concentration of insulin.

As compared to normal circumstances, the glucose tolerance test represents a rather artificial situation. The usual pattern of mixed meal ingestion does not involve consumption of a 100-gm concentrated carbohydrate load. Furthermore, the postprandial blood glucose fluctuations during the course of the day (15–50 mg/100 ml) (43) are far less than those observed during a GTT (glucose tolerance test). Thus, from the standpoint of normal glucose homeostasis, a more germane question concerns the relative importance of hypoglucagonemia and hyperinsulinemia in the control of hepatic glucose output in response to small increments (10–20 mg/100 ml) in blood glucose concentration. When small doses of glucose (150 mg/min) are infused intravenously to normal subjects, blood glucose rises by 15 mg/100 ml and splanchnic glucose output falls by 85% (44). Glucose homeostasis is thus stimulating peripheral glucose uptake (44). Under these conditions of mild hyperglycemia and profound inhibition of hepatic glucose output, peripheral insulin levels rise by 60–80%, where as arterial glucagon concentration remains unchanged (44). Although a decline in portal glucagon levels cannot be excluded, the small portal-peripheral gradient for this hormone (7, 8) makes this possibility unlikely. These findings indicate that the fine tuning of hepatic glucose regulation in response to small changes in blood glucose is determined by β-cell secretion rather than by a combined α- and β-cell response. In accord with this conclusion are the data demonstrating that plasma insulin and glucose fluctuate in concert in response to mixed meal ingestion, whereas plasma glucagon remains static throughout the day (9).

Inasmuch as a fall in glucagon is not essential for the metabolism of large (100 gm) carbohydrate loads (34) and inasmuch as glucagon levels fail to change in response to small carbohydrate loads (44), one may question the precise role of this hormone in normal physiology. The importance of glucagon clearly emerges when one considers the response to protein ingestion. Following a protein meal, peripheral levels of insulin increase by 60–100% (10, 14, 45). Such a rise in insulin would be expected to suppress hepatic glucose output by 85% (44) and result in hypoglycemia. However, direct observations in man indicate that splanchnic glucose output is maintained at basal values after protein feeding (45). The maintenance of euglycemia in the face of hyperinsulinemia accompanying a protein meal was initially attributed by Unger and co-workers to the concomitant release of glucagon (10). This hypothesis has recently been tested by simulating the hyperinsulinemia and hyperglucagonemia of a protein meal (35). In these studies, glucose was infused at a rate of 150 mg/min, resulting in a

60–80% rise in plasma insulin and virtually complete inhibition of splanchnic glucose output. The glucose infusion was then continued and glucagon was infused (3 ng/kg/min) in order to achieve increments in plasma glucagon comparable to those observed after protein feeding. The effect of addition of glucagon was a prompt increase in splanchnic glucose output to basal levels (35). These data indicate that physiological hyperglucagonemia can at least transiently overcome the suppressive effects of small increments in insulin on hepatic glucose output. Glucagon thus may be viewed as providing a rapid means whereby euglycemia is maintained in the face of noncarbohydrate (e.g., protein)-mediated stimulation of insulin secretion. Glucagon may also contribute to the reversal of acute (insulin-induced) hypoglycemia. However, the time course of the hormonal response to hypoglycemia suggests that catecholamines may be of greater importance than glucagon (46).

GLUCAGON-INSULIN INTERACTIONS
IN GLUCOSE METABOLISM IN DIABETES

The concept that glucagon and insulin jointly regulate glucose homeostasis is particularly attractive regarding the pathogenesis of the diabetic syndrome. It has been suggested that diabetes results not from insulin lack by itself, but rather from a bihormonal disturbance of α- and β-cell function (39, 47, 48). The importance of glucagon in the development of the diabetic syndrome is suggested by the demonstration that 1) suppression of glucagon by glucose is lost in diabetes (1, 11); 2) protein-stimulated glucagon secretion is augmented (1, 11, 49); 3) diabetes is characterized by absolute or relative basal hyperglucagonemia (1, 11, 49); 4) the hyperglycemia accompanying insulin withdrawal is associated with increasing glucagon levels (50); and 5) a reduction in plasma glucagon induced by infusion of somatostatin results in a reduction of diabetic hyperglycemia (51–53). On the basis of these data, an essential role for glucagon in the pathogenesis of diabetic hyperglycemia has been postulated (48). However, with the exception of the somatostatin studies, these data are indirect and fail to prove that glucagon of itself is a primary contributing factor to abnormal glucose regulation in diabetes. The questions that need to be addressed are 1) whether hyperglucagonemia of the magnitude observed in diabetes is a sufficient hormonal alteration to cause worsening of diabetes in the absence of changes in insulin availability and 2) whether the presence of basal glucagon secretion is required for the development of fasting hyperglycemia in diabetes.

Sherwin et al. (34) evaluated the effect of physiological infusions of glucagon for periods of 2–4 days in adult-onset (noninsulin-dependent) diabetics and in juvenile-onset diabetics in whom insulin was administered in the usual amounts. The infusion of glucagon (3–9 ng/kg/min) resulted in elevations in plasma glucagon (250–800 pg/ml) which were comparable to or in excess of that observed in most patients with diabetic ketoacidosis (26). Despite ongoing hyperglucagonemia, fasting and postprandial blood glucose levels, as well as ketonemia, were unchanged from those observed during a pre- and postcontrol period. Furthermore, urinary glucose excretion in these patients was also unaffected by glucagon administration (54). In contrast, when similar amounts of glucagon were given to insulin-withdrawn, juvenile-onset diabetics, the rise in blood glucose was 5–15-fold greater than in normal subjects (34).

These findings indicate that in diabetics with substantial endogenous insulin secretion or in more severe juvenile-onset diabetics given exogenous insulin, a rise in plasma glucagon is insufficient of itself to bring about deterioration in blood glucose regulation. The diabetogenic effects of physiological increments in glucagon secretion are manifest only in circumstances of insulin deficiency. These results, together with the observations in normal subjects made hyperglucagonemic, underscore the primary role of insulin deficiency rather than glucagon excess in the pathogenesis of diabetes.

These observations do not, however, exclude the possibility of a diabetogenic effect of glucagon at higher dose levels. Using intermittent injections of glucagon in doses up to 3 mg/day, Raskin and Unger (55) have observed deterioration of blood glucose regulation in insulin-treated diabetics (55). It should, however, be noted that such doses are 20–30-fold greater than the 24-hr secretory rate of glucagon (0.10–0.15 mg/day) observed in normal (7, 23) or diabetic patients (34, 56) and 5–10-fold greater than the amounts infused by Sherwin et al. (34). Thus, it is likely that endogenous glucagon secretion rates in diabetic man rarely approach such values in the absence of a glucagonoma syndrome. It is of interest in this regard that, even in patients with the glucagonoma syndrome in whom plasma glucagon levels generally exceed 1,000 pg/ml, glucose intolerance is mild and inconsistent (57).

The foregoing observations on the response to exogenous glucagon indicate that hyperglucagonemia (of the magnitude encountered in human health or disease) is not sufficient to bring about diabetes so long as insulin is available. A second major question regarding the pathogenesis of diabetes is whether glucagon is necessary for the development of the diabetic syndrome. As noted above, evidence suggesting an essential role for glucagon in diabetes has largely derived from studies with somatostatin (51–53). This tetradecapeptide originally isolated from the hypothalamus (58) has subsequently been identified in the D-cells of the islets of Langerhans using immunofluorescent techniques (59). In addition to suppressing growth hormone release (58), somatostatin is a potent inhibitor of glucagon (51, 52, 60–62) and insulin secretion (62, 63). In normal (64, 65) as well as diabetic patients (52. 53), administration of somatostatin results in a prompt fall in blood glucose at a rate of 0.5–1.0 mg/100 ml/min. This effect of somatostatin is a consequence of a marked reduction in hepatic glucose production and is not associated with enhanced peripheral glucose uptake (66). Infusion of physiological doses of exogenous glucagon (but not growth hormone), together with somatostatin, prevents the decline in blood glucose normally observed, suggesting that the hypoglycemic effect is mediated by suppression of endogenous glucagon secretion (64, 67). On the basis of the ameliorative effect of this agent in experimental (51) and human diabetes (52, 53), it has been suggested that glucagon is essential for the development of hyperglycemia in diabetes (47, 48). Furthermore, a therapeutic role for somatostatin in the management of diabetes has been suggested on the basis of its effects in lowering the fasting blood glucose and its ability to markedly reduce the blood glucose rise following ingestion of carbohydrate-containing meals by diabetic subjects (52).

More recent studies with somatostatin involving prolonged infusions (5–6 hr) rather than brief administration (1–2 hr) have, however, seriously eroded, rather than substantiated, the concept of glucagon essentiality in diabetes. When somatostatin is infused for prolonged periods to normal subjects, the decline in blood glucose persists for 90–120 min (Figure 5). Beyond 2 hr the hypoglycemic effect wanes, and hyperglycemia (140–150 mg/100 ml) develops within 3–5 hr, despite persistent suppression of glucagon secretion (68) (Figure 5). The increase in blood glucose during prolonged infusion of somatostatin is a consequence of an increase in hepatic glucose output (68). Glucose production, initially reduced by 40–50%, rises progressively to values 15–20% above basal, preinfusion levels. The rise in glucose production, coupled with a reduction in glucose utilization, results in hyperglycemia. The condition produced with somatostatin is thus analogous to the situation in spontaneous diabetes. In spontaneously diabetic patients, as in the subjects given somatostatin, glucose

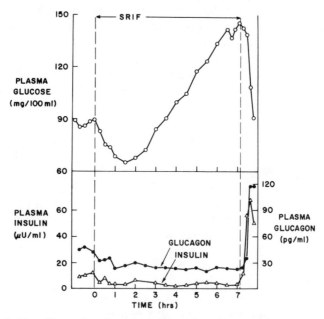

Figure 5. The effects of prolonged administration of somatostatin (SRIF) on glucose homeostasis in normal man. Despite ongoing suppression of plasma glucagon, fasting hyperglycemia develops within 3–5 hr. Based on the data of Sherwin et al. (68).

production is slightly increased or normal but inappropriate for the accompanying hyperglycemia (69).

With respect to the mechanism of these changes in glucose homeostasis produced by prolonged somatostatin infusion, insulin deficiency appears to be the primary factor. This is indicated by the prompt decline in blood glucose in association with restoration of insulin levels either by cessation of the somatostatin infusion (Figure 5) or by administration of physiological replacement doses of insulin (68). In contrast, it is unlikely that counter-regulatory hormones are responsible for the delayed hyperglycemia inasmuch as prevention of the initial somatostatin-induced hypoglycemia by infusion of intravenous glucose fails to prevent the delayed hyperglycemia (68).

The findings with prolonged somatostatin indicate that hypoglycemia is only transient and that fasting hyperglycemia develops in circumstances of ongoing insulin deficiency in normal subjects despite persistent suppression of glucagon. Basal secretion of glucagon is, therefore, not essential for the development of the diabetic syndrome (fasting hyperglycemia) (68). A similar conclusion has been reached on the basis of observations in depancreatized patients (postpancreatectomy). Clinical diabetes with fasting hyperglycemia develops in this condition in the absence of detectable, circulating pancreatic glucagon (70). These findings support the conclusion that insulin deficiency rather than glucagon excess is the primary hormonal disturbance in the pathogenesis of diabetes mellitus.

The effects of prolonged administration of somatostatin have implications regarding its potential usefulness in the treatment of diabetes. In addition to maturity-onset diabetes, residual endogenous insulin secretion has been demonstrated in many juvenile-onset diabetics (71). To the extent that prolonged administration of somatostatin induces fasting hyperglycemia in normal subjects, intensification rather than amelioration of diabetes may occur with prolonged infusion in patients with residual insulin secretion. Recent studies in our laboratory have in fact demonstrated that prolonged somatostatin administration in maturity-onset diabetics results in worsening of diabetic control (72).

The observation that somatostatin has a salutory effect in reducing postprandial hyperglycemia in diabetes (52) is seemingly at odds with the above data demonstrating the hyperglycemic effects of somatostatin on fasting blood glucose levels. The explanation for these apparently conflicting findings becomes evident, however, when the effects of somatostatin on oral and intravenous glucose tolerance and on xylose tolerance are examined in diabetic patients (73). Whereas infusion of somatostatin markedly blunts the rise in blood glucose after oral glucose administration, intravenous glucose tolerance is unchanged by somatostatin despite comparable inhibition of glucagon secretion (73). This dissociation between oral and intravenous glucose tolerance raised the possibility of an effect on carbohydrate absorption. Indeed, somatostatin dramatically reduced blood xylose levels after ingestion of this pentose, and the peak increment was delayed by 1–2 hr (73). Administration of glucagon (3 ng/kg/min) or intraduodenal administration of xylose failed to reverse the effect of somatostatin on xylose absorption. These observations suggest that somatostatin reduces postprandial hyperglycemia in diabetes primarily by decreasing and/or delaying carbohydrate absorption, rather than by enhancing carbohydrate disposal. The failure to improve glucose disposal provides further evidence for the primary role of insulin deficiency rather than glucagon excess in the pathogenesis of glucose intolerance in diabetes.

ALTERED SENSITIVITY TO GLUCAGON IN UREMIA

In addition to the importance of insulin deficiency, recent studies suggest that under certain circumstances altered tissue responsiveness to glucagon may contribute to the diabetogenic effect of this hormone. The importance of augmented tissue sensitivity to glucagon in the pathogenesis of glucose intolerance is suggested by observations in uremic man (23). Chronic renal failure is characterized by an increased incidence of glucose intolerance (74), insulin resistance (75, 76), and a 3–4-fold increase in circulating glucagon (3, 21, 23). Following chronic dialysis, glucose tolerance and insulin sensitivity return to normal (75) in the absence of changes in plasma glucagon (21, 23). On the basis of these observations, hyperglucagonemia did not appear to contribute to uremia-induced glucose intolerance. However, the role of glucagon in uremia is evident when tissue responsiveness to this hormone is examined. When glucagon is infused to uremic subjects (nondialyzed) in physiological doses, the glycemic effect is increased 3–4-fold when compared to healthy controls (23) (Figure 6). Furthermore, a direct linear correlation is observed between performance on glucose tolerance testing and the glycemic response to glucagon infusion (23). This augmented glycemic response to glucagon returns to normal following dialysis (Figure 6), thereby accounting for improved glucose tolerance despite persistence of the hyperglucagonemia (23). Recent studies with the use of the uremic rat model provide a cellular mechanism for these changes in responsiveness to glucagon. In 70% and 90% nephrectomized rats, glucagon binding to liver membranes and cyclic AMP generation in response to glucagon are increased 2–3-fold (77). Thus, changes in glucagon responsiveness in uremia may result from augmented binding of this hormone by target cells. These findings provide evidence of an important role of glucagon receptors in a syndrome of carbohydrate intolerance.

GLUCAGON-INSULIN INTERACTIONS IN KETONE METABOLISM

The development of ketosis in diabetes and fasting is a consequence of three distinct metabolic events: 1) increased delivery of free fatty acids from adipose tissue to the liver; 2) hepatic conversion of free fatty acids to ketone acids rather than triglycerides (ketogenic capacity) (78); and 3) a reduction in ketone utilization by peripheral tissues (79). Activation of both steps 1 and 2 appears to be a prerequisite for the development ketosis, whereas step 3 influences the magni-

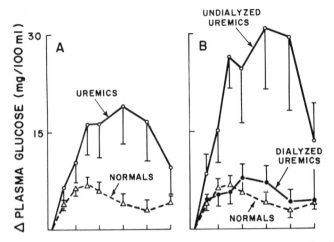

Figure 6. The glycemic response to physiological doses of glucagon (3 ng/kg/min) in undialyzed and dialyzed uremic patients and in healthy control subjects. In the undialyzed uremics, sensitivity to the hyperglycemic effect of glucagon is increased and returns to normal after dialysis. Based on the data of Sherwin et al. (23).

tude of the hyperketonemic response. The essential role for insulin deficiency in all ketotic states derives from the important influence of this hormone on lipolysis (80) as well as on ketone turnover (79). In addition, the ketogenic capacity of the liver may be affected by insulin deficiency inasmuch as in vivo administration of anti-insulin serum enhances the ability of rat livers to synthesize ketones when perfused with oleic acid (78).

The contribution of glucagon to hyperketonemia derives solely from the effect of this hormone on the ketogenic capacity of the liver (78). Livers obtained from rats given physiological doses of glucagon demonstrate augmented ketone production from oleic acid, despite the absence of detectable increments in plasma free fatty acids (78). On the basis of these findings a bihormonal hypothesis similar to that proposed by Unger and co-workers (47, 48) for glucose homeostasis has been suggested for the control of ketone body production (81). Ketosis, according to this concept, results from increased mobilization of free fatty acids secondary to insulin deficiency, coupled with simultaneous enhancement of the capacity of the liver to convert these substrates to ketones as a consequence of glucagon excess (81). Support for this concept derives from observations with somatostatin. Administration of this agent to acutely insulin-withdrawn, juvenile-onset diabetics markedly delays and reduces the magnitude of hyperketonemia (53).

Other studies have, however, cast doubt on the primacy or essentiality of glucagon in the development or maintenance of hyperketonemia. Schade and Eaton (82) infused glucagon into normal subjects at a rate of 3 ng/kg/min to produce hyperglucagonemia and after 30 min induced marked elevations of plasma free fatty acid concentration by administration of heparin. Despite physiological increments in plasma glucagon (300 pg/ml) and marked increases in free fatty acids and despite stable insulin levels, plasma ketones failed to exceed concentrations observed during a saline solution control infusion (82). These observations suggest that hyperglucagonemia, even in the presence of elevated free fatty acids, cannot of itself bring about hyperketonemia in normal man (82). It is of interest in this regard that patients with the glucagonoma syndrome in which plasma glucagon levels of 1,000–3,000 pg/ml are achieved characteristically do not develop hyperketonemia even when diabetes is present (57).

With respect to the ketogenic role of glucagon in diabetes, pharmacological infusions of exogenous glucagon stimulate splanchnic ketone production by 75–90% (83). However, increases in blood ketones have not been observed in diabetics in whom insulin is available when physiological doses of this hormone have been employed (34). Prolonged (2–4 days) physiological increments in plasma glucagon have no effect on ketosis in maturity-onset diabetes and in juvenile-onset diabetes treated with insulin (34). Furthermore, in patients with already manifest diabetic ketoacidosis, glucagon suppression by somatostatin fails to diminish ketosis or to improve the response to insulin (84). On the other hand, a diabetogenic effect of physiological hyperglucagonemia is demonstrable in insulin-deficient diabetics when simultaneous elevations in plasma free fatty acids are induced by heparin administration (85). In contrast to normal subjects, diabetic patients receiving glucagon demonstrate a 3–4-fold greater increment in blood ketones after plasma free fatty acids are increased to 1.5–2 mM (85). These findings suggest that hyperglucagonemia is insufficient to cause augmented ketone production in normal man (even if free fatty acid delivery is increased) or in diabetics in whom insulin is available. Glucagon can, however, bring about a worsening of the ketotic state in circumstances of absolute insulin lack. Overall, the prime factor governing the severity of ketoacidosis in diabetes appears to be insulin deficiency rather than glucagon excess.

REFERENCES

1. Unger, R. H., Aguilar-Parada, E., Müller, W. A., and Eisentraut, A. M. (1970). Studies of pancreatic alpha cell function in normal and diabetic subjects. J. Clin. Invest. 49:837.
2. Valverde, I., Villaneuva, M. L., Lazano, I., and Marco, J. (1974). Presence of glucagon immunoreactivity in the globulin fraction of human plasma (big plasma glucagon). J. Clin. Endocrinol. Metab. 39:1090.
3. Kuku, S. F., Jaspan, J. B., Emmanouel, D. S., Zeidler, A., Katx, A. L., and Rubinstein, A. H. (1976). Heterogeneity of plasma glucagon: circulating components in normal subjects and patients with chronic renal failure. J. Clin. Invest. 58:742.
4. Weir, G. C., Knowlton, S. D., and Martin, D. B. (1975). High molecular weight glucagon-like immunoreactivity in plasma. J. Clin. Endocrinol. Metab. 40:296.

5. Recant, L., Perrino, P. V., Bhathena, S. J., Danforth, D. N., Jr., and Lavine, R. L. (1976). Plasma immunoreactive glucagon fractions in four cases of glucagonoma: increased "large glucagon-immunoreactivity." Diabetologia 12:319.
6. Fisher, M., Sherwin, R. S., Hendler, R., and Felig, P. (1976). Kinetics of glucagon in man: effects of starvation. Proc. Natl. Acad. Sci. U. S. A. 73:1735.
7. Felig, P., Gusberg, R., Hendler, R., Gump, F. E., and Kinney, J. M. (1974). Concentration of glucagon and the insulin: glucagon ratio in the portal and peripheral circulation. Proc. Soc. Exp. Biol. Med. 147:88.
8. Blackard, W. G., Nelson, N. C., and Andrews, S. S. (1974). Portal and peripheral vein immunoreactive glucagon concentrations after arginine or glucose infusions. Diabetes 23:199.
9. Tasaka, Y., Sekine, M., Wakatsuki, M., Lhgawara, H., and Shizume, K. (1975). Levels of pancreatic glucagon, insulin and glucose during twenty-four hours of the day in normal subjects. Horm. Metab. Res. 7:205.
10. Unger, R. H., Ohneda, A., Aguilar-Parada, E., and Eisentraut, A. M. (1969). The role of aminogenic glucagon secretion in blood glucose homeostasis. J. Clin. Invest. 48:810.
11. Müller, W. A., Faloona, G. R., Aguilar-Parada, E., and Unger, R. H. (1970). Abnormal alpha-cell function in diabetes: response to carbohydrate and protein ingestion, N. Engl. J. Med. 283:109.
12. Ohneda, A., Aguilar-Parada, E., Eisentraut, A. M., and Unger, R. H. (1969). Control of pancreatic glucagon secretion by glucose. Diabetes 18:1.
13. Felig, P., Wahren, J., Hendler, R., and Ahlborg, G. (1972). Plasma glucagon levels in exercising man. N. Engl. J. Med. 287:184.
14. Wise, J. K., Hendler, R., and Felig, P. (1973). Influence of glucocorticoids on glucagon secretion and plasma amino acid concentrations in man. J. Clin. Invest. 52:2774.
15. Frohman, L. A., and Bernardis, L. L. (1971). Effect of hypothalamic stimulation on plasma glucose, insulin, and glucagon levels. Am. J. Physiol. 221:1596.
16. Gerich, J. E., Langlois, M., Noacco, C., Schneider, V., and Forsham, P. H. (1974). Adrenergic modulation of pancreatic glucagon secretion in man. J. Clin. Invest. 53:1441.
17. Lefebvre, P. J., Luyckx, A. S., and Nizet, A. H. (1974). Renal handling of endogenous glucagon in the dog: comparison with insulin. Metabolism 23:753.
18. Forrest, J. N., Fisher, M., Hendler, R., Sherwin, R., and Felig, P. (1976). Contrasting roles of the kidney in the disposal and hormonal action of physiologic concentrations of glucagon. Clin. Res. 24:400A.
19. Bastl, C., Finkelstein, F. A., Sherwin, R. S., Hendler, R., Felig, P., and Hayslett, J. R. Renal extraction of glucagon in rats with normal and reduced renal function. Am. J. Physiol. In press.
20. Lefebvre, P. J., Luyckx, A. S., and Nizet, A. H. (1974). Kidney function as a major factor regulating peripheral glucagon levels. Diabetes (Suppl. 1) 23:343.
21. Bilbrey, G. L., Faloona, G. R., White, M. G., and Knochel, J. P. (1974). Hyperglucagonemia of renal failure. J. Clin. Invest. 53:841.
22. Bilbrey, G. L., Faloona, G. R., White, M. G., Atkins, C., Hull, A. R., and Knochel, J. (1975). Hyperglucagonemia in uremia: reversal by renal transplantation. Ann. Intern. Med. 82:525.

23. Sherwin, R. S., Bastl, C., Finkelstein, F. O., Fisher, M., Black, H., Hendler, R., and Felig, P. (1976). Influence of uremia and hemodialysis on the turnover and metabolic effects of glucagon. J. Clin. Invest. 57:722
24. Lindsey, A., Santeusania, F., Braaten, J., Faloona, G. R., and Unger, R. H. (1974). Pancreatic alpha-cell function in trauma. JAMA 227:757.
25. Willerson, J. T., Hutcheson, D. R., Leshin, S. J., Faloona, G. R., and Unger, R. H. Serum glucagon and insulin levels and their relationship to blood glucose values in patients with acute myocardial infarction and acute coronary insufficiency. Am. J. Med. 57:747.
26. Müller, W. A., Faloona, G. R., and Unger, R. H. (1973). Hyperglucagonemia in diabetic ketoacidosis: its prevalence and significance. Am. J. Med. 54:52.
27. Lindsey, C. A., Faloona, G. R., and Unger, R. H. (1974). Plasma glucagon in nonketotic hyperosmolar coma. JAMA 229:1771.
28. Duckworth, W. C., Heineman, C. M., and Kemp, K. (1975). Insulin and glucagon degradation by kidney. Clin. Res. 23:318A.
29. Charles, M. A., Imagawa, W., Forsham, P. H., and Grodsky, G. M. (1976). Islet transplantation into rat liver: in vitro secretion of insulin from the isolated perfused liver and in vivo glucagon suppression. Endocrinology 98:738.
30. Sherwin, R., Fisher, M., Bessoff, J., Synder, N., Hendler, R., Conn, H. O., and Felig, P. (1976). Glucagon in cirrhosis: altered secretion and sensitivity and evidence of a feedback relationship. Clin. Res. 24:487A.
31. Marliss, E. B., Aoki, T. T., Unger, R. H., Soeldner, J. B., and Cahill, G. F., Jr. (1970). Glucagon levels and metabolic effects in fasting man. J. Clin. Invest. 49:2256.
32. Park, C. R., and Exton, J. H. (1972). Glucagon and the metabolism of glucose. In R. J. Lefebvre and R. H. Unger (eds.). Glucagon. Pergamon Press, Oxford.
33. Liljenquist, J. E., Bomboy, J. D., Lewis, S. B., Sinclair-Smith, B. C., Felts, P. W., Lacy, W. W., Crofford, O. B., and Liddle, G. W. (1974). Effect of glucagon on net splanchnic cyclic AMP production in normal and diabetic man. J. Clin. Invest. 53:198.
34. Sherwin, R. S., Fisher, M., Hendler, R., and Felig, P. (1976). Hyperglucagonemia and blood glucose regulation in normal, obese and diabetic subjects. N. Engl. J. Med. 294:455.
35. Felig, P., Wahren, J., and Hendler, R. (1976). Influence on physiologic hyperglucagonemia on basal and insulin-inhibited splanchnic glucose output in normal man. J. Clin. Invest. 58:761.
36. Sherwin, R., Wahren, J., and Felig, P. (1976). Evanescent effects of hypo and hyperglucagonemia on blood glucose homeostasis. Metabolism (Suppl. 1) 25:1381.
37. Sherwin, R. S., Kramer, K. J., Tobin, J. D., Insel, P. A., Liljenquist, J. E., Berman, M., and Andres, R. (1974). A model of the kinetics of insulin in man. J. Clin. Invest. 53:1481.
38. Insel, P. A., Liljenquist, J. E., Tobin, J. D., Sherwin, R. S., Watkins, P., Andres, R., and Berman, M. (1975). Insulin control of glucose metabolism in man: a new kinetic analysis. J. Clin. Invest. 55:1057.
39. Unger, R. H. (1974). Alpha- and beta-cell interrelationships in health and disease. Metabolism 23:581.
40. Felig, P., Wahren, J., and Hendler, R. (1975). Influence of oral glucose ingestion on splanchnic glucose and gluconeogenic substrate metabolism in man. Diabetes 24:468.

41. Sherwin, R., Joshi, P., Hendler, R., Felig, P., and Conn, H. O. (1974). Hyperglucagonemia in Laennec's cirrhosis: the role of portal-systemic shunting. N. Engl. J. Med. 290:239.
42. Unger, R. H. (1976). Glucagon and blood sugar. N. Engl. J. Med. 294:1239.
43. Service, F. S., Molnar, G. D., Rosevear, J. M., Ackerman, E., Gatewood, L. C., and Taylor, W. F. (1970). Mean amplitude of glycemic excursions, a measure of diabetic stability. Diabetes 19:644.
44. Felig, P., and Wahren, J. (1971). Influence of endogenous insulin secretion on splanchnic glucose and amino acid metabolism in man. J. Clin. Invest. 50:1702.
45. Wahren, J., Felig, P., and Hagenfeldt, L. (1976). Effect of protein ingestion on splanchnic and leg metabolism in normal man and in patients with diabetic mellitus. J. Clin. Invest. 57:987.
46. Garber, A. J., Cryer, P. E., Santiago, J. V., Haymond, M. W., Pagliara, A. S., and Kipnis, D. M. (1976). The role of adrenergic mechanisms in the substrate and hormonal response to insulin-induced hypoglycemia in man. J. Clin. Invest. 58:7.
47. Unger, R. H. (1976). Diabetes and the alpha cell. Diabetes 25:136.
48. Unger, R. H., and Orci, L. (1975). The essential role of glucagon in the pathogenesis of the endogenous hyperglycemia of diabetes. Lancet 1:14.
49. Wise, J. K., Hendler, R., and Felig, P. (1973). Evaluation of alpha-cell function by infusion of alanine in normal, diabetic and obese subjects. N. Engl. J. Med. 288:487.
50. Gerich, J. E., Tsalikian, E., Lorenzi, M., Karman, J. H., and Bier, D. M. (1975). Plasma glucagon and alanine responses to acute insulin deficiency in man. J. Clin. Endocrinol. Metab. 40:526.
51. Dobbs, R., Sakurai, H., Sasaki, H., Faloona, G., Valverde, I., Baetens, D., Orci, L., and Unger, R. (1975). Glucagon: role in the hyperglycemia of diabetes mellitus. Science 187:544.
52. Gerich, J. E., Lorenzi, M., Schneider, V., Karam, J. H., Rivier, J., Guillemin, R., and Forsham, P. H. (1974). Effects of somatostatin on plasma glucose and glucagon levels in human diabetes mellitus. N. Engl. J. Med. 291:544.
53. Gerich, J. E., Lorenzi, M., Bier, D. M., Schneider, V., Tsalikian, E., Karam, J. M., and Forsham, P. H. (1975). Prevention of human diabetic ketoacidosis by somatostatin: evidence for an essential role for glucagon. N. Engl. J. Med. 292:985.
54. Sherwin, R. S., Hendler, R., and Felig, P. (1977). Influence of physiologic hyperglucagonemia on urinary glucose, nitrogen, and electrolyte excretion in diabetes. Metabolism 26:53.
55. Raskin, P., and Unger, R. H. (1976). Effects of exogenous glucagon in insulin-treated diabetics. Diabetes 25 (Suppl. 1) 341.
56. Felig, P., and Sherwin, R. (1976). Glucagon and blood sugar. N. Engl. J. Med. 295:452.
57. Mallinson, C. N., Bloom, S. R., Warin, A. P., Salmon, P. R., and Cox, B. (1974). A glucagonoma syndrome. Lancet 2:1.
58. Brazeau, P., Vale, W., Burgus, R., Ling, N., Butcher, M., Rivier, J., and Guillemin, R. (1973). Hypothalamic polypeptide that inhibits the secretion of immunoreactive pituitary growth hormone. Science 179:77.
59. Orci, L., Baeten, D., and Rufener, C. (1975). Evidence for the D-cell of the pancreas secreting somatostatin. Horm. Metab. Res. 7:400.
60. Koerker, D., Ruch, W., Chideckel, E., Palmer, J., Goodner, C., Ensinck, J., and Gale, C. (1974). Somatostatin: hypothalamic inhibitor of the endocrine pancreas. Science 184:482.

61. Iversen, J. (1974). Inhibition of pancreatic glucagon release by somatostatin: in vitro. Scand. J. Clin. Lab. Invest. 33:125.
62. Leblanc, H., Anderson, J. R., Sigel, M. B., and Yen, S. S. C. (1974). Inhibitory action of somatostatin on pancreatic α and β cell functions. J. Clin. Endocrinol. Metab. 40:568.
63. Alberti, K. G., Christensen, S. E., Iversen, J., Hansen, A. P., Christensen, N. J., Sayer-Hansen, K., Lundbaek, K., and Orskov, H. (1973). Inhibition of insulin secretion by somatostatin. Lancet 2:1299.
64. Alford, F., Bloom, S., Nabarro, J., Hall, R., Besser, G., Coy, D., Kastin, A., and Schally, A. V. (1974). Glucagon control of fasting glucose in man. Lancet 2:974.
65. Gerich, J. E., Lorenzi, M., Hane, S., Gustafson, G., Guillemin, R., and Forsham, P. H. (1975). Evidence for a physiologic role of pancreatic glucagon in human glucose homeostasis: studies with somatostatin. Metabolism 24:175.
66. Altszuler, N., Gottlieb, Hampshire, J. (1976). Interaction of somatostatin, glucagon, and insulin on hepatic glucose output in the dog. Diabetes 25:116.
67. Gerich, J. E., Lorenzi, M., Bier, D. M., Tsalikian, E., Schneider, V., Karam, J. H., and Forsham, P. H. (1976). Effects of physiologic levels of glucagon and growth hormone on human carbohydrate and lipid metabolism: studies involving administration of exogenous hormone during suppression of endogenous hormone secretion with somatostatin. J. Clin. Invest. 57:875.
68. Sherwin, R. S., Hendler, R., DeFronzo, R. A., Wahren, J., and Felig. P. (1977). Glucose homeostasis during prolonged suppression of glucagon and insulin secretion by somatostatin. Proc. Natl. Acad. Sci. U. S. A. 74:348.
69. Wahren, J., Felig, P., Cerasi, E., and Luft, R. (1972). Splanchnic and peripheral glucose and amino acid metabolism in diabetes mellitus. J. Clin. Invest. 51:1870.
70. Barnes, A. J., and Bloom, S. R. (1976). Pancreatectomized man: a model for diabetes without glucagon. Lancet 1:219.
71. Block, M. B., Mako, M. E., Steiner, D. E., and Rubinstein, A. H. (1972). Circulating C-peptide immunoreactivity: studies in normals and diabetic patients. Diabetes 21:1013.
72. Sherwin, R., Tamborlane, W., Hendler, R., and Felig, P. (1977). Hyperglycemic effects of somatostatin in maturity onset diabetes and normal man: primacy of insulin deficiency rather than glucagon excess in diabetes. Clin. Res. 25:523A.
73. Wahren, J., and Felig, P. (1976). Influence of somatostatin on carbohydrate disposal and absorption in diabetes mellitus. Lancet 2:1213.
74. DeFronzo, R. A., Andres, R., Edgar, P., and Walker, W. G. (1973). Carbohydrate metabolism in uremia: a review. Medicine (Baltimore) 52:469.
75. Hampers, C. L., Soeldner, J. S., Doak, P. B., and Merrill, J. P. (1966). Effect of chronic renal failure and hemodialysis on carbohydrate metabolism. J. Clin. Invest. 45:1719.
76. Westervelt, F. B., Jr. (1969). Insulin effect in uremia. J. Lab. Clin. Med. 74:79.
77. Soman, V., and Felig, P. (1977). Altered glucagon and insulin binding to hepatic receptors: Cellular mechanism of glucose intolerance in uremia. Clin. Res. 25:401A.
78. McGarry, J. D., Wright, P., and Foster, D. (1975). Hormonal control of

ketogenesis: rapid activation of hepatic ketogenic capacity in fed rats by anti-insulin serum and glucagon. J. Clin. Invest. 55:1202.
79. Sherwin, R. S., Hendler, R. G., and Felig, P. (1976). Effect of diabetes mellitus and insulin on the turnover and metabolic response to ketones in man. Diabetes 25:776.
80. Foster, D. W. (1967). Studies in the ketosis of fasting. J. Clin. Invest. 46:1283.
81. McGarry, J. D., and Foster, D. W. (1977). Hormonal control of ketogenesis: biochemical considerations. Arch. Intern. Med. 137:495.
82. Schade, D. S., and Eaton, R. P. (1976). Modulation of fatty acid metabolism by glucagon in man. IV. Effects of a physiologic hormone infusion in normal man. Diabetes 25:978.
83. Liljenquist, J. E., Bomboy, J. D., Lewis, S. B., Sinclair-Smith, B. C., Felts, P. W., Lacy, W. W., Crofford, O. B., and Liddle, G. W. (1974). Effects of glucagon on lipolysis and ketogenesis in normal and diabetic men. J. Clin. Invest. 53:190.
84. Lundbaek, K., Hansen, A., Orskov, H., Christensen, S., Iversen, J., Sayer-Hansen, K., Alberti, S., and Whitefoot, R. (1976). Failure of somatostatin to correct manifest diabetic ketoacidosis. Lancet 1:215.
85. Schade, D. S., and Eaton, R. P. (1975). Glucagon regulation of plasma ketone body concentration in human diabetes. J. Clin. Invest. 56:1340.

International Review of Physiology
Endocrine Physiology II, Volume 16
Edited by S. M. McCann
Copyright 1977　　　University Park Press　　　Baltimore

5

The Hormonal Control of Sodium Excretion

F. G. KNOX and J. A. DIAZ-BUXO

Mayo Medical School, Rochester, Minnesota

The hormonal control of sodium excretion by the kidneys involves the extrarenal modulation of hormone levels in the blood and the intrarenal response of the kidneys. The extrarenal control of hormone activity, of which regulation of aldosterone secretion is the most important, was emphasized by Reid and Ganong (1) in the first edition of this series. In the present chapter, the emphasis will be on the intrarenal regulation of sodium excretion.

The renal excretion of sodium is the net result of two basic processes, the formation of an ultrafiltrate of plasma at the glomerulus and the ultimate reabsorption of most of that filtrate by the renal tubules. Although filtration is an obvious prerequisite for sodium excretion and, therefore, important in renal failure, it is probably not an important factor in the normal regulation of sodium excretion. Lindheimer et al. (2) showed that marked increases in filtration rate were accompanied by trivial and statistically significant increases in sodium excretion. Furthermore, DeWardener et al. (3, 4) showed that the natriuresis of saline loading could be maintained after reduction of glomerular filtration rate to values below those in hydropenia.

REGULATION OF SODIUM REABSORPTION BY PROXIMAL TUBULE

The bulk of glomerular filtrate, 70–80%, is reabsorbed in the proximal tubule; however, the role of the proximal tubule in the regulation of sodium excretion is relatively small. This conclusion contrasts with earlier interpretations indicating a major role for the proximal tubule in the regulation of sodium excretion. Dirks et al. (5) showed that, in the dog, intravenous infusions of isotonic saline solution significantly decreased sodium reabsorption by the proximal tubule. The resulting increases in sodium delivery from the proximal tubule were more than sufficient to account for the increases in sodium excretion in the urine. It, therefore, was accepted that a decrease in sodium reabsorption by the proximal tubule was the mechanism by which sodium excretion increased after saline solution infusions. Defects in this mechanism have been held responsible for the sodium retention in edema states (6). The role of the proximal tubule was questioned, however, after it had been shown that marked decreases in sodium reabsorption by the proximal tubule were not accompanied by a pronounced increase in sodium excretion. In these studies by Howards and associates (7), infusion of hyperoncotic albumin solution decreased sodium reabsorption by the proximal tubule with only a very small increase in sodium excretion. Similarly, Knox et al. (8) and Burke et al. (9) demonstrated decreased sodium reabsorption by the proximal tubule after hemodilution without significant changes in sodium excretion. Finally, Knox et al. (10) demonstrated that increased delivery of sodium from the proximal tubule is not a prerequisite for the natriuresis of saline loading. In these three-part experiments, Ringer's infusion decreased sodium reabsorption by the proximal tubule and markedly increased sodium excretion. Albumin was then infused into the renal artery; through an oncotic effect in the peritubule microcirculation, sodium reabsorption was restored to below hydropenic control levels. Despite a restoration of proximal sodium reabsorption to below control levels, natriuresis was sustained (Figure 1). Since

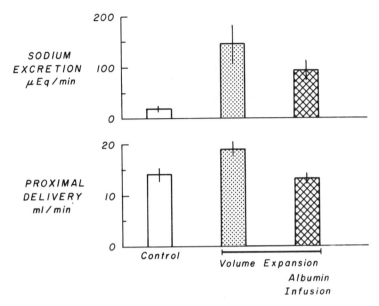

Figure 1. Effect of volume expansion on sodium excretion in the presence and absence of increased delivery from the proximal tubule (six dogs ± SE).

approximately 70% of the natriuresis of volume expansion persisted despite the absence of increased delivery from the proximal tubule, it was concluded that the proximal tubule plays a relatively minor role in the mediation of the increased sodium excretion accompanying volume expansion. Willis et al. (11) compared two groups of dogs with approximately 300 mEq differences in sodium balance and found no difference in sodium reabsorption by the proximal tubule.

The role of the proximal tubule in the pathogenesis of sodium retention has also been extensively studied. Continued sodium retention is a feature of models of heart failure and is characterized by the inability to excrete a saline load. Schneider et al. (12) have evaluated the role of the proximal tubule in dogs in which aorta-vena cava (AV) fistulas were created in order to produce high output heart failure. These dogs retained virtually all the dietary intake of sodium and became grossly edematous. Sodium reabsorption by the proximal tubule did not differ significantly from that of control animals. Furthermore, when saline solution was infused, the normal inhibition of proximal reabsorption occurred so that delivery from the proximal tubule was markedly increased, yet sodium excretion was increased very little. Stumpe and associates (13) reported similar findings in rats with AV fistulas. Auld et al. (14) and Levy (15) also found that sodium reabsorption by the proximal tubule was not significantly altered in dogs with chronic sodium retention due to obstruction of the thoracic vena cava. Thus, these findings illustrate the limited importance of the proximal tubule in the final regulation of sodium excretion.

Physical Factors

Although alterations in oncotic and hydrostatic forces in the peritubular micro-circulation have been conclusively shown to affect sodium reabsorption by the proximal tubule (16–18), recent studies by Ott et al. (19) show that volume expansion is a prerequisite for this effect. In contrast to results in volume-expanded dogs, increases in peritubular oncotic pressure had no effect in hydropenic dogs. Similarly, Strandhoy et al. (20) have shown that increases in hydrostatic pressures in peritubular capillaries had no effect on sodium reabsorption by the proximal tubule in hydropenic dogs. Thus, peritubular physical factors may play only a minor role in the normal regulation of sodium reabsorption by the proximal tubule.

Hormonal Regulation

In addressing the role of hormones in the regulation of sodium reabsorption by the proximal tubule, it is interesting to note that those hormones known to regulate sodium transport per se, for example, aldosterone, have no effect on sodium reabsorption by the proximal tubule. Aldosterone-stimulated sodium reabsorption in the proximal tubule has been reported in rats (21–29). However, Lynch et al. (28) and Martin and Berliner (29) were unable to find any effects of mineralocorticoids on sodium reabsorption in the proximal tubules of adrenalectomized dogs and rats, respectively, even though urinary sodium and potassium excretion rates were affected. It may be that the impaired sodium reabsorption in the proximal tubules of adrenalectomized rats observed by Hierholzer (22) reflected the general deterioration of the hemodynamic state associated with adrenalectomy. Similarly, Lowitz et al. (30) found no effect of angiotensin II on sodium reabsorption by the proximal tubule.

In contrast, those hormones primarily regulating anion reabsorption in the proximal tubule have significant effects on sodium reabsorption. For example, parathyroid hormone modulates fluid reabsorption by the proximal tubules through the regulation of anion transport (31–34).

These findings do not mean that parathyroid hormone is important in the final regulation of sodium excretion. What they do indicate is that the humoral regulation of anion reabsorption has secondary effects on proximal sodium reabsorption. Agus et al. (31) have shown that the increased delivery of sodium from the proximal tubule is almost completely reabsorbed in the distal nephron segments. Thus, consideration of parathyroid hormone is of particular interest in the regulation of sodium reabsorption by the proximal tubule but not for final regulation of sodium excretion.

Parathyroid hormone decreases isotonic reabsorption by the proximal tubule perhaps secondary to the regulation of phosphate and bicarbonate transport. Recent studies indicate that the normal regulation of phosphate reabsorption by parathyroid hormone occurs in part by an alteration in the phosphate concentration achieved in the proximal tubule (31–35). These primary alterations in phosphate regulation may secondarily affect sodium reabsorption by the proximal tubule.

Parathyroid hormone has also been postulated to inhibit the proximal tubular reabsorption of bicarbonate since the hormone causes a bicarbonaturia (36–38). In support of this thesis, there is a qualitative similarity between the alterations of the proximal tubular reabsorption of sodium, phosphate, and water after parathyroid hormone (PTH) administration and after administration of acetazolamide, a carbonic anhydrase inhibitor. Beck and Goldberg (39) administered acetazolamide to thyroparathyroidectomized dogs and found an inhibition of sodium, phosphate, and water reabsorption in the proximal tubule. They concluded that acetazolamide has an inhibitory effect on electrolyte reabsorption by the proximal tubule much like that of PTH.

Beck and co-workers (40) observed that PTH inhibited carbonic anhydrase specifically in renal cortex in vitro, possibly through the cyclic AMP system. They and Bank et al. (41) suggested that the inhibition of proximal tubular reabsorption of sodium, bicarbonate, phosphate, and water after the administration of PTH might be at least in part mediated through the subsequent increases in intraluminal pH.

Although the precise mechanisms involved are in need of further study, it is clear that parathyroid hormone inhibits sodium reabsorption by the proximal tubule. Furthermore, the effects of the hormone are probably mediated through the adenylate cyclase system, as supported by a review edited by Talmage and Belanger (42). Indeed, both micropuncture and clearance studies have demonstrated that infusion of dibutyrl cyclic AMP results in inhibition of sodium and phosphate reabsorption by the proximal tubule (31).

REGULATION OF SODIUM REABSORPTION IN LOOP OF HENLE

Much of the increased delivery of sodium from the proximal tubule is reabsorbed in the loop of Henle. The primary driving force for reabsorption in the ascending limb of the loop of Henle is active chloride transport with sodium following passively (43). Landwehr et al. (44) reported increased fractional and absolute reabsorption of sodium in the loop of Henle after infusion of saline solution in the rat. Dirks and Seely (45) found no change in fractional reabsorption but did find increased absolute sodium reabsorption after saline loading in the dog.

Stein et al. (46) also found enhanced sodium reabsorption in the loop of Henle after volume expansion in the rat. Microperfusion studies by Morgan and Berliner (47) indicate that sodium transport in the loop of Henle responds to load and is not affected by changes in extracellular fluid volume per se.

Sodium reabsorption by the loop of Henle is increased in models of chronic sodium retention. Stumpe et al. (13) found increased loop reabsorption in rats with AV fistulas, and Levy (15) found increased loop reabsorption in dogs with chronic obstruction of the vena cava. Stein and Reineck (48) have pointed out that in both of these studies arterial blood pressure was significantly reduced. When considered in light of studies showing decreased loop reabsorption in hypertension (49, 50), these studies suggest an inverse relationship between arterial blood pressure and reabsorption by the loop of Henle.

These findings suggest that it is not necessary to postulate a role for hormones in the regulation of sodium reabsorption by the loop of Henle. In contrast, evidence of effects of mineralocorticoids on the excretion of solute-free water, the concentration of urine, and the development of corticomedullary concentration gradients has been interpreted to indicate effects on the ascending limb of the loop of Henle (51–53). However, no direct evidence exists for an effect of mineralocorticoids on the loop of Henle. Furthermore, the recent demonstration of the marked diluting capacity of the collecting duct obviates the necessity to postulate an effect of aldosterone on the loop to account for changes in urine concentration and free water excretion (54). Thus, the major role for the loop of Henle in regulation of sodium excretion is to buffer the increased delivery of sodium from the proximal tubule.

REGULATION OF SODIUM REABSORPTION BY DISTAL CONVOLUTED TUBULE

In the distal convoluted tubule, the primary driving force is active sodium transport (55). In other respects, the transport characteristics resemble the loop of Henle. Strieder et al. (56), and Knox and Gasser (57) found increased absolute, but decreased fractional, reabsorption along the distal tubule after Ringer's infusions. In micropuncture studies, Morgan and Berliner (47) found that the rate of sodium reabsorption paralleled the rate of delivery of sodium to the distal tubule.

The commonly held concept that a principal, if not only, site of action of aldosterone is the distal tubule is open to serious question. As discussed subsequently, aldosterone has a marked effect on sodium transport in the collecting system. Studies by Vander et al. (58, 59) with the use of stop-flow techniques identified the distal nephron as a principal site of action of aldosterone. However, in light of more recent evidence indicating the collecting system as a site of urinary dilution, these data can be reinterpreted to define the site of action of aldosterone in the collecting system. Micropuncture studies by Hierholzer and associates (60) reported that the ability of the late distal tubule to establish concentration gradients for sodium was diminished in adrenalectomized rats. Two considerations of these studies are important. First, data from the adrenalectomized rats were compared with intact rats. It is possible that differences in blood pressure between the groups of rats due to the adrenalectomy are responsible for the results rather than direct effects of the hormone on transport. Second, Woodhall and Tisher (61) have recently shown that the late distal tubule, as identified by micropuncture localization techniques, is often the cortical collecting duct when identified with histological techniques. Furthermore, Malnic et al. (62) have shown that dietary sodium depletion, which would be expected to increase aldosterone concentrations in the blood, does not alter sodium concentrations in the distal tubule as might be expected. Finally, recent studies of isolated perfused tubules by Gross et al. (63) indicate that mineralocorticoids have no effect on the distal convoluted tubule.

REGULATION OF COLLECTING DUCT SODIUM REABSORPTION

The primary driving force for reabsorption in the collecting duct is active sodium transport. Hilger et al. (64) and Jamison et al. (65) clearly demonstrated the sodium reabsorptive capacity of the papillary collecting duct. Windhager (66), Laurence and Marsh (67), and Rau and Frömter (68, 69) have demonstrated that the reabsorption of sodium occurs against an electrochemical gradient in the papillary collecting duct. The cortical collecting duct has similar transport properties as demonstrated with the isolated tubule preparation (70–73).

The response of the collecting system to increased delivery of sodium is similar to that of more proximal nephron segments. Diezi et al. (74) have shown that after volume expansion fractional sodium reabsorption decreases and absolute sodium reabsorption increases. Stein et al. (46) and Knox and Gasser (57) have demonstrated diminished sodium reabsorption in the collecting duct after Ringer's infusion when compared with a similar delivery of sodium after albumin infusion. Sonnenberg (75) and Stein et al. (76) have also reported inhibited sodium reabsorption by the collecting duct after chronic volume expansion.

Gross et al. (63), using the isolated tubule, have shown a significant effect of mineralocorticoids on the cortical collecting duct. Diezi and colleagues (74) concluded that the enhanced sodium reabsorption by the papillary collecting duct in sodium-deprived rats was due to effects of aldosterone. Furthermore, Uhlich et al. (77) have provided direct evidence for a stimulatory effect of the mineralocorticoids on sodium reabsorption at the level of the papillary collecting ducts (Figure 2). In these studies, aldosterone administration mimicked the

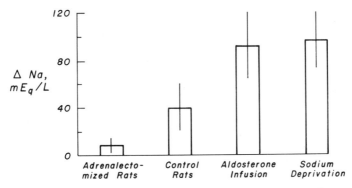

Figure 2. Effect of aldosterone on transtubule sodium gradients across papillary collecting duct. Data from Uhlich et al. (77).

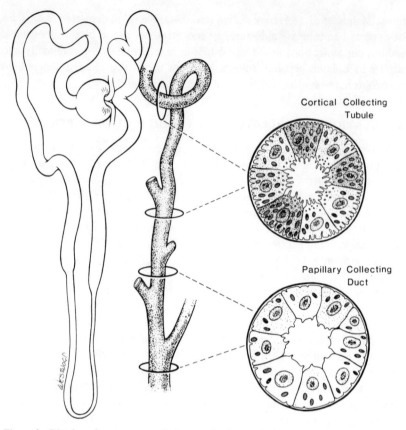

Figure 3. Distal nephron segments important in the regulation of sodium excretion.

effect of a low salt diet on the sodium concentration gradient across the papillary duct. It was concluded that aldosterone increased the intrinsic capacity of the collecting duct to reabsorb sodium and decreased the backleak of sodium from interstitium to tubule lumen. These findings indicate that the collecting system may be the primary site of action of mineralocorticoids on sodium transport (Figure 3).

HORMONAL REGULATION OF SODIUM EXCRETION

Mineralocorticoids

Aldosterone plays a central role in the hormonal regulation of sodium transport. The effects of aldosterone to decrease sodium excretion were described by Barger et al. in 1958 (78). The intracellular mechanism of action has been extensively reviewed elsewhere (79–81).

In brief, aldosterone binds to cytoplasmic receptors, and the resultant complex is then transferred to the nucleus where it binds to chromatin acceptor sites (82–85). Induction of RNA and protein synthesis at the transcriptional level are apparently necessary for stimulation of sodium transport (86, 87). These phenomena may account for the full effect of administered aldosterone on sodium transport in adrenalectomized animals (87).

Mineralocorticoids have been recognized as mediators of hypertension through their sodium-retaining effects. However, actual measurements of aldosterone and other known mineralocorticoids have failed to document elevated levels of these steroids in the pathogenesis of low renin hypertension in most of these patients. Nevertheless, patients with low renin hypertension share characteristics similar to hyperaldosteronism (88). Thus, aminoglutethimide, an inhibitor of adrenal steroid biosynthesis, decreases blood pressure in these patients, whereas patients with normal renin essential hypertension had no effect from the drug (89). In addition, low renin essential hypertensives have significantly higher exchangeable body sodium than patients with normal renal essential hypertension (90). Similarly, treatment with spironolactone, an antagonist of mineralocorticoids, decreases the blood pressure of patients with low renin essential hypertension. Finally, patients with low renin hypertension showed decreased blood pressure following adrenalectomy.

Patients with this syndrome, unlike most patients with currently recognized hypermineralocorticoid syndrome, i.e., primary aldosteronism, hypertensive congenital adrenal hyperplasia, licorice intoxication, etc., are usually not hypokalemic (90), nor do they have a measurable reduction in total body potassium (89).

The role of mineralocorticoids in regulating collecting duct potassium transport has not been clearly established. Although it is widely held that aldosterone stimulates potassium secretion, Malnic et al. (62) found net potassium reabsorption by the collecting duct of sodium-depleted animals in which aldosterone was presumably elevated. Similarly, Diezi et al. (74) found potassium reabsorption in the papillary collecting duct of sodium-depleted rats. These authors speculated that net potassium reabsorption might occur in sodium-depleted animals as a result of decreased delivery of sodium to the papillary collecting duct. In support of this concept, in the isolated cortical collecting tubule, potassium secretion was dependent upon sodium reabsorption (70). On the other hand, Stewart (91) has concluded from genetic studies in mice that the effect of aldosterone on potassium excretion is separable from and not directly a consequence of sodium retention. Thus, it is possible that a mineralocorticoid with sodium-retaining properties, but without potassium-losing properties, is responsible for low renin essential hypertension.

Sennett and co-workers (92) have recently isolated a new mineralocorticoid from the urine of patients with low renin hypertension. In these studies, urine extracts were assayed for mineralocorticoid activity in adrenalectomized rats. More activity was found than could be accounted for by the known mineralocorticoids. The factor responsible for the remaining activity was identified as 16β-hydroxydehydroepiandrosterone (16β-OH-DHEA). Synthetic 16β-OH-DHEA had a mineralocorticoid potency of approximately one-fortieth that of aldosterone, as tested with bioassay procedures. Although the urinary Na to K ratio was decreased following 16β-OH-DHEA, specific effects on potassium secretion were not differentiated from an effect primarily on sodium reabsorption.

Although only recently identified as a mineralocorticoid, 16β-OH-DHEA was first identified in human infant urine in 1968 (93). In addition, an isomer of 16β-OH-DHEA, 16-oxoandrostenediol, has also been found to have mineralocorticoid activity in adrenalectomized rats and is found in infant urine.

Recently, another 16-oxygenated steroid, 16α,18-dihydroxydeoxycorticosterone (16α,18-OH-DOC), has been implicated in the pathogenesis of low renin essential hypertension (94). Large amounts of this steroid were formed when 18-OH-DOC was incubated with adrenal tissue obtained from two patients with low renin essential hypertension, whereas only minimal conversion occurred when 18-OH-DOC was incubated with normal adrenals. This steroid exerted no effect on sodium metabolism in adrenalectomized rats and in the toad bladder assay, but it markedly enhanced activity of subthreshold doses of aldosterone. Thus, this steroid may be important in the genesis of low renin hypertension, functioning as a positive allosteric effector of aldosterone. In addition, the effect of mineralocorticoids on potassium secretion may be altered by sex steroids. In experiments designed to investigate why pregnant women do not become hypokalemic despite markedly increased aldosterone, normal men were administered progesterone (95). Abolishment of 11-deoxycorticosterone acetate (DOCA)-induced kaliuresis was noted, whereas sodium excretion was virtually unaltered. Thus, another mechanism by which low renin essential hypertensives might remain normokalemic, even in the presence of excess mineralocorticoid activity, is that many essential hypertensives have elevated progesterone levels (96).

Estrogens

An association between estrogens and sodium metabolism has been suspected for many years. Clinical evidence pointing to this relationship includes premenstrual edema, edema of late pregnancy, and edema observed following administration of high doses of estrogenic compounds for the treatment of metastatic carcinoma. The interpretation of these data is difficult since during pregnancy and the premenstrual phase of the cycle both estrogen and progesterone secretions are increased. The possibility that the sodium and water retention seen in these circumstances may be mediated by increased secretion of mineralocorticoids has been considered (97). However, the fact that progesterone levels are concomitantly increased and progesterone itself may stimulate aldosterone production prevents definite conclusions. Additional evidence to suggest a mineralocorticoid-like effect of estrogen on sodium metabolism includes experiments by Rogoff and Stewart (98) in which pregnancy prolonged the survival of adrenalectomized dogs. However, Thorn and Engel (99) did not find estrogen or progesterone effective in prolonging the lives of adrenalectomized animals.

The possibility of a diminished filtered load of sodium as the potential factor responsible for sodium retention in estrogen excess has been raised by studies by

Richardson and Houck (100) in which a fall in glomerular filtration rate (GFR) was seen in intact dogs after estrogen administration. In the light of a constant plasma concentration of sodium, a diminished GFR will result in decreased filtered load with possibly enhanced sodium reabsorption. On the other hand, other studies have shown increases in GFR following administration of stilbesterol (101).

A third possibility to explain the sodium and fluid retention of estrogenic compounds is an extrarenal action of the hormone. Some have suggested that this may result from an increase in fluid content of the tissues in general (101, 102), and others have shown increased fluid transfer by the rat intestinal mucosa (103). These effects may or may not be mediated by mineralocorticoid action.

In man, the evidence suggests that estrogen produces a moderate sodium-retaining effect (104, 105). Whether this action is mediated through the renin-aldosterone system remains to be established. Some evidence exists to defend both positions. Crane and Harris (106) observed a significant increase in aldosterone secretion following a 1-week administration of estradiol, but falling values were observed by the 3rd week, suggesting a direct effect of estrogens on aldosterone secretion, at least during acute administration. However, long-term estrogenic stimulation has been shown to produce no rise in aldosterone secretion (107). Christy and Shaver (108), in a comprehensive review of this subject, propose that the best evidence against a role for estrogen-induced aldosteronism is that estrogen-induced sodium retention is not accompanied by increased urinary potassium excretion.

Progesterone

Progesterone may influence sodium metabolism through its influence on aldosterone secretion. Most of the information to date comes from observations during pregnancy, when progesterone secretion significantly increases aldosterone secretion rate. In normal pregnant women, Jones et al. (109) observed a direct correlation between excretion of pregnanediol in the urine and the secretion rate of aldosterone, and administration of progesterone is known to increase aldosterone secretion in normal males (110). The role of the increased secretion of aldosterone seen in pregnancy was addressed by Ehrlich and Lindheimer (111). They observed sodium retention in pregnant women after administration of mineralocorticoids and ACTH with a concomitant decrease in aldosterone excretion. Natriuresis was observed following discontinuance of exogenous steroids. These observations are in agreement with the concept of a physiological role of increased aldosterone production in pregnancy. However, at the renal level, Landau and Lugibihl (112) demonstrated inhibition of the sodium-retaining effects of aldosterone by progesterone.

A relationship between hypertension and oral contraceptives containing estrogen-progesterone combinations has been recognized for several years (113). Marked increases in renin-substrate concentration were soon noted in women on oral contraceptive therapy (113–115). Other reports have also provided evidence for an increase in plasma renin activity and aldosterone excretion rate (116–118) as a result of oral contraceptive therapy. However, the significance of these abnormalities in the development of arterial hypertension remains obscure in view of similar findings in women treated with oral contraceptives who remain normotensive (113). It is likely that estrogenic compounds and not progesterone are responsible for the increased synthesis of plasma renin substrate (117, 119–122). The mechanism by which estrogen stimulates the renin system has been investigated and the evidence to date points toward stimulation of hepatic biosynthesis of the substrate (122), which in turn may result in an elevation of plasma renin activity and accelerated angiotensinogen conversion (113, 117, 121, 122).

Angiotensin II

In addition to the role of angiotensin II in the regulation of aldosterone secretion, the peptide may have direct effects on sodium transport. However, the dose-related effect of angiotensin II on sodium excretion is exceedingly variable (123). In the rat, low doses decrease sodium excretion, whereas larger doses increase sodium excretion (124). In man, infusions of angiotensin reduce sodium excretion (125, 126). In addition, it has been difficult to distinguish between the possible direct effects on tubular transport of sodium from hemodynamic effects. Several studies support a direct effect of angiotensin, however. Leyssac et al. (127) found that angiotensin II inhibits active sodium efflux from renal cortical slices. Using the stop-flow technique, Vander (128) showed that angiotensin injected into the renal artery inhibited sodium transport in the distal nephron. Cuypers (129) found that angiotensin infused into the renal portal system in the chicken kidney caused an increase in sodium excretion from that kidney. Lowitz et al. (30) perfused peritubular capillaries with angiotensin II and found that distal tubular sodium reabsorption as measured with the split-drop technique was significantly reduced.

On the other hand, it is doubtful that angiotensin is directly responsible for sodium retention in those pathological conditions associated with high levels of circulating angiotensin. Spielman and colleagues (130) have shown that blockade of circulating angiotensin with angiotensin antagonists has little effect on sodium reabsorption. Specifically, Spielman et al. (130) have shown that blockade of angiotensin II in dogs with experimental high output heart failure and massive sodium retention does not significantly effect sodium excretion even though there were increases in renal blood flow associated with the angiotensin II blockade. Thus, although the trophic role of angiotensin II on aldosterone secretion is relatively clear in the regulation of sodium excretion, the role of a direct effect of the peptide has not been completely elucidated.

Prostaglandins

Prostaglandins may also have a role in the intrarenal regulation of sodium excretion. Prostaglandins have been isolated from the renal medulla and the renal medullary interstitial cells in particular (131). These cells can be grown in tissue culture and prostaglandin E_2 and neutral lipid precursor extracted from them. The interstitial cells, in turn, are strategically located adjacent to the collecting ducts, where they may play a role in regulation of sodium transport (132).

Johnston et al. (133) and Vander (134) have infused prostaglandin E_1 directly into the renal artery. Sodium excretion and total renal blood flow rose although glomerular filtration rate did not change. Similarly, Strandhoy and co-workers (20) have infused prostaglandin E_2 in the renal artery and found that, although sodium excretion was increased, there were no changes in proximal sodium reabsorption. Thus, to account for the natriuresis it was concluded that prostaglandins inhibited sodium transport at some distal nephron site. The vasodilation is accompanied by a marked increase in peritubular capillary and renal interstitial pressure, thereby raising the possibility that the natriuresis may be mediated by the vasodilatation per se. This speculation does not rule out a direct effect of prostaglandins on sodium transport. In the toad bladder, Lipson and Sharp (135) have demonstrated that prostaglandin E_1 stimulates sodium transport, an effect opposite to that expected for a natriuretic hormone.

Bradykinin

The kinins have also been found in the renal parenchyma and have an effect on sodium excretion. The intrarenal distribution of kallikrein in the kidney resembles that for renin. Whereas prostaglandins are found in abundance in the papilla of the kidney, kallikrein is found predominantly in the cortex with only 4% of total enzyme activity found in the papilla (136). Thus, a direct effect of the kallikrein system on sodium transport in the collecting system is less likely than for prostaglandins. The interrelationships between the kinins and other systems have yet to be fully resolved. Barraclough and Mills (137) have infused bradykinin into the renal artery and found increased renal blood flow and sodium excretion. Schneider, Stein, Willis, and respective co-workers (33, 138, 139) found that bradykinin increases sodium excretion without changes in reabsorption by superficial proximal tubules, suggesting a site of action in the distal nephron. In additional studies by Willis et al. (140), bradykinin increased pressures in peritubular capillaries; therefore, it is difficult to separate the possible effects of increased renal interstitial pressures from direct effects of the peptide on sodium excretion.

Catecholamines

Renal denervation results in a prompt natriuresis, as first demonstrated by Marshall and Kolls (141). It is also well known that infusions of catecholamines cause renal vasoconstriction, increased filtration fraction, and decreased urinary sodium excretion (142). Although several workers have concluded that the fall in urinary sodium excretion is due to the altered renal hemodynamics, recent evidence suggests that catecholamines may have a direct effect on tubular reabsorption of sodium. Smythe et al. (143) infused very small amounts of catecholamines into man. They obtained a fall in sodium excretion despite an unchanged filtration rate and a rise in arterial pressure. Strandhoy et al. (144) have shown that blockade with phenoxybenzamine results in a natriuresis without changes in perfusion pressure or renal hemodynamics. In these studies there were no changes in proximal sodium reabsorption, suggesting that the adrenergic nervous system stimulates distal sodium transport. It should be noted that, in the frog skin, epinephrine and norepinephrine have direct effects on sodium transport (145).

Intravenous or renal arterial infusion of dopamine increases the excretion of sodium (146–148). It has been hypothesized that an increase in renal dopamine could decrease sodium reabsorption via dopaminergic receptors and play a physiological role in sodium regulation (149, 150). Alexander and co-workers (149) measured urinary dopamine in seven normal subjects on a 9 mEq/day sodium diet and then on a 209–259 mEq/day sodium diet. Urinary dopamine increased from 136 ± 18 to 195 ± 20 μg/day, whereas urinary norepinephrine decreased reciprocally.

Gill and Bartter (151) have found that in four subjects adrenergic blockade with guanethidine inhibited the usual reduction in urinary sodium excretion that occurs with sodium deprivation. The greater urinary sodium excretion during adrenergic blockade could not be accounted for by changes in blood pressure or glomerular filtration rate. Perhaps conservation of sodium during sodium deprivation depends upon both increased aldosterone and sympathetic nerve activity.

Glucagon

Since Staub et al. (152) first reported an enhanced excretion of sodium, as well as other electrolytes, following glucagon infusion in dogs, multiple similar observations have been made by others in dogs (153–157) as well as in man (158–160). The precise mechanism by which glucagon increases sodium excretion has not been characterized, but three possibilities should be considered: 1) hemodynamic alterations resulting in an increased filtered load of sodium; 2) a direct tubular effect of the hormone, resulting in decreased net sodium reabsorption; or 3) the alteration of the secretion of other hormones or substances in plasma that would influence sodium reabsorption in an indirect manner. Staub (152), Dalle (154), Pullman (155), and Saudek (159) and respective collaborators were unable to attribute the increased sodium excretion which follows administration of glucagon to a significant change in glomerular filtration rate. However, Serratto and Earle (153) and Stowe and Hook (156) concluded that increased glomerular filtration rate induced by exogenous glucagon accounts for the natriuresis observed. Elrick et al. (158), from their experiments in normal men, concluded that the effect of glucagon on the clearance of sodium is probably due to a direct tubular action, although a glomerular effect is not excluded by their data. The controversy has not been resolved, but others (153) have suggested differences in glucagon preparations as a possible explanation for the differences in glucagon-induced hemodynamic effects. If impurities prove to be responsible for the increased GFR seen by some after infusion of glucagon, it will not be surprising, taking into account the technical difficulties in purifying the hormone and the similar observations reported by others with parathyroid hormone.

The thesis that glucagon acts directly on the renal tubules to decrease reabsorption of sodium is supported by experiments performed by Pullman et al. (155) in dogs by injecting glucagon into one renal artery. Clearances were calculated before and after infusion of glucagon, and collections were obtained from the control and experimental kidneys. Glucagon infusion increased glomerular filtration rate and filtration fraction; however, the differences between the control and experimental kidneys were similar and insignificant. Glucagon, on the other hand, produced a marked differential increase in sodium excretion. Therefore, even though filtered load increased bilaterally, only the glucagon-infused kidney showed a marked and significant natriuresis, favoring the conclusion of a direct renal tubular effect of glucagon.

Multiple observations suggest that the effect of glucagon on glucose metabolism does not mediate the increased sodium excretion. In support of this conclusion, Staub et al. (152) elevated the plasma glucose concentration of dogs to 300–500 mg per cent prior to glucagon administration and found that, in the presence of hyperglycemia, glucagon increased urinary excretion of sodium. Elrick et al. (158) noted no significant effect in sodium excretion following glucose administration, concluding that the glucagon-induced natriuresis is not secondary to the hyperglycemic action of the hormone. Finally, it is possible that glucagon acts as a mineralocorticoid antagonist (160) by increasing cyclic AMP production (157) or by affecting the secretion of other hormones.

Thyroid

The broad relationships between thyroid hormone and renal function have recently been reviewed by Bradley et al. (161). Although complicated by the general metabolic effects of thyroid hormone, the hormone may have direct effects on tubular sodium transport. Holmes and DiScala (162) have shown that hypertonic NaCl infusion to hypothyroid rats results in fractional sodium excretions of 45% of the filtered load, whereas control rats excreted less than 10% (162). Furthermore, micropuncture studies by Michael and co-workers (163) have demonstrated reduced sodium reabsorption by the proximal tubule in hypothyroid rats. Distal sodium reabsorption is probably diminished as well to account for the magnitude of the natriuresis. In the context of the metabolic effects of the hormone, it is likely that thyroid hormone is necessary for sodium transport when stressed, as with infusion of hypertonic sodium chloride. On the other hand, myxedematous patients excrete sodium normally (164), suggesting that thyroid hormone may have little or no role in the daily regulation of sodium excretion.

Vasopressin

In addition to its primary antidiuretic action, vasopressin increases sodium excretion when administered during a water diuresis (165–169). This subject has been covered by Reid and Ganong (1) in a previous edition and extensively reviewed by Hays and Levine (170). The natriuretic effect of the hormone seems to be independent of alterations in mineralocorticoid secretion (169) and hemo-dynamic changes (168). The site of action has been postulated to lie in the proximal segments of the nephron (168, 171). However, in a recent communication describing recollection micropuncture in dogs, Wen (1972) concludes that vasopressin inhibits sodium reabsorption in the distal nephron. Further studies are necessary to determine the precise location of vasopressin effects on sodium reabsorption.

Natriuretic Hormone

The growing body of circumstantial evidence in support of the existence of a natriuretic hormone has recently been reviewed by DeWardener (4) and Lee and DeWardener (173). The search for the elusive hormone was formalized by Smith's (174) review of salt and water volume receptors in which he proposed natriuretic and antinatriuretic systems. Given the critical role of the distal nephron in sodium regulation, it is reasonable to postulate that such a system affects the distal nephron (175). On the other hand, the very existence of a natriuretic hormone has been open to serious question (176), not because of conclusive evidence against the hypothesis, but because of the incomplete nature of the evidence for it to date.

REFERENCES

1. Reid, I. A., and Ganong, W. F. (1974). The hormonal control of sodium excretion. *In* S. McCann (ed.), MTP International Review of Science, Physiology Series 1, Vol. 1, Endocrine Physiology. Medical and Technical Publishing Company, London.
2. Lindheimer, M. D., Lalone, R. C., and Levinsky, N. G. (1967). Evidence that an acute increase in glomerular filtration has little effect on sodium excretion in the dog unless extracellular volume is expanded. J. Clin. Invest. 46:256.
3. DeWardener, H. E., Mills, I. H., Clapham, W. F., and Hayter, C. J. (1961). Studies on the efferent mechanism of the sodium diuresis which follows the administration of intravenous saline in the dog. Clin. Sci. 21:249.
4. DeWardener, H. E. (1973). The control of sodium excretion. *In* J. Orloff and R. Berliner (eds.), Handbook of Physiology, p. 677. American Physiological Society, Washington, D.C.
5. Dirks, J., Circksena, W., and Berliner, R. (1965). The effect of saline infusion on sodium reabsorption by the proximal tubule of the dog. J. Clin. Invest. 44:1160.
6. Cirksena, W. J., Dirks, J. H., and Berliner, R. W. (1966). Effect of thoracic cava obstruction on response of proximal tubule sodium reabsorption to saline infusion. J. Clin. Invest. 45:179.

7. Howards, S., Davis, B., Knox, F., Wright, F., and Berliner, R. (1968). Depression of fractional sodium reabsorption by the proximal tubule of the dog without sodium diuresis. J. Clin. Invest. 47:1561.

8. Knox, F. G., Howards, S., Wright, F. S., Davis, B. B., and Berliner, R. W. (1968). Effect of dilution and expansion of blood volume on proximal sodium reabsorption. Am. J. Physiol. 215:1041.

9. Burke, T., Robinson, R., and Clapp, J. (1971). Effect of arterial hematocrit on sodium reabsorption by the proximal tubule. Am. J. Physiol. 220:1536.

10. Knox, F. G., Schneider, E. G., Willis, L. R., Strandhoy, J. W., and Ott, C. E. (1973). Effect of volume expansion on sodium excretion in the presence and absence of increased delivery from superficial proximal tubules, J. Clin. Invest. 52:1642.

11. Willis, L. R., Schneider, E. G., Lynch, R. E., and Knox, F. G. (1972). Effect of chronic alteration of sodium balance on reabsorption by proximal tubule of the dog. Am. J. Physiol. 223:34.

12. Schneider, E. G., Dresser, T. P., Lynch, R. E., and Knox, F. G. (1971). Sodium reabsorption by proximal tubule of dogs with experimental heart failure. Am. J. Physiol. 220:952.

13. Stumpe, K. O., Solle, H., Klein, H., and Kruck, F. (1973). Mechanism of sodium and water retention in rats with experimental heart failure. Kidney Int. 4:309.

14. Auld, R., Alexander, E., and Levinsky, N. (1971). Proximal tubular function in dogs with thoracic caval constriction. J. Clin. Invest. 50:2150.

15. Levy, M. (1972). Effects of acute volume expansion and altered hemodynamics on renal tubular function in chronic caval dogs. J. Clin. Invest. 51:922.

16. Earley, L. E., Humphreys, M. H., and Bartoli, E. (1972). Capillary circulation as a regulator of sodium reabsorption and excretion. Circ. Res. 31:1.

17. Windhager, E. E., Lewy, J. E., and Spitzer, A. (1969). Intrarenal control of proximal tubular reabsorption of sodium and water. Nephron 6:247.

18. Brenner, B. M., Falchuk, K. H., Keimpwitz, R. I., and Berliner, R. W. (1969). The relationship between peritubule capillary protein concentration and fluid reabsorption by the renal proximal tubule. J. Clin. Invest. 48:1519.

19. Ott, C. E., Haas, J. A., Cuche, J. L., and Knox, F. G. (1975). Effect of increased peritubule protein concentration on proximal tubule reabsorption in the presence and absence of extracellular volume expansion. J. Clin. Invest. 55:612.

20. Strandhoy, J. W., Ott, C. E., Schneider, E. G., Willis, L. R., Beck, N. P., Davis, B. B., and Knox, F. G. (1974). Effects of prostaglandins E_1 and E_2 on renal sodium reabsorption and Starling forces. Am. J. Physiol. 226:1015.

21. Wiederholt, M., Hierholzer, K., and Brecht, J. P. (1964). Die Wirkung von Aldosteron und cortison auf den tubularen Na-Transport adrenalektomierter Ratten. Pfluegers Arch. 281:85.

22. Hierholzer, K., Wiederholt, M., and Stolte, H. (1966). Hemmung der Natriumresorption im proximalen und distalen Konvolut adrenalektomierter Ratten. Arch. Ges. Physiol. 291:43.

23. Wiederholt, M., Stolte, H., Brecht, J. P., and Hierholzer, K. (1966). Micropuncture research on the effect of aldosterone, cortisone and dexamethasone on renal sodium reabsorption in adrenalectomized rats. Arch. Ges. Physiol. 292:316.

24. Hierholzer, K., and Stolte, H. (1969). The proximal and distal tubular action of adrenal steroids on sodium reabosrption. Nephron 6:188.
25. Hierholzer, K. (1969). Intrarenal action of steroid hormones on sodium transport. In K. Thurau and H. Jahrmarker (eds.), Renal Transport and Diuretics, p. 153. Springer, Berlin.
26. Wiederholt, M., Schoormans, W., Hansen, L., and Behn, C. (1974). Sodium conductance changes by aldosterone in the rat kidney. Pfluegers Arch. 248:155.
27. Stumpe, K. O., and Ochwadt, B. (1968). Effect of aldosterone on proximal tubular sodium and water reabsorption in chronically salt-loaded rats. Arch. Ges. Physiol. 300:148.
28. Lynch, R. E., Schneider, E. G., Willis, L. R., and Knox, F. G. (1972). Absence of mineralocorticoid dependent sodium reabsorption in the dog proximal tubule. Am. J. Physiol. 223:40.
29. Martin, D. G., and Berliner, R. W. (1969). The effect of aldosterone on proximal tubular sodium reabsorption in the rat (Abstr.), p. 45. Third Annual Meeting of the American Society of Nephrology, Washington, D.C.
30. Lowitz, H. D., Stumpe, K. O., and Ochwadt, B. (1969). Micropuncture study of the action of angiotensin II on sodium reabsorption and water reabsorption in the rat. Nephron 6:173.
31. Agus, Z. S., Puschett, J. B., Senesky, D., and Goldberg, M. (1971). Mode of action of parathyroid hormone and cyclic adenosine $3',5'$-monophosphate on renal tubular phosphate reabsorption in the dog. J. Clin. Invest. 50:617.
32. Agus, Z. S., Gardner, L. B., Beck, L. H., and Goldberg, M. (1973). Effects of parathyroid hormone on renal tubular reabsorption of calcium, sodium, and phosphate. Am. J. Physiol. 224:1143.
33. Schneider, E. G., Strandhoy, J. W., Willis, L. R., and Knox, F. G. (1973). Relationship between proximal sodium reabsorption and excretion of calcium, magnesium and phosphate. Kidney Int. 4:369.
34. Wen, S. F. (1974). Micropuncture studies of phosphate transport in the proximal tubule of the dog. J. Clin. Invest. 53:143.
35. Knox, F. G., and Lechene, C. (1975). Distal site of action of parathyroid hormone on phosphate reabsorption in the thyroparathyroidectomized dog. Am. J. Physiol. 229:1556.
36. Crumb, C. K., Maldonado-Martinez, M., Eknoyan, G., and Suki, W. N. (1974). Effects of volume expansion, purified parathyroid extract, and calcium on renal bicarbonate absorption in the dog. J. Clin. Invest. 54:1287.
37. Karlinsky, M. L., Sager, D. S., Kurtzman, N. A., and Pillay, V. K. G. (1974). Effect of parathormone and cyclic adenosine monophosphate on renal bicarbonate reabsorption. Am. J. Physiol. 227:1226.
38. Diaz-Buxo, J. A., Ott, C. E., Cuche, J. L., Marchand, G. R., Wilson, D. M., and Knox, F. G. (1975). Effects of extracellular fluid volume contraction and expansion on the bicarbonaturia of parathyroid hormone. Kidney Int. 8:105.
39. Beck, L. H., and Goldberg, M. (1973). Effects of acetazolamide and parathyroidectomy on renal transport of sodium, calcium, and phosphate. Am. J. Physiol. 224:1136.
40. Beck, N. P., Kim, K. S., Wolak, M., and Davis, B. B. (1975). Inhibition of carbonic anhydrase by parathyroid hormone and cyclic AMP in rat renal cortex in vitro. J. Clin. Invest. 55:149.

41. Bank, N., Aynedjian, H. S., and Weinstein, S. W. (1974). A microperfusion study of phosphate reabsorption by the rat proximal renal tubule. J. Clin. Invest. 54:1040.

42. Talmage, R. V., and Belanger, L. F. (eds.) (1968). Parathyroid Hormone and Thyrocalcitonin (Calcitonin). Excerpta Medica Foundation, New York.

43. Burg, M. B., and Green, N. (1973). Function of the thick ascending limb of Henle's loop. Am. J. Physiol. 224:659.

44. Landwehr, D. M., Klose, R. M., and Giebisch, G. (1967). Renal tubular sodium and water reabsorption in the isotonic sodium chloride-induced rat. Am. J. Physiol. 212:1327.

45. Dirks, J. H., and Seely, J. F. (1970). Effect of saline infusions and furosemide on the dog distal nephron. Am. J. Physiol. 219:114.

46. Stein, J. H., Osgood, R. W., Boonjarern, S., and Ferris, T. (1973). A comparison of the segmental analysis of sodium reabsorption during Ringer's and hyperoncotic albumin infusion in the rat. J. Clin. Invest. 52:2312.

47. Morgan, T., and Berliner, R. (1969). A study by continuous microperfusion of water and electrolyte movements in the loop of Henle and distal tubule of the rat. Nephron 6:386.

48. Stein, J. H., and Reineck, H. J. (1975). Effect of alterations in extracellular fluid volume on segmental sodium transport. Physiol. Rev. 55:127.

49. Bank, N., Aynedjian, H. S., Bansal, V. K., and Goldman, D. M. (1970). Effect of acute hypertension on sodium transport by the distal nephron. Am. J. Physiol. 219:275.

50. Stumpe, K., Lowitz, H., and Ochwadt, B. (1970). Fluid reabsorption in Henle's loop and urinary excretion of sodium and water in normal rats and rats with chronic hypertension. J. Clin. Invest. 49:1200.

51. Thorn, G. W., Jenkins, D., Laidlaw, J. C., Goetz, F. C., Dingman, J. F., Arons, W. L., Streeten, D. H. P., and McCracken, B. H. (1953). Pharmacologic aspects of adrenocortical steroids and ACTH in man. N. Engl. J. Med. 248:232; 284; 323; 369; 414; 588; 632.

52. Crabbe, J. (1961). The role of aldosterone in the renal concentration mechanism in man. Clin. Sci. 23:39.

53. Sonnenblick, E. H., Cannon, P. J., and Laragh, J. H. (1961). The nature of the action of intravenous aldosterone, evidence for a role of the hormone in urinary dilution. J. Clin. Invest. 40:903.

54. Jamison, R. L., and Lacy, F. B. (1972). Evidence for urinary dilution by the collecting tubule. Am. J. Physiol. 223:898.

55. Burg, M. B., and Stoner, L. (1974). Sodium transport in the distal nephron. Fed. Proc. 33:31.

56. Strieder, U., Khuri, R., and Giebisch, G. (1969). Recollection micropuncture study of distal tubular sodium reabsorption during graded extracellular volume expansion in the rat. Abstracts of American Society of Nephrology, p. 64. Washington, D.C.

57. Knox, F. G., and Gasser, J. (1974). Altered distal sodium reabsorption in volume expansion. Mayo Clin. Proc. 49:775.

58. Vander, A. J., Malvin, R. L., Wilde, W. S., Lapides, J., Sullivan, L. P., and McMurray, V. M. (1958). Effects of adrenalectomy and aldosterone on proximal and distal tubular sodium reabsorption. Proc. Soc. Exp. Biol. Med. 99:323.

59. Vander, A. J., Wilde, W. S., and Malvin, R. L. (1960). Stop-flow analysis of

aldosterone and steroidal antagonist SC 8109 on renal tubular sodium transport kinetics. Proc. Soc. Exp. Biol. Med. 103:525.
60. Hierholzer, K., Wiederholt, M., Holgreve, H., Giebisch, G., Klose, R. M., and Windhager, E. E. (1965). Micropuncture study of renal transtubule concentration gradients of sodium and potassium in adrenalectomized rats. Arch. Ges. Physiol. 283:193.
61. Woodhall, P. B., and Tisher, C. C. (1973). Response of the distal tubule and cortical collecting duct to vasopressin in the rat. J. Clin. Invest. 52:3095.
62. Malnic, G., Klose, R. M., and Giebisch, G. (1966). Micropuncture study of distal tubular potassium and sodium transport in rat nephron. Am. J. Physiol. 211:529.
63. Gross, J. B., Imai, M., and Kokko, J. P. (1974). Functional comparison of the distal convoluted tubule and the cortical collecting tubule. Am. Soc. Neph. 7:34.
64. Hilger, H., Kluemper, J., and Ullrich, K. (1958). Wasserruckresorption und ionentransport durch die Sammel rohrzellen der Saugelierniere. Pfluegers Arch. 267:238.
65. Jamison, R. L., Buerkert, J., and Lacy, F. (1971). A micropuncture study of collecting tubule function in rats with hereditary diabetes insipidus. J. Clin. Invest. 50:2444.
66. Windhager, E. E. (1964). Electrophysiological study of renal papilla of golden hamsters. Am. J. Physiol. 206:694.
67. Laurence, R., and Marsh, D. J. (1971). Effect of diuretic states on hamster collecting duct electrical potential differences. Am. J. Physiol. 220:1610.
68. Rau, W. S., and Frömter, E. (1974). Electrical properties of the medullary collecting ducts of the golden hamster kidney. I. The transepithelial potential difference. Pfluegers Arch. 351:99.
69. Rau, W. S., and Frömter, E. (1974). Electrical properties of the medullary collecting ducts of the golden hamster kidney. II. The transepithelial resistance. Pfluegers Arch. 351:113.
70. Grantham, J. J., Burg, M. B., and Orloff, J. (1970). The nature of transtubular Na and K transport in isolated rabbit renal collecting tubules. J. Clin. Invest. 49:1815.
71. Burg, M. B., Isaacson, L., Grantham, J. J., and Orloff, J. (1968). Electrical properties of isolated perfused rabbit renal tubules. Am. J. Physiol. 215:788.
72. Frindt, G., and Burg, M. B. (1972). Effect of vasopressin on sodium transport in renal cortical collecting tubules. Kidney Int. 1:224.
73. Helman, S. I., Grantham, J. J., and Burg, M. B. (1971). Effect of vasopressin on electrical resistance of renal cortical collecting tubules. Am. J. Physiol. 220:1825.
74. Diezi, J., Michoud, P., Aceves, J., and Giebisch, G. (1973). Micropuncture study of electrolyte transport across papillary collecting duct of the rat. Am. J. Physiol. 224:623.
75. Sonnenberg, H. (1973). Proximal and distal tubular function in salt-deprived and in salt-loaded deoxycorticosterone acetate-escaped rats. J. Clin. Invest. 52:263.
76. Stein, J. H., Osgood, R. W., Boonjarern, S., Cox, J., and Ferris, T. F. (1974). Segmental analysis of sodium reabsorption in rats with mild and severe extracellular fluid volume depletion: studies before and after volume depletion. Am. J. Physiol. 227:351.

77. Uhlich, E., Baldamus, C., and Ullrich, K. (1969). Einfluss vons aldosteron auf den natriumtransport in den sämmelrohren der saugetierneire. Pfluegers Arch. 308:111.
78. Barger, A. C., Berlin, R. D., and Tulenko, J. F. (1958). Infusion of aldosterone, 9α-fluorhydrocortisone and antidiuretic hormone into the renal artery of normal and adrenalectomized, unanesthetized dogs: effect on electrolyte and water excretions. Endocrinology 62:804.
79. Sharp, G. W. G., and Leaf, A. (1966). Studies on the mode of action of aldosterone. Recent Prog. Horm. Res. 22:431.
80. Edelman, I. S., and Fanestil, D. D. (1970). Mineralocorticoids. In G. Litwack (ed.), Biochemical Actions of Hormones, Vol. 1, p. 321. Academic Press, New York.
81. Pelletier, M., Ludens, J. H., and Fanestil, D. D. (1972). The role of aldosterone in active sodium transport. Arch. Intern. Med. 129:248.
82. Herman, T. S., Fimognari, G. M., and Edelman, I. S. (1968). Studies on renal aldosterone-binding proteins. J. Biol. Chem. 243:3849.
83. Marver, D., Goodman, D., and Edelman, I. S. (1972). Relationship between renal cytoplasmic and nuclear aldosterone receptors. Kidney Int. 1:210.
84. Chu, L. L. H., and Edelman, I. S. (1972). Cordycepin and α-amanitin: inhibitors of transcription as probes of aldosterone action. J. Membr. Biol. 10:291.
85. Lahav, M., Dietz, T., and Edelman, I. S. (1973). The action of aldosterone on sodium transport: further studies with inhibition of RNA and protein synthesis. Endocrinology 92:1685.
86. Fimognari, G. M., Fanestil, D. D., and Edelman, I. S. (1967). Induction of RNA and protein synthesis in the action of aldosterone in the rat. Am. J. Physiol. 213:954.
87. Wiederholt, M., Aguilan, S. K., and Khuri, R. N. (1974). Intracellular potassium in the distal tubule of the adrenalectomized and aldosterone treated rat. Pfluegers Arch. 347:117.
88. Biglieri, E. G., and Forsham, P. H. (1961). Studies on the expanded extracellular fluid and the responses to various stimuli in primary aldosteronism. Am. J. Med. 30:564.
89. Woods, J. W., Liddle, G. W., Stant, E. G., Jr., Michelakis, A. M., and Brill, A. B. (1969). Effect of an adrenal inhibitor in hypertensive patients with suppressed renin. Arch. Intern. Med. 123:366.
90. Carey, R. M., Douglas, J. G., Schweikert, J. R., and Liddle, G. W. (1972). The syndrome of essential hypertension and suppressed plasma renin activity. Arch. Intern. Med. 130:849.
91. Stewart, J. (1975). Genetic studies on the mechanism of action of aldosterone in mice. Endocrinology 96:711.
92. Sennett, J. A., Brown, R. D., Island, D. P., Yarbro, L. R., Watson, J. T., Slaton, P. E., Hollifield, J. W., and Liddle, G. W. (1975). Evidence for a new mineralocorticoid in patients with low-renin essential hypertension. Circ. Res. 36 (Suppl. I) I–2.
93. Shackleton, C. H. L., Kelly, R. W., Adhikary, P. M., Brooks, C. J. W., Harkness, R. A., Sykes, P. J., and Mitchell, F. L. (1968). The identification and measurement of a new steroid 16β-hydroxydehydroepiandrosterone in infant urine. Steroids 12:705.
94. Dale, S., and Melby, J. (1974). Altered adrenal steroidogenesis in "low renin" essential hypertension. Clin. Res. 22:557A.

95. Ehrlich, E. N., and Lindheimer, M. D. (1972). Effect of administered mineralocorticoids or ACTH in pregnant women: attenuation of kaliuretic influence of mineralocorticoids during pregnancy. J. Clin. Invest. 51:1301.
96. Sasaki, C., Nowacznyski, W., Kuchel, O., Chavex, C., Ledoux, F., Gauthier, S., and Genest, J. (1972). Plasma progesterone in normal subjects and patients with benign essential hypertension on normal low and high sodium intake. J. Clin. Endocrinol. Metab. 34:650.
97. Hinsull, S. M., and Crocker, A. D. (1970). The effects of ovarian hormones on the activity of the adrenal cortex and on water and sodium transport. J. Endocrinol. 48:29.
98. Rogoff, J. M., and Stewart, G. N. (1927). Studies on adrenal insufficiency: influence of pregnancy upon survival period in adrenalectomized dogs. Am. J. Physiol. 79:508.
99. Thorn, G. W., and Engel, L. L. (1938). The effect of sex hormones on the renal excretion of electrolytes. J. Exp. Med. 68:299.
100. Richardson, J. A., and Houck, C. R. (1951). Renal tubular excretory mass and the reabsorption of sodium, chloride and potassium in female dogs receiving testosterone propionate or estradiol benzoate. Am. J. Physiol. 165:93.
101. Dance, P., Lloyd, S., and Pickford, M. (1959). The effects of stilbestrol on the renal activity of conscious dogs. J. Physiol. 145:225.
102. Deis, R. P., Lloyd, S., and Pickford, M. (1963). The effects of stilbestrol and progesterone, and of renal denervation on the response of the kidneys to vasopressin and oxytocin. J. Physiol. 165:348.
103. Crocker, A. D. (1971). Variations in mucosal water and sodium transfer associated with the rat oestrus cycle. J. Physiol. 214:257.
104. Dignam, W. S., Voskian, J., and Assali, N. S. (1956). Effects of estrogens on renal hemodynamics and excretion of electrolytes in human subjects. J. Clin. Endocrinol. 16:1032.
105. Preedy, J. R. K., and Aitken, E. H. (1956). The effect of estrogen on water and electrolyte metabolism. I. The normal. J. Clin. Invest. 35:423.
106. Crane, M. G., and Harris, J. J. (1969). Plasma renin activity and aldosterone excretion rate in normal subjects. I. Effect of ethinyl estradiol and medroxyprogesterone acetate. J. Clin. Endocrinol. 29:550.
107. Laidlaw, J. C., Ruse, J. L., and Gornall, A. G. (1962). The influence of estrogen and progesterone on aldosterone excretion. J. Clin. Endocrinol. 22:161.
108. Christy, N. P., and Shaver, J. C. (1974). Estrogens and the kidney. Kidney Int. 6:366.
109. Jones, K. M., Lloyd-Jones, R., Riondel, A., Tait, J. F., Tait, S. A. S., Bulbrook, R. D., and Greenwood, F. C. (1959). Aldosterone secretion and metabolism in normal men and women and in pregnancy. Acta Endocrinol. 20:321.
110. Laidlaw, J. C., Ruse, J. L., and Gornall, A. G. (1961). The influence of estrogen and progesterone on aldosterone excretion. J. Clin. Endocrinol. Metab. 22:161.
111. Ehrlich, E. N., and Lindheimer, M. (1972). Effect of administered mineralocorticoids or ACTH in pregnant women: attenuation of kaluretic influence of mineralocorticoids during pregnancy. J. Clin. Invest. 51:1301.
112. Landau, R. L., and Lugibihl, K. (1958). Inhibition of the sodium-retaining influence of aldosterone by progesterone. J. Clin. Endocrinol. Metab. 18:1237.

113. Laragh, J. H., Sealey, J. E., Ledingham, J. G. G., and Newton, M. A. (1967). Oral contraceptives: renin, aldosterone, and high blood pressure. J.A.M.A. 201:918.
114. Swaab, L. I. (1966). Blood pressure and oral contraception. Proceedings of Second International Congress on Hormonal Steroids, Milan, Italy, p. 198. Excerpta Medica Foundation, Amsterdam.
115. Skinner, S. L., Lumbers, E. R., and Symonds, E. M. (1969). Alteration by oral contraceptives of normal menstrual changes in plasma renin activity, concentration and substrate. Clin. Sci. 36:67.
116. Layne, D. S., Meyer, C. J., Vaishwanar, P. S., and Pincus, G. (1962). The secretion and metabolism of cortisol and aldosterone in normal and in steroid-treated women. J. Clin. Endocrinol. 22:107.
117. Crane, M. G., Heitsch, J., Harris, J. J., and Johns, V. J. (1966). Effect of ethinyl estradiol (Estinyl) on plasma renin activity. J. Clin. Endocrinol. 26:1403.
118. Helmer, O. M., and Judson, W. E. (1967). Influence of high renin substrate levels on renin-angiotensin system in pregnancy. Am. J. Obstet. Gynecol. 99:9.
119. Helmer, O. M., and Griffith, R. S. (1952). The effect of the administration of estrogens in the renin-substrate (hypertensinogen) content of rat plasma. Endocrinology 51:421.
120. Crane, M. G., and Harris, J. J. (1969). Plasma renin activity and aldosterone excretion rate in normal subjects. I. Effects of ethinyl estradiol and medroxyprogesterone acetate. J. Clin. Endocrinol. 29:550.
121. Crane, M. G., and Harris, J. J. (1969). Plasma renin activity and aldosterone excretion rate in normal subjects. II. Effect of oral contraceptive agents. J. Clin. Endocrinol. 29:558.
122. Weir, R. J., Tree, M., Fraser, R., Chime, R. H., Davies, D. L., Düsterdieck, G. O., Robertson, J. I. S., Horne, C. H. W., and Mallinson, A. C. (1971). The effect of continued oestrogen-progesterone oral contraceptives, and of their separate components, on plasma levels of renin, renin-substrate, angiotensin, and aldosterone, and on blood pressure. In V. H. T. James and C. Martini (eds.), Proceedings of the Third International Congress on Hormone Steroids, p. 929. Excerpta Medica, Amsterdam.
123. Peart, W. S. (1965). The renin-angiotensin system. Pharmacol. Rev. 17:143.
124. Barraclough, M. A., Jones, N. F., and Mardsen, C. D. (1967). Effect of angiotensin on renal function in the rat. Am. J. Physiol. 212:1153.
125. Jones, N. F., Barraclough, M. A., Perriello, V. A., and Mardsen, C. D. (1967). Effect of angiotensin on urea reabsorption in man. Clin. Sci. 32:257.
126. Louis, W. J., and Doyle, A. E. (1966). The effects of aldosterone and angiotensin on renal function. Clin. Sci. 30:179.
127. Leyssac, P. P., Lassen, U. V., and Thaysen, J. H. (1961). Inhibition of sodium transport in isolated renal tissue by angiotensin. Biochim. Biophys. Acta 48:602.
128. Vander, A. J. (1963). Inhibition of distal tubular sodium reabsorption by angiotensin II. Am. J. Physiol. 205:133.
129. Cuypers, Y. (1965). L'action tubulaire rénale de l'α-angiotensine II-amide chez le coq. Arch. Intern. Pharmacodyn. 155:495.
130. Spielman, W. S., Davis, J. O., Freeman, R. H., and Lohmeier, T. R. E. (1974). Systemic and intrarenal arteriolar action of angiotensin II in dogs with experimental high output heart failure. Physiologist 17:335.

131. Hickler, R. B., Lauler, D. P., Saravis, C. A., Vagnucci, D. I., Steiner, G., and Thorn, G. W. (1964). Vasodepressor lipid from the renal medulla. Can. Med. Assoc. J. 90:280.
132. Tobian, L. (1974). How sodium and the kidney relate to the hypertensive arteriole. Fed. Proc. 33:138.
133. Johnston, H. H., Herzog, J. P., and Lauler, D. P. (1967). Effect of prostaglandin-E_1 on renal hemodynamics, sodium and water excretion. Am. J. Physiol. 213:939.
134. Vander, A. J. (1968). Direct effects of prostaglandin on renal function and renin release in anesthetized dog. Am. J. Physiol. 214:218.
135. Lipson, L. C., and Sharp, G. W. G. (1971). Effect of prostaglandin E_1 on sodium transport and osmotic water flow in the toad bladder. Am. J. Physiol. 220:1046.
136. Scicli, A. G., Oza, N. B., and Carretero, O. A. (1974). Distribution of kallikrein in the kidney. Physiologist 17:327A.
137. Barraclough, M. A., and Mills, I. H. (1965). Effect of bradykinin on renal function. Clin. Sci. 28:69.
138. Stein, J. H., Congbalay, R. C., Karsh, D. L., Osgood, R. W., and Ferris, T. F. (1972). The effect of bradykinin on proximal tubular sodium reabsorption in the dog: evidence for functional nephron heterogeneity. J. Clin. Invest. 51:1709.
139. Willis, L. R., Schneider, E. G., Strandhoy, J. W., and Knox, F. G. (1972). Comparison of the effects of two vasodilator drugs upon peritubule capillary hydrostatic pressure and proximal sodium reabsorption in the dog. Clin. Res. 20:616.
140. Willis, L. R., Schneider, E. G., Strandhoy, J. W., and Knox, F. G. (1972). Comparison of the effects of two vasodilators on peritubule Starling forces and proximal sodium reabsorption in the dog. Abstracts of the Fifth International Congress of Nephrology, Vol. 333, p. 65.
141. Marshall, E. K., and Kolls, A. C. (1919). Studies on the nervous control of the kidney in relation to diuresis and urinary secretion. II. A comparison of the changes caused by unilateral splanchnotomy with those caused by unilateral compression of the renal artery. Am. J. Physiol. 49:317.
142. Jacobson, W. E., Hammarsten, J. F., and Heller, B. I. (1951). The effects of adrenaline upon renal function and electrolyte excretion. J. Clin. Invest. 30:1503.
143. Smythe, C. M., Nickel, J. F., and Bradley, S. E. (1952). The effect of epinephrine (USP) 1-epinephrine and 1-norepinephrine on glomerular filtration rate, renal plasma flow and the urinary excretion of sodium, potassium and water in normal man. J. Clin. Invest. 31:499.
144. Strandhoy, J. W., Schneider, E. G., Willis, L. R., and Knox, F. G. (1974). Intrarenal effects of phenoxybenzamine on sodium reabsorption. J. Lab. Clin. Med. 83:263.
145. Watlington, C. O. (1965). The nature of adrenergic influence on sodium transport in frog skin. J. Clin. Invest. 44:1108.
146. Davis, B. B., Walter, M. J., and Murdaugh, H. V. (1965). The mechanism of the increase in sodium excretion following dopamine infusion. Proc. Soc. Exp. Biol. Med. 129:210.
147. McDonald, R. H., Jr., Goldberg, L. I., McNay, J. L., and Tuttle, E. P., Jr. (1964). Effects of dopamine in man: augmentation of sodium excretion, glomerular filtration rate and renal plasma flow. J. Clin. Invest. 43:1116.
148. Meyer, M. B., McNay, J. L., and Goldberg, L. I. (1967). Effects of

dopamine on renal function and hemodynamics in the dog. J. Pharmacol. Exp. Ther. 156:186.

149. Alexander, R. W., Gill, J. R., Jr., Yambe, H., Lovenberg, W., and Keiser, H. R. (1974). Effects of dietary sodium and of acute saline infusion on the interrelationship between dopamine excretion and adrenergic activity in man. J. Clin. Invest. 54:194.

150. Yeh, B. K., McNay, J. L., and Goldberg, L. I. (1969). Attenuation of dopamine renal and mesenteric vasodilator by haloperidol. evidence for a specific dopamine receptor. J. Pharmacol. Exp. Ther. 168:303.

151. Gill, J. R., and Bartter, F. C. (1966). Adrenergic nervous system in sodium metabolism. II. Effects of guanethidine on the renal response to sodium deprivation in normal man. N. Engl. J. Med. 275:1466.

152. Staub, A., Springs, V., Stoll, F., and Elrick, H. (1957). A renal action of glucagon. Proc. Soc. Exp. Biol. Med. 94:57.

153. Serratto, M., and Earle, D. P. (1959). Effect of glucagon on renal function in the dog. Proc. Soc. Exp. Biol. Med. 102:701.

154. Dalle, X., and Gryspeerdt, J. T. W. (1959). Influence du glucagon sur l'excretion renale des electrolytes. Arch. Int. Pharmacodyn. 120:505.

155. Pullman, T. N., Lavender, A. R., and Aho, I. (1967). Direct effects of glucagon on renal hemodynamics and excretion of inorganic ions. Metabolism 16:358.

156. Stowe, N. T., and Hook, J. B. (1970). Role of alterations in renal hemodynamics in the natriuretic action of glucagon. Arch. Int. Pharmacodyn. 183:65.

157. Schwille, P. O., and Barth, B. (1972). Clearance and stop-flow studies in glucagon mediated hyperelectrolyturia. Acta Endocrinol. (Suppl.) 159:92.

158. Elrick, H., Huffman, E. R., Hlad, C. J., Jr., Whipple, N., and Staub, A. (1958). Effects of glucagon on renal function in man. J. Clin. Endocrinol. Metab. 18:813.

159. Saudek, C. D., Boulter, P. R., and Arky, R. A. (1973). The natriuretic effect of glucagon and its role in starvation. J. Clin. Endocrinol. Metab. 36:761.

160. O'Brian, J. T., Saudek, C. D., Spark, R., and Arky, A. (1973). Glucagon: a potent mineralocorticoid antagonist. Clin. Res. 21:499.

161. Bradley, S. E., Stephan, F., Coelho, J. B., and Reville, P. (1974). The thyroid and the kidney. Kidney Int. 6:346.

162. Holmes, E. W., Jr., and DiScala, V. A. (1970). Exaggerated natriuresis in the hypothyroid rat. Clin. Res. 18:502.

163. Michael, U. F., Barenburg, R. L., Chavez, R., Vaamonde, C. A., and Papper, S. (1972). Renal handling of sodium and water in the hypothyroid rat. J. Clin. Invest. 51:1405.

164. Davies, C. E., MacKinnon, J., and Platts, M. M. (1952). Renal circulation and cardiac output in "low-output" heart failure and in myxedema. Br. Med. J. 2:595.

165. Ali, M. N. (1958). A comparison of some activities of arginine vasopressin and lysine vasopressin on kidney function in conscious dogs. Br. J. Pharmacol. 13:131.

166. Chan, W. Y., and Sawyer, W. H. (1961). Saluretic actions of neurohypophyseal peptides in conscious dogs. Am. J. Physiol. 201:799.

167. Chan, W. Y., and Sawyer, W. H. (1962). Natriuresis in conscious dogs

during arginine vasopressin infusion and after oxytocin injection. Proc. Soc. Exp. Biol. Med. 110:697.

168. Humphreys, M. H., Friedler, R. M., and Earley, L. E. (1970). Natriuresis produced by vasopressin or hemorrhage during water diuresis in the dog. Am. J. Physiol. 219:658.

169. Jones, N. F., Barraclough, M. A., and Mills, I. H. (1963). The mechanism of increased sodium excretion during water loading with 2.5% dextrose and vasopressin. Clin. Sci. 25:449.

170. Hays, R. M., and Levine, S. D. (1974). Vasopressin. Kidney Int. 6:307.

171. Martinez-Maldonado, M., Eknoyan, G., and Suki, W. N. (1971). Natriuretic effects of vasopressin and cyclic AMP: possible site of action in the nephron. Am. J. Physiol. 220:2013.

172. Wen, S. F. (1974). The effect of vasopressin on phosphate transport in the proximal tubule of the dog. J. Clin. Invest. 53:660.

173. Lee, J., and DeWardener, H. E. (1974). Neurosecretion and sodium excretion. Kidney Int. 6:323.

174. Smith, H. W. (1957). Salt and water volume receptors. Am. J. Med. 23:623.

175. Knox, F. G. (1973). Role of proximal tubule in the regulation of urinary sodium excretion. Mayo Clin. Proc. 48:656.

176. Levinsky, N. G. (1972). A critical appraisal of some of the evidence for a natriuretic hormone. Proceedings of the Fifth International Congress on Nephrology, Mexico City, Mexico, p. 162.

International Review of Physiology
Endocrine Physiology II, Volume 16
Edited by S. M. McCann
Copyright 1977   University Park Press   Baltimore

6
Hormonal Regulation
of Mineral Metabolism

L. G. RAISZ, G. R. MUNDY, J. W. DIETRICH, and E. M. CANALIS
University of Connecticut Health Center, Farmington, Connecticut

---

During the past 15 years, the study of the regulation of calcium and phosphorus metabolism has been considerably extended by the discovery of several new regulatory systems. In addition to regulation by parathyroid hormone (PTH), there is important regulation by the hypocalcemic hormone, calcitonin or thyrocalcitonin (CT), and by the active metabolites of vitamin D. These systems are under intense study, and their physiological role is not yet fully understood. The vitamin D system includes at least one compound, 1,25-dihydroxycholecalciferol ($1,25\text{-}(OH)_2 D_3$), which is recognized as a new calcium regulatory hormone but may also include additional metabolites which have a regulatory role.

There have also been further studies on the role in mineral metabolism of hormones with more generalized regulatory roles such as glucocorticoids, gonadal hormones, thyroxine, and growth hormone and its intermediates. Finally, several new humoral factors such as prostaglandins and the osteoclast-activating factor (OAF) secreted by normal human peripheral blood leukocytes have been identified which have powerful effects on bone metabolism. These factors have not been shown to regulate calcium metabolism systemically and may be more important for their local influence.

Since PTH and CT were extensively reviewed in the previous volume of this series, only recent advances in the study of these hormones are covered in this chapter. In general, material published since 1972 is emphasized and all papers available up to September 1, 1975, are included.

PARATHYROID HORMONE

Chemistry

Structures After further information concerning the chemical composition of PTH was obtained, a controversy developed concerning the specific amino acid sequences, particularly for human PTH. The amino acid sequence for bovine PTH reported in 1970 was initially confirmed, but recent re-examination by Brewer et al. (1) has suggested that amino acid 22 is not glutamic acid but glutamine, which becomes deaminated during the analytic procedure. The amino acid sequence for porcine PTH was recently published and found to have several amino acids different from bovine PTH, three of which occurred in the first 34 NH_2-terminal amino acids (2). Chick PTH has been partially purified and resembles bovine PTH in molecular size and charge as well as in biological activity (3).

Amino acid sequences have been published for the NH_2-terminal third of human PTH by two different laboratories with differing results. Both groups used human parathyroid adenomas rather than normal tissue as the starting material. Both the sequences published by Brewer et al. (1) and that published by Niall et al. (4) have been synthesized. Recently the Niall sequence was reinvestigated by the same laboratory and their identification confirmed (5). Moreover, there are two publications indicating that the immunoreactivity and biological activity of the material synthesized with the Niall sequence closely resemble human PTH in their behavior (6, 7).

Active Fragments Although previous studies indicated that the major form of bovine PTH, both in extracts of the parathyroid glands and in the effluent venous blood, was of the 84-amino-acid size, there is evidence that smaller, biologically active fragments of the hormone may be present either in the gland or produced after secretion. Such a fragment has been isolated from glands which represent bovine PTH 1-65 (8). This material could result from a tryptic-like cleavage of the molecule between lysine and serine; it could also represent incomplete synthesis. Its biological role is not known. It is now clear that the first 34 amino acids from the amino terminus in bovine PTH are sufficient for nearly complete biological activity (9). Studies of the cleavage products of bovine PTH in dogs (10) suggest that there may be a specific cleavage at amino acid 33. Studies with the use of isolated perfused liver have suggested that an active NH_2-terminal fragment is generated from the 1–84 molecule in the liver and that this phenomenon is under calcium control (11); that is, high calcium level inhibits and low calcium level stimulates this presumed activation step.

Proparathyroid Hormone   The existence of a precursor form of PTH is now well established. The form of proparathyroid hormone (pro-PTH) that was originally isolated from the parathyroid glands has been analyzed chemically, and the six additional amino acids of the amino terminus have been identified (12,13). It is not established whether this is the only extension of the pro-PTH molecule or whether there are additional amino acids at the COOH-terminal end which are cleaved to form 1–84 PTH.

Recently, Kemper et al. (14) reported a "pre-pro-PTH." This material was synthesized in vitro by using ribosomes and cofactors from nonparathyroid tissue and messenger RNA from bovine parathyroid glands. It contains at least 115 amino acids and includes an extension on the NH_2-terminal end. It has not been found in extracts of bovine parathyroid glands and, therefore, was presumed to be a short-lived form of the molecule. These amino acids may be important in initiating translation or in the transport of the pre-pro-PTH from the ribosomes to the endoplasmic reticulum. Subsequently, the pro-PTH is probably the form in which the hormone is taken up by the vesicles of the Golgi apparatus to form secretory granules. Studies of the conversion of pro-PTH to PTH output established the precursor-product relationship (15), and chronic studies have suggested that this conversion may be a point at which PTH is regulated (16,17). However, in acute studies, no effect of calcium on conversion of pro-PTH to PTH could be demonstrated (18). Studies showing that colchicine and vinblastine increase the ratio of pro-PTH to PTH in bovine parathyroid glands suggested that microtubules may be involved in the intracellular conversion (19). Ordinarily, pro-PTH is completely converted to PTH before secretion; however, it is possible that under pathological circumstances conversion may be incomplete. The release of a large molecule which could be pro-PTH has been demonstrated in cultures of human parathyroid adenomas (20) and in cases of ectopic hyperparathyroidism produced by nonparathyroid malignancies (21).

Secreted, Circulating, and Active Molecular Species   Even if we accept that the major active hormone secreted by the parathyroid glands is 1–84 PTH, it is clear that other material can be released by the parathyroids. A small glycoprotein with a molecular weight of about 3,000 has been found in the medium of cultured rat parathyroid glands (22), and a larger 50,000-molecular-weight parathyroid secretory protein (PSP) has been identified in the incubation fluid of bovine parathyroid slices (23). Both materials appeared to be released under calcium control. It is possible that these materials are derived from components of the secretory granules or the cell membrane that are released during secretion.

A number of laboratories have confirmed that circulating immunoreactive PTH represents several different molecular species (24–28). Of these, the most persistent appears to be a 7,500-molecular-weight COOH-terminal peptide which is presumed to be biologically inactive although its activity has not been studied in all systems. The presence of low molecular weight, biologically active fragments in the circulation has been reported (29), but there may also be biologically inactive, low molecular weight end products.

Immunoassays

Because of the heterogeneity of circulating immunoreactive PTH referred to above, there has been some uncertainty in the interpretation of radioimmunoassays, although these have been developed to a considerable degree of precision and sophistication. Since PTH receptors in the kidney have been identified, it should be possible to develop a specific radioreceptor assay with the use of renal membranes. Such an assay has not yet reached general application. Bioassays have been improved both in sensitivity and precision, but are still not able to detect circulating PTH.

Biological Assays Bioassays based on the hypercalcemic response of the intact chick or quail to PTH appear to be more sensitive and rapid than the classic Munson assay using parathyroidectomized rats (30,31). Assays based on PTH stimulation or renal adenylate cyclase are rapid and widely used but of relatively low sensitivity and specificity. Analysis of the structural requirements for this effect suggests that different portions of the molecule may be involved in binding to renal membrane and in activating adenylate cyclase (32). In addition to the earlier in vitro bioassays based on the ability of PTH to mobilize previously incorporated radiocalcium from cultured bones, assays which use PTH inhibition of citrate oxidation (33) and increased stable calcium in the medium (34) have been presented. At best, these assays can detect PTH at concentrations of 10^{-9} M, which is certainly not sufficient to measure circulating, biologically active material. Nevertheless, such a bioassay would be most useful since it is apparent that the biological and immunological activity of parathyroid hormone can be dissociated; for example, oxidation of methionine will inactivate PTH biologically but not immunologically (35).

Radioimmunoassay Recent development of more sequence-specific antibodies to PTH should permit more precise identification of circulating forms. The data continue to support the concept that the chronic state of parathyroid activity is better reflected by circulating concentrations of inactive COOH-terminal fragments than by concentrations of whole PTH or smaller NH_2-terminal fragments (36). A new method has been presented for labeling parathyroid hormone which does not inactivate the molecule biologically (37). A novel method for measuring bound hormone has also been described (38). Nevertheless, there have been no major advances in the methodology or in the application of PTH immunoassay since the subject was reviewed in 1973 (39).

Sites and Modes of Action

Recent studies have reinforced the concept that bone and kidney are the major target organs for PTH. On the other hand, in both of these tissues the effects of the hormones are complex and probably involve multiple sites and mechanisms. The effects of PTH on other tissues are less well defined and their biological importance uncertain. Nevertheless, it is possible that PTH has an important role in regulating intracellular calcium concentration in many tissues.

Bone   The actions of PTH on bone probably involve at least two completely separate systems. The following list represents the major direct effects of the hormone. It is presented in the approximate time sequence in which the effects occur. This sequence may be more of a reflection of ability to measure a particular change than of the actual sequence of events.

1. Binding to a specific cell surface receptor.
2. Activation of adenylate cyclase.
3. Increased entry of calcium into cells.
4. Increased synthesis of hyaluronic acid.
5. Increased relative volume of ruffled borders in osteoclasts.
6. Decreased oxidation of citrate to CO_2.
7. Decreased collagen synthesis.
8. Increase in the number and size of osteoclasts.
9. Proliferation of endosteal fibroblasts and conversion of periosteal osteoblasts to fibroblast-like cells.

The relationships among these phenomena are difficult to determine. It is likely that different populations of PTH-responsive cells are involved. For example, hyaluronic acid synthesis appears to be associated with bone resorption and may be a function of osteoclasts or their precursors (40,41). Collagen synthesis is clearly a function of osteoblasts (42). It is not clear whether osteoclasts and osteoblasts derive from the same cell line or have separate precursors. Because of the tight linkage between osteoclastic bone resorption and osteoblastic bone formation in vivo, it was recently postulated that there is a direct conversion of bone-resorbing cells to bone-forming cells. However, there is little experimental evidence to support this view (43).

The relationship between early effects of parathyroid hormone and the subsequent changes in bone resorption and formation remains obscure. The idea that cyclic AMP (cAMP) mediates the resorptive response has been challenged by recent studies (44) which show substantial differences between effects of agents which increase the concentration of cyclic nucleotides such as dibutyryl-cAMP and theophylline and the effect of PTH itself. It is possible that cAMP concentration is increased differentially in different cell populations from bone in response to PTH or CT (45). Whatever its effects on bone metabolism, the increase of cAMP concentration is one of the most sensitive indicators of PTH action on bone cells. It can be observed at much lower concentrations of PTH in vitro than are required to produce changes in bone resorption or formation (46,47). Recently, it has been found that adenosine enhances the cAMP response of isolated bone cells to PTH (48).

The quantitative role of osteocytic osteolysis in PTH-stimulated bone resorption is not established, although morphological studies have shown an increase in osteocytic lacunar size and changes suggestive of resorption (49). Quantitative morphological studies of a different resorption model, namely, hypervitaminosis D, indicated that only a small proportion of bone loss could be accounted for by osteocytes and that the major mechanism was probably osteoclastic resorption (50).

Kidney   Recent attempts to determine the precise sites and mechanisms of action of PTH on the kidney have suggested that, as in bone, the hormone has different effects on different cell types and systems. In the proximal tubule, PTH decreases the reabsorption of sodium, calcium, and phosphate (51). This effect is mimicked by dibutyryl-cAMP. PTH can also inhibit the secretion of hydrogen ions and increase the excretion of bicarbonate (52). This effect resembles that of carbonic anhydrase inhibitors, and it has been suggested that PTH and cAMP work by inhibiting this enzyme (53). However, in a subsequent study no such effect could be demonstrated (54).

The net effects of PTH on calcium and phosphate excretion probably depend upon effects beyond the proximal tubule. A similar inhibition of sodium and phosphate reabsorption is produced by either volume expansion with saline solution infusions or PTH administration, but after PTH the fraction of phosphate excreted in the urine is much higher than after treatment with saline solution (55). This is presumably due to inhibition of phosphate reabsorption in the Henle loop and beyond (56). PTH probably also stimulates calcium reabsorption distally, although the precise site has not been identified.

Increased tubular reabsorption of calcium may play an important role in the regulation of serum calcium by PTH in older animals and calcium-loaded animals in whom bone turnover is decreased, but in calcium deprivation the bone effect must predominate (57,58). The renal mechanism for serum calcium regulation by PTH appears to be particularly important in the hamster (59). It may also be the predominant factor in the hypercalcemia produced by low doses of PTH, whereas excessive bone resorption could play a greater role at high PTH concentrations.

Intestine   The issue of whether PTH has important, direct effects on the intestine has not been resolved. Evidence has been presented to show that parathyroid hormone can alter calcium release from mucosal cells as well as the activity of a calcium-dependent phosphatase (60,61), apparently independent of changes in vitamin D metabolism. On the other hand, the effect of parathyroid hormone to stimulate the synthesis of the active metabolite of vitamin D $(1,25\text{-}(OH)_2 D_3)$ could mediate the changes seen in calcium absorption in hyper-

and hypoparathyroidism (62). The physiological importance of endogenous PTH in regulating intestinal absorption of calcium was relatively small in nutritional studies in the rat (63).

The secretion of acid and pepsin by the stomach may also be increased in hyperparathyroidism. This may be an indirect effect of hypercalcemia, which is known to stimulate gastric secretion, rather than a direct effect of PTH on gastric mucosal cells (64).

Other Tissues   In addition to the major target organ systems—bone, kidney, and intestine—PTH probably affects the metabolism of many other body tissues. However, no physiological or regulatory role for the hormone has been established in other target organs. In the liver, PTH is not only degraded but, as noted above, may be split to release an active, low molecular weight metabolite. PTH can increase adenylate cyclase activity in liver although high concentrations are required (65). Even higher concentrations have been used to increase glucose and urea production in isolated cells (66). PTH may affect cell proliferation, not only in the liver (67) but in many other cells, particularly in the lymphoid and hematopoietic systems (68). These effects have been largely demonstrated in vitro and represent complex interactions between cell calcium, cyclic nucleotides, and calcium regulatory hormones. Such interactions are probably also involved in the stimulation of lipolysis by PTH which is accompanied by increased tissue calcium (69) and opposed by CT (70). Calcium may also mediate the effect of hyperparathyroidism to increase the insulin response to glucose (71). The effects of PTH on the nervous system were originally thought to largely represent indirect results of changes in serum calcium concentration. However, PTH may also affect intracellular calcium in the brain, possibly mediating the electroencephalographic changes in uremia (72) and the degenerative changes in motor neurons seen in hyperparathyroidism (73). The neuromuscular defect in hyperparathyroidism appears to involve the nerves of type II or slow muscle fibers selectively and to be related more to the chronicity of the disorder than to the severity of hypercalcemia.

Mechanisms of Action   The current concept of the action of peptide hormones and catecholamines is that there is a specific receptor for each hormone on the target cell membrane. This receptor is linked to a membrane-bound adenylate cyclase. However, the link may contain intermediate steps which could represent additional control points. Ordinarily, binding of hormone to the receptor activates adenylate cyclase and increases the production of cAMP. Increased cyclic nucleotide production in turn can alter cell metabolism through the activation of specific protein kinases by the binding of cAMP to regulatory subunits. These protein kinases may phosphorylate or dephosphorylate key enzymes in the cell and hence affect specific metabolic reactions. In the case of parathyroid hormone, the first step of binding to the cell surface has now been reasonably well demonstrated for the kidney (74,75), and the activation of adenylate cyclase has been demonstrated in kidney, bone, and other systems. Definitive evidence for a protein kinase has not yet been presented. As noted above, some of the changes in bone metabolism in response to PTH are not easily explained by adenylate cyclase activation alone, and the existence of additional mediators, possibly involving other cyclic nucleotides, has been suggested. Modulation of parathyroid hormone responses by changes in ionic environment or by other hormones can occur, and it has been suggested that these factors exert their influence by affecting cyclic nucleotide responses (43).

Whatever the initial effects of parathyroid hormone on cyclic nucleotide metabolism, it is not yet possible to connect its effect to specific physiological responses. In particular, there is no direct evidence linking adenylate cyclase activation to alterations in cell transcription in the nucleus, although earlier studies suggested that PTH did effect transcription, particularly in bone. This problem may now be easier to study with the use of isolated populations of bone cells with different response to PTH.

Regulation of Secretion

Recent studies have reinforced the concept that PTH secretion is under exquisitely precise control by circulating ionized calcium concentration. Changes of as little as 1% can alter PTH secretion in seconds (76). This initial effect probably involves a small pool of PTH and may be separate from effects on hormone synthesis and even on the release of hormone that has been stored for a long time. In vitro studies suggest that newly synthesized hormone can bypass the secretory granule and be secreted almost immediately in a stimulated gland (77). The inhibitory effects of hypercalcemia may involve accelerated degradation of PTH stores as well as decreased synthesis and secretion (78). There have been few additional studies on the mechanism of calcium regulation. Evidence that the microtubule system is involved has been obtained by morphological studies which show that parathyroid microtubule content is increased in stimulated glands (79). In addition to inhibiting the conversion of pro-PTH to PTH, as noted above, colchicine can increase the number of secretory granules in the parathyroid, and vinblastine, another inhibitor of microtubules, can decrease PTH secretion in vitro (80). It was also reported that vitamin A and cytochalasin B enhance PTH secretion in bovine gland slices. This could point to roles for lysosomal enzyme activation and microfilaments in the secretory process, although their precise role is not known. A role for cAMP in regulating parathyroid gland secretion has been suggested but not established. Additional evidence that high concentrations of dibutyryl-cAMP and theophylline can enhance PTH release has been presented (81), but no calcium-sensitive adenylate cyclase has been reported.

The role of magnesium in regulating parathyroid function has been clarified by several recent studies. Contrary to earlier concepts, magnesium appears to be much less effective than calcium in inhibiting PTH secretion (82). Moreover, there is recent evidence that the development of hypocalcemia in magnesium deficiency is due to impairment of PTH synthesis and secretion (83,84). This may not explain hypocalcemia entirely since there is also evidence for impaired end organ response to PTH in magnesium deficiency (85). Moreover, it does not explain the hypercalcemia observed in magnesium-deficient rats. Presumably in this species, magnesium deficiency is associated either with increased PTH secretion, increased end organ sensitivity, or the formation of an unrelated hypercalcemic factor.

There is now evidence in vivo (86,87), as well as in vitro (81), that β-adrenergic agents, such as epinephrine, can stimulate PTH secretion. This phenomenon is of uncertain physiological significance but could explain the association between pheochromocytoma and hypercalcemia (88), although the alternative possibility of production of a PTH-like substance by pheochromo-cytomas has also been postulated (89). Parathyroid gland metabolism may also be influenced by glucocorticoids, vitamin A, and vitamin D. In vivo administration of glucocorticoids can cause a rapid increase in serum PTH concentration, which could be an indirect effect mediated by the inhibition of bone resorption or decreased calcium absorption in the intestine (90,91). However, evidence for direct stimulation of the parathyroid glands has recently been presented (92). The effect of vitamin D on the parathyroids appears to be inhibitory. In vivo vitamin D-deficient individuals often have high serum PTH concentrations, and the administration of vitamin D can reduce these values (93). Vitamin D could act indirectly by increasing calcium absorption or bone resorption. However, $1,25(OH)_2D_3$ is localized in the parathyroid glands (94), and a calcium binding protein has been isolated from the parathyroids (95). Recently, evidence for a direct inhibitory effect of $1,25(OH)_2D_3$ on PTH secretion has been obtained both in vitro and in vivo (96). As noted above, vitamin A may have a nonspecific stimulatory effect on PTH secretion related to its ability to activate lysosomal enzymes (97).

Metabolism

The metabolism of PTH is complex and may involve both inactivation and activation processes. The major sites are the liver and kidney. As noted above, the generation of PTH fragments in isolated perfused livers may be under calcium control. If high calcium levels inhibited and low calcium levels stimulated the generation of active fragment, this could represent an additional control point. However, such control has not yet been demonstrated with the use of homologous hormone. Renal degradation appears to be largely to inactive products. A heat-labile enzyme which hydrolyzes parathyroid hormone has been identified but not purified (98). In the rat, this enzyme appears to be associated with the binding site for PTH, but this association was not found in bovine tissue (99).

The metabolic clearance of PTH is rapid and represents the sum of several different removal rates. The disappearance of PTH has been measured after stopping a constant intravenous infusion of bovine PTH in the dog (100). A complex multiexponential curve was obtained. The first two half-times were 4–8 and 50–100 min, respectively. Both the liver and the kidney showed large arteriovenous differences in PTH concentration.

The role of the kidney in degradation has been studied in both normal dogs and in animals with renal failure (101). In these animals, the renal clearance represented 60% of the total removal of hormone for natural 1–84 bovine PTH and even more for the 1–34 synthetic active fragment. In renal failure, not only the renal, but also the extrarenal, clearance was depressed (102). As in man, dogs with renal failure show increased accumulation of fragments of PTH in the blood, particularly the large, presumably inactive, COOH-terminal moiety. Renal membranes prepared from canine kidneys can degrade PTH to produce a COOH-terminal fragment similar to the circulating material (102). In renal failure, there may be enough tissue to form this fragment but not enough function to clear it from the blood.

CALCITONIN (THYROCALCITONIN)

Since calcitonin was extensively reviewed in the preceding volume of this series and since there have been few major changes in our understanding of this hormone, only a brief update is provided in this section.

Cellular and Embryonic Origin

The neural crest origin of calcitonin-producing or C-cells which belong to the so-called APUD series (cells which are capable of amine precursor uptake and decarboxylation), first described by Pearse (103), is now well established (104). The well recognized clinical association of medullary carcinoma of the thyroid (a tumor of thyroid C-cells) with pheochromocytoma and parathyroid adenoma or hyperplasia may be related to the neural crest origin of these cells. This common origin may account for the recent finding of biologically active and immunoreactive CT in pheochromocytomas, and of catecholamines in metastatic medullary carcinoma cells (105). However, because it is now apparent that a wide variety of neoplastic tissues can release materials which cross-react with CT antibodies (106–108), the specificity of these findings is still not clear.

In the chick, a close relationship between PTH and CT-secreting cells has been suggested by studies which show that not only do ultimobranchial bodies contain parathyroid tissue but that calcitonin-like activity may be secreted by the parathyroid (109). Interestingly, the secretion of this calcitonin-like activity by the parathyroid appears to be stimulated by low calcium concentration. The relevance of these findings to mammalian systems is unknown.

Chemistry and Structure-Activity Relationships

Several calcitonins have now been added to the series of five molecules whose amino acid sequences were reviewed in the previous volume. CT from rats has been isolated and purified (110). In addition, a number of analogs of human CT have now been synthesized, including compounds with alterations in amino acids 29 and 31 which are more potent than the native molecule (111).

Receptors

The relative potency of different forms of CT has been demonstrated not only in bioassays but also by their relative affinity for receptors prepared from either kidney or bone tissue (112). Competitive binding studies in these tissues showed that salmon CT has a higher affinity for the receptors than the other forms. The high biological potency of salmon CT in vivo may be due to both this greater affinity to receptors and a slower rate of degradation (113). In rats, but not in man, cow, or dog, the CT receptor and CT-activated adenylate cyclase can be isolated together in renal membrane preparations and show parallel sensitivity to different forms of CT (114).

Preliminary evidence has also been presented for CT receptors on lymphoid cells growing in continuous culture (115). Inhibitory effects of CT on the lymphocyte mitogenic response have been demonstrated in vitro (116–118). Although the relationship between the lymphoid cell lines studied by Marx and his co-workers and normal lymphocytes is unclear, it is possible that these receptors on lymphoid cells may have physiological importance. The recent finding of CT receptors on marrow cells has been related to bone-resorbing cells or their precursors, but could represent a lymphoid cell receptor as well (119).

Biological and Radioimmunological Assays

Biological Assays As radioimmunoassays have been undergoing intensive study, less attention has been paid to biological assays. Nevertheless, highly sensitive bioassays for CT are available. For example, with the use of an in vitro bioassay, it was possible to demonstrate increased CT concentration in the sera of patients with medullary carcinoma of the thyroid (120). This bioassay measures an upper limit of approximately 0.5 ng/ml of biologically active CT in the blood. The fact that such concentrations are not observed in normal subjects even after calcium infusion suggests that some of the immunoassays which record higher levels may be measuring biologically inactive material (see below).

Radioimmunoassays Many radioimmunoassays for different forms of CT have now been presented. All of these are sensitive and show increases in immunoreactive CT in response to physiological stimuli such as calcium or gastrointestinal peptides. Recent studies suggest that the material being measured in the plasma in normal people (121,122) and in medullary carcinoma of the thyroid (123) is quite heterogeneous and may involve either large molecules which cross-react with CT or aggregated forms of CT. There is still considerable controversy concerning the normal concentrations of CT in the serum. Some assays, particularly those which use extraction procedures (124), report substantially lower levels than others (125). It seems likely that true CT may be present at concentrations of 50 pg/ml or less in the circulating blood. The higher levels reported by other immunoassays could represent cross-reactivity with other plasma proteins or degradation products.

Sites and Modes of Action   The inhibition of bone resorption remains the most clear cut and physiologically interpretable effect of CT. Nevertheless, other effects of CT are clearly important and may be physiologically more important than the inhibition of bone resorption in man. There are clearly powerful effects on the intestine, and there may be general effects on cell transport of calcium (126) and phosphate (127). The latter could explain why phosphate concentrations can be lowered in animals under conditions in which calcium is not affected (128). The renal effects of CT have not received much further study and are probably less important than its effects on bone and intestine.

Bone   The effect of calcitonin on bone resorption appears to be due to a rapid and almost complete inhibition of the activity of osteoclasts (129–131). The loss of osteoclast ruffled borders has been reported as early as 15 min after calcitonin administration and is quantitatively significant at 1 hr. In tissue culture, the inhibition of ruffled border activity has paralleled the inhibition of ^{45}Ca release, and when the escape phenomenon occurs the number of ruffled borders increases (131). Escape is not a universal response of osteoclasts; for example, colchicine causes prolonged inhibition of bone resorption and ruffled border activity in the same model system.

The inability of continuous high concentrations of calcitonin to maintain inhibition of bone resorption is supported by certain in vivo observations (132). In hyperparathyroid subjects, calcitonin produces only a transient decrease in serum calcium (133). In patients with medullary carcinoma of the thyroid, serum calcium regulation appears to be normal. However, it is possible that calcitonin exerts a chronic inhibitory effect on osteoclasts which is masked by the slow bone turnover in this condition. In patients with Paget's disease, CT produces a powerful inhibitory effect on osteoclasts quite rapidly, but this effect also can be transient and escape has been reported (134). Here, loss of response is much slower than in hyperparathyroidism and usually takes several months.

Other effects of CT on bone metabolism have not really been established. For example, there are almost an equal number of studies suggesting increased bone formation and decreased bone formation as the primary calcitonin response (135). The simplest resolution of this problem might be to suggest that calcitonin does not have any direct effect on osteoblasts. An indirect effect mediated through its effects on osteoclasts has been suggested to explain the decrease in bone-forming cells as well as bone-resorbing cells following calcitonin treatment of Paget's disease (136). However, the nature of this coupling has not been established.

Kidney   Since CT has been shown to bind to renal tissue and to elevate cyclic AMP concentrations (137) and since the receptor differs from that of PTH or vasopressin, which also increases AMP in the kidney, it is likely the hormone has some effect on renal tubular transport. Multiple effects on ion excretion have been reported (138,139), but these may represent nonspecific inhibition of tubular transport and have little importance in the regulation of mineral metabolism (140).

Gastrointestinal Tract   The multiple and complex interactions between CT and the gastrointestinal system point increasingly to a major role for CT as a gastrointestinal hormone. CT has been shown to be a powerful inhibitor of gastric acid and pepsin secretion (141,142). Although gastrin release is also inhibited by calcitonin (143), the effect on gastric acid secretion is probably not mediated through an inhibitory effect on gastrin secretion (144). A feedback system involving gastrin stimulation of calcitonin and calcitonin inhibition of gastrin would provide an important regulatory system.

Recent evidence strongly supports a role for physiological levels of calcitonin in regulating small intestinal secretion. Calcitonin causes an increase in intestinal secretion in man (145). It does not appear to affect mineral transport specifically, although there may be a decrease in phosphate absorption (146). The general effect on intestinal secretion may resemble that of other agents such as cholera toxin and prostaglandins which increase cyclic AMP concentration and enhance intestinal secretion. The question of a specific effect on calcium absorption has not been resolved, although recent studies suggest that CT does not have an important direct influence on calcium transport (147).

Mechanisms of Action   It is now well established that both calcitonin and parathyroid hormone increase intracellular cAMP concentrations in bone and kidney, but that the receptors are distinct (75,137,148). It is easier to accept the hypothesis that all the effects of CT are mediated through cAMP than it is to accept this hypothesis for PTH. Most calcitonin effects are acute and can be mimicked by either cAMP analogs or other agents which increase cAMP concentration. On the other hand, the role of calcium as a modulator of cAMP response to CT may also be important. Recent evidence supports the concept that CT increases cell calcium content (126,149,150). However, PTH is also supposed to increase calcium entry into bone cells, and it is difficult to explain how parathyroid hormone and calcitonin have opposite effects on osteoclasts if their actions are related to intracellular calcium. One possibility is that there may be a biphasic effect of intracellular calcium; from low to intermediate concentrations, bone resorption is stimulated, but at higher concentrations, bone resorption is inhibited. Earlier studies of the relationship of medium calcium concentration to the ability of PTH to induce prolonged resorptive responses are consistent with this possibility (151).

Regulation of Secretion

Although calcium is a potent secretagogue for CT and both magnesium and strontium also stimulate secretion (152), the regulation of this hormone is quite different from that of PTH in the extent to which nonionic factors affect secretion. The regulatory effects of the gastrointestinal hormones on CT secretion were reviewed in the previous volume. Recent evidence serves largely to reinforce the importance of this regulation. Under any circumstances in which serum gastrin concentrations are increased, CT secretion appears to be enhanced (153). A feedback system exists whereby calcitonin in turn inhibits gastrin secretion. Elevations in serum gastrin may increase CT secretion early during the ingestion of a meal. This could explain the fact that serum calcium concentrations may actually fall during feeding (154). An increase in CT could also occur in anticipation of feeding through neurological stimulation of gastrin secretion, although there is conflict concerning this possibility (154,155). Although gastrin is a potent CT secretagogue, many other hormones as well as cAMP analogs have been shown to stimulate calcitonin secretion at high concentrations (156—159). The physiological importance of these stimuli is not known.

Metabolism

Although some further data on the metabolism of CT have been presented (160,161), these largely confirm that a number of organs can inactivate the various calcitonins and that there are important differences in the half-life between hormones of different species. The fact that multiple forms of immunoreactive CT are found in the blood could indicate that metabolic transformations other than simple degradation take place. However, this area has not yet been explored.

Physiological Role

The major effect of CT is probably to prevent hypercalcemia following food ingestion. CT secreted before or during feeding would decrease bone resorption so that the absorbed calcium would not lead to hypercalcemia or hypercalciuria and could be deposited in bone. The increase in intestinal secretion may represent an additional aid in absorption. Such mechanisms would be most important in growing animals and might be relatively unimportant in adults with fully developed skeletons in whom bone turnover is less important for calcium regulation than intestinal absorption and renal excretion. However, there is some evidence that in older rats calcitonin may exert tonic physiological control of serum calcium concentration (162,163). In such animals, thyroparathyroidectomy and thyroidectomy produced an increase in serum calcium concentration, whereas in younger animals only a decrease in serum calcium concentration was observed after thyroparathyroidectomy. Evidence reviewed in the previous volume also suggests that calcitonin has an important role in calcium regulation during other stages of high mineral demands such as egg laying, pregnancy, and lactation, as well as during rapid growth; recent immunoassay measurements support this view (164—167).

VITAMIN D

It is now established that the activation of vitamin D in the liver and kidney involves a controlled hormonal system vital for the regulation of calcium and phosphate metabolism. The rapid progress in this area has resulted in many publications. Since these have been summarized in several reviews (168-172), this section outlines the major advances by using a few key references.

Chemistry

A number of natural and synthetic forms of vitamin D and its active metabolites have now been synthesized and tested biologically. Vitamin D_2 (ergocalciferol), the plant form, is synthesized by irradiation of ergosterol. Vitamin D_3 (cholecalciferol), the natural form, is synthesized by irradiation of 7-dehydrocholesterol in the skin. Both undergo 25-hydroxylation in the liver. 25-(OH)D_3 and probably D_2 can undergo further hydroxylation to $1\alpha,25$-(OH)$_2 D_3$ or 24R,25-(OH)$_2 D_3$ in the kidney. An additional form which combines these hydroxylations (1,24,25-(OH)$_3 D_3$) has been identified (173). Other compounds which have been synthesized but presumably are not formed naturally include isomers of the natural forms, such as *trans*-25-(OH)D_3, instead of the natural *cis* isomer, and compounds in which one of the hydroxyl groups has been deleted (1α-(OH)D_3 and $1\alpha,3$-deoxy-D_3) (174,175). Both of these compounds are biologically active in vivo, but this may depend upon their being 25-hydroxylated in the liver (176).

Synthesis

Vitamin D is unique among hormones because its synthesis involves three steps in different organs and because of the importance of the dietary supply of active material. The emergence of rickets and osteomalacia as a major clinical problem and the discovery of vitamin D as an essential food factor could be ascribed to environmental factors. In the industrial revolution, the combination of limited sunlight in the temperate zone, long working hours, and poor intakes of calcium or phosphate which might increase the requirement for active forms of vitamin D made supplementation essential.

Skin Even though there is now substantial supplementation of the Western diet with vitamin D_2, most of the active vitamin D in the body is probably D_3 formed in the skin by irradiation of 7-dehydrocholesterol with ultraviolet light; 70-90% of 25-(OH)D in the blood is in the form of D_3 when large loads of D_2 are administered (177). Increased exposure to ultraviolet irradiation either from sunlight or artificial ultraviolet light can increase the levels of 25-(OH)D_3 in the plasma (178,179). Since such changes can be accompanied by changes in intestinal calcium absorption, they are presumably of physiological importance. However, the skin does not appear to be an important regulatory site. Differences in skin pigmentation, either genetic or in response to ultraviolet radiation, probably do not have a large effect on ultimate vitamin D activity.

Liver The liver is the site of both inactivation and activation of vitamin D. There are probably several different inactivation steps. Only one activation step has been identified: 25-hydroxylation. The enzyme or enzymes which carry out this process differ from the microsomal, mixed function oxidases which generally convert endogenous steroids and many exogenous drugs to inactive products. There may be separate enzymes or differences in the regulation of 25-hydroxylation for D_2, D_3, and dihydrotachysterol (DHT) (180,181). There is no evidence for a long loop or physiological feedback regulation of 25-$(OH)D_3$ formation. The major control appears to be by product inhibition. As a result, 25-$(OH)D_3$ concentration in the blood may increase only 2-fold as D_3 intake is increased by several orders of magnitude (181). Hydroxylation of DHT is not limited to the same extent. This may account for the ability of this compound to produce greater calcium mobilization in man and experimental animals.

Kidney On the basis of current knowledge, the true "endocrine organ" for vitamin D is the kidney. It is here that the activation step of 1,25-$(OH)_2D_3$ occurs, as well as hydroxylation at position 24. Both processes appear to be under physiological control. The 1α-hydroxylase in the kidney has been studied extensively. It is a mitochondrial enzyme containing cytochrome P_{450} and resembles the specific adrenal hydroxylases which are involved in activation of cholesterol to biologically active glucocorticoids. This enzyme has been extensively studied in the chick, where it can readily be extracted from kidney tissue (182,183). Its regulation has also been studied in vitro with the use of isolated renal tubules and mitochondria. The results are complex and difficult to relate to in vivo observations; enzyme activity can be influenced by other hormones, by the product 1,25-$(OH)_2D_3$, and by the concentrations of calcium, phosphate, and other ions (184–186). The enzyme can hydroxylate 25-$(OH)D_3$ and probably also 25-$(OH)D_2$. 24,25-$(OH)_2D_3$ can also be hydroxylated at position 1, presumably by the same enzyme. The enzyme appears early in fetal life; it is found in the 9-day fetal embryonic chick mesonephros (187), although the amounts are greater later in development. The enzyme which hydroxylates 25-$(OH)D_3$ on the side chain to form 24,25-$(OH)_2D_3$ has not been extensively studied. There is evidence that the two hydroxylations may be coupled to the extent that, as 1-hydroxylase activity increases, 24-hydroxylase decreases and vice versa (171,172).

Physiological Regulation of Synthesis and Secretion

Vitamin D differs from the peptide hormones PTH and CT in that it does not appear to be stored in the form of secretory granules. There is abundant storage of the lipid-soluble inactive forms. Both D_3 and D_2 can accumulate not only in fat but in muscle and liver. As noted above, activation in the skin and 25-hydroxylation in the liver have not been shown to be under feedback physiological control. An enterohepatic circulation for 25-$(OH)D_3$ has been postulated, but this is more likely to be an excretory than a regulatory mechanism. 25-$(OH)D_3$ is the major circulating form of the hormone and is to this extent the storage form since the blood concentration is high relative to the amount needed for activation in the kidney. This high blood level exists in the form of 25-$(OH)D_3$ bound to a specific plasma binding protein with selective affinity for this metabolite (188,189). The amount of binding protein is not affected by variations in intake of calcium and phosphate, which would influence activation in the kidney (190).

The major site for physiological regulation appears to be the kidney. The formation of 1,25-$(OH)_2D_3$ responds to changes in parathyroid function or calcium and phosphate intake. It has been difficult to correlate these changes with enzyme activity in the rat because the 1α-hydroxylase cannot be extracted due to an inhibitor in rat renal tissue. The importance of parathyroid function has been demonstrated in man as well as rat (191). When intact animals are calcium-depleted, 1,25-$(OH)_2D_3$ formation is increased, but parathyroidectomy can abolish this response. The increased intestinal absorption of calcium which occurs on low intakes presumably depends upon PTH stimulation of metabolite activation since animals on a constant intake of 1,25-$(OH)_2D_3$ do not show this response to calcium deficiency (192). This suggests that 1,25-$(OH)_2D_3$ is Nicolaysen's endogenous factor, that is, the substance which mediates the absorptive response to dietary calcium intake and links it with bone turnover. It is likely that the regulation will be more complex when fully elucidated. The formation of 24,25-$(OH)_2D_3$ is generally reciprocally related to 1α-hydroxylase activity. However, this relationship is not always precise, and the amount of 24,25-metabolite may influence the response. Finally, it is possible that 1,24,25-$(OH)_3D_3$ is an important physiological form, which would further complicate the regulatory system.

PTH is a major regulator of 1-hydroxylation (193,194), but this may not represent a direct effect of the hormone. Parathyroidectomized animals can increase 1-hydroxylation and decrease 24-hydroxylation when given diets deficient in phosphate (195). This result led DeLuca and Tanaka to postulate that intracellular phosphate concentration controls 1-hydroxylation. In calcium deficiency, secondary hyperparathyroidism would inhibit tubular reabsorption of phosphate and hence decrease cell phosphate concentration. In phosphate depletion, this would occur as a direct effect. The latter would be more marked in the absence of parathyroid hormone since phosphate depletion inhibits PTH secretion, which would result in increased tubular reabsorption of phosphate. The acquisition of new knowledge in this field is so rapid that this theory, like its predecessors, may soon require revision.

Metabolism

Inactivation of vitamin D probably occurs in the liver. Inactive metabolites include a wide variety of polar forms (196). The inactivation of vitamin D can be stimulated by enzyme induction in the liver. Phenobarbitol and diphenylhydantoin are particularly effective inducers of the nonspecific microsomal, mixed function oxidase systems which inactivate steroid hormones. This may explain the effect of chronic anticonvulsive therapy to decrease serum 25-$(OH)D_3$ concentrations in the blood and increase the incidence of subclinical or clinical rickets and osteomalacia in epileptic patients (197).

Little is known about the metabolic inactivation of the hydroxylated active forms of vitamin D. 25-$(OH)D_3$ is found in the bile and undergoes enterohepatic recirculation (198), probably in the form of an inactive glucuronide or sulfate conjugate. The inactivation of the dihydroxy and trihydroxy metabolites is probably relatively rapid. This, together with the fact that much less is bound to a circulating plasma protein, probably accounts for a shorter half-life in the blood. Little is known about the degradation of $1,25\text{-}(OH)_2 D_3$, although there is some evidence that it can be affected by glucocorticoids (199).

Mechanisms of Action

Although the data are not as extensive as those for glucocorticoids and estrogens, there is evidence that $1,25\text{-}(OH)_2 D_3$ has a specific cytosol receptor and like other steroid hormones is carried into the nucleus where it interacts with chromatin to produce changes in transcription (200–202). The specificity of this receptor system has not been completely worked out. Other metabolites can be bound by rat intestinal cytosol (203) and can have biological effects on chick intestine in organ culture (204). The data are even more fragmentary for bone, but evidence for nuclear localization for $1,25\text{-}(OH)_2 D_3$ has been presented (205). Nuclear binding of the active forms of vitamin D could result in many transcriptional changes. One of these is the synthesis of calcium-binding protein (CaBP). Isolated chick intestinal polyribosomes from vitamin D-treated chick can synthesize CaBP, but polyribosomes from vitamin D-deficient animals cannot (206). Additional effects of vitamin D directly on cell membranes have been postulated on the basis of the resemblance of its effects to those of the polyene antibiotic filipin in increasing cellular calcium uptake (207). This could represent a nonspecific high dose effect on lipid membranes, such as has been described for other steroid hormones. An interaction between vitamin D and adenylate cyclase has also been postulated on the basis of increased cAMP content in vitamin D-treated cultured chick intestine (208) and an increase in the amount of cAMP produced in response to PTH in bone cells treated with either 25-$(OH)D_3$ or $1,25\text{-}(OH)_2 D_3$ (209). However, direct stimulation of membrane-bound adenylate cyclase through a surface receptor has not been demonstrated.

Effects on Intestine

The most extensively studied biochemical effect of vitamin D is the stimulation of intestinal synthesis of CaBP. This protein has now been identified in a large number of species (210). Most of the mammalian proteins isolated are similar in molecular size (about 10,000 daltons), electrophoretic mobility, amino acid composition, and affinity for calcium. The role of CaBP in intestinal absorption of calcium is still not established. Earlier data localized the protein to the brush border of mucosal cells and cytoplasm of goblet cells. More recently, CaBP has been identified inside the mucosal cells as well as in kidney tubule and pancreatic islet cells (211). Electron probe analysis suggests that calcium transport may occur in packets intracellularly, but it is not known whether this is in association with CaBP or some other subcellular moiety (212). This localization could represent uptake by mitochondria since it has been shown that intestinal cells from vitamin D-deficient animals show impaired mitochondrial calcium uptake which is improved by vitamin D treatment (213). Another possible mechanism for the effect of vitamin D on intestinal calcium transport is an increase in the activity or synthesis of a divalent cation-dependent ATPase (214). Vitamin D also increases phosphate absorption in the intestine. This effect appears to be on an active transport system which can be stimulated independent of changes in calcium transport (215–217). Vitamin D may have a general tropic effect on the intestinal mucosa. The effect of vitamin D deficiency on some enzymes can be duplicated by starvation (214). Moreover, the rate of growth of intestinal mucosal cells is increased after vitamin D repletion (218,219).

Effects on Bone

The ability of active metabolites of vitamin D to stimulate bone resorption directly is now well established (220–222). This effect resembles that of PTH in that a short period of exposure to the vitamin produces prolonged resorptive responses (151). Since $1,25\text{-}(OH)_2D_3$ is by far the most active form of vitamin D in resorbing bone in tissue culture, it is possible that other forms may be converted to this metabolite by the bone cells. However, this would not account for all biological activities. For example, *trans*-25-(OH)DHT$_3$ which is not 1-hydroxylated is also capable of stimulating bone resorption directly (223). Just as earlier data showed that PTH was less effective in the absence of vitamin D, the bone resorptive effects of $1,25\text{-}(OH)_2D_3$ are blunted in parathyroidectomized animals. This does not appear to be the case for the intestinal effects of the active vitamin D metabolites (224).

The effects of vitamin D on bone formation remain uncertain. Any indirect effect on mineralization would occur because of increased calcium and phosphate absorption in the gut as well as calcium and phosphate release from resorbing bone. There are no in vitro studies demonstrating a direct effect of vitamin D on either bone matrix formation or mineralization that have been reported. Differences in collagen composition have been described between vitamin D-deficient and vitamin D-repleted animals, but these could represent alterations in the relative proportion of cartilage or immature osteoid and mature bone matrix.

Effects on Kidney

Despite extensive study, it is not certain whether vitamin D and its metabolites have important regulatory effects on mineral transport in the kidney (225). Interactions between PTH and vitamin D have been reported, and the effect of PTH on phosphate excretion is enhanced in vitamin D-repleted animals (226). Direct stimulation of tubular reabsorption of phosphate has been reported (227–229), as well as effects on renal transport of sodium and calcium. These effects are small relative to those of PTH. Moreover, they are similar for $25\text{-}(OH)D_3$ and $1,25\text{-}(OH)_2D_3$ and require large doses of both compounds. In intact animals, the effect of vitamin D repletion on the kidney is probably largely due to the diminution of secondary hyperparathyroidism as a result of increased calcium supply. Hence, the PTH-induced phosphaturia seen in the vitamin D-deficient animals decreases after repletion.

As Growth Hormone for Bone

A reasonable teleological explanation for the existence of vitamin D is that it is essential for the regulation of skeletal growth and hence differs from PTH and CT, which are largely concerned with regulating calcium and phosphate concentrations in blood and soft tissues. Skeletal growth requires supplies of calcium and phosphate from the intestine and bone turnover, that is, resorption of old bone so that bone can be remodeled and mineralized. During periods of rapid skeletal growth, both formation and resorption of bone are accelerated. The coupling between these two processes persists, but formation slightly exceeds resorption so that a net increase in skeletal mass occurs. It seems likely that, as new knowledge concerning the complex metabolism of vitamin D is acquired, new effects will be uncovered. If direct stimulation of bone matrix synthesis or mineralization, which has been suggested from in vivo studies, can be demonstrated with some form of vitamin D, this would provide further support for the role of vitamin D as a growth hormone for bone.

INTERACTIONS OF IONS AND HORMONES

The hormones described above not only influence the movements of calcium, phosphate, magnesium, hydrogen ions, and bicarbonate, but these ions in turn can alter hormonal responses and affect the hormonally responsive end organs. Space does not permit a complete review but a few examples should indicate the complexity and importance of these interactions.

The role of calcium as a mediator of PTH response, as well as the regulator of secretion, was discussed above. The interaction between intracellular calcium and cyclic nucleotides may provide a means of modulating hormone responses (230). Extracellular calcium may influence hormonal responses as well. Hypercalcemia can inhibit the actions of PTH on phosphate excretion (231) but does not block the phosphaturic effect of dibutyryl cyclic AMP, suggesting an inhibitory effect on adenylate cyclase. Calcium may also influence the renal response to vasopressin and to volume expansion. Although extracellular calcium concentration appears to have little effect on bone resorption in organ culture, it does appear to be important in bone matrix formation and mineralization (232–234). This may not represent a selective effect on skeletal tissues, but rather a part of a general effect of calcium to enhance cell proliferation.

Changes in extracellular phosphate concentration can have an even more striking effect on bone metabolism. Both bone matrix formation and mineralization appear to be phosphate-dependent (232–235). This effect is probably more important than the inhibitory effect of phosphate on bone resorption which was described earlier (236). In vivo, these effects may be obscured by an indirect hormonal response to phosphate. For example, phosphate loading is known to produce secondary hyperparathyroidism and loss of bone mass (237). Nevertheless, phosphate depletion is associated with impaired growth and with increased bone resorption. The latter might be due to alterations in vitamin D metabolism rather than to direct effects.

The hormones regulating calcium and phosphate metabolism also have important effects on hydrogen ion and bicarbonate transport. Indeed, PTH has been considered as a regulatory hormone for acid-base homeostasis. This concept seems unlikely, however, since PTH has opposite effects on hydrogen ion movement in bone and kidney. PTH-stimulated bone resorption would release carbonate and phosphate and tend to buffer hydrogen ion excess. In the kidney, PTH decreases hydrogen ion secretion and increases bicarbonate excretion. In adults with primary hyperparathyroidism, the latter effect appears to predominate since mild hyperchloremic acidosis often develops. Changes in hydrogen ions also affect the response to PTH. In bone, acidosis enhances the response to parathyroid hormone and may increase serum calcium concentration (238). In the kidney, acidosis tends to impair the response to PTH, perhaps by interfering with adenylate cyclase, since the response to dibutyryl-cAMP is not affected (239).

Other ions can influence hormonal regulation of mineral metabolism. The complex interactions between PTH and magnesium have been discussed above. Magnesium can also act as an inhibitor of mineralization. This is probably more important in the urinary tract, where high magnesium concentration may reduce the likelihood of formation of calcium containing renal stones. Pyrophosphate also has a powerful effect on bone metabolism. This is difficult to demonstrate in vivo because of the rapid hydrolysis of pyrophosphate to inorganic phosphate. The effect may be demonstrated by the use of the less easily hydrolyzed diphosphonates which are long lasting inhibitors of the deposition and removal of bone mineral (240). Recently, the renal response to PTH was also found to be decreased in potassium depletion (241). However, this could represent nonspecific impairment of renal function.

OTHER HORMONES INFLUENCING MINERAL METABOLISM

In addition to the three major regulatory systems described above, many other hormones act on calcium and phosphate transport and on skeletal metabolism. Because these hormones are important for their effects on other tissues and are discussed elsewhere, this section is limited to effects on skeletal metabolism. Moreover, since this subject was reviewed recently (242), only selected recent references are cited.

Glucocorticoids

Normal amounts of glucocorticoids are essential for skeletal development and growth; on the other hand, glucocorticoid excess is associated with loss of bone mass. Direct effects may be less important than indirect effects in producing these changes. For example, high doses of glucocorticoids can impair growth hormone responses and somatomedin generation (243, 244). As noted, glucocorticoids can increase parathyroid hormone secretion and decrease calcium absorption in the gut. These effects would tend to decrease bone formation and increase bone resorption. Although there is some evidence that glucocorticoids act by interfering with vitamin D metabolism (199), other studies indicate that glucocorticoids inhibit calcium transport in the intestine directly independent of vitamin D (245–248). The direct effects of glucocorticoids on bone have not been studied extensively. Inhibition of bone resorption can be demonstrated under certain circumstances, but the effect is not sufficiently powerful to overcome an established stimulation of resorption by PTH (249). In bone cell cultures, glucocorticoids decrease the synthesis of protein and RNA (250), but it has been found that low concentrations of glucocorticoids can actually enhance collagen synthesis in organ cultures of fetal rat bone (J. W. Dietrich, E. M. Canalis, and L. G. Raisz, unpublished observations). Whatever the mechanism is, it appears likely that glucocorticoids have a specific role in skeletal metabolism since receptors with selective affinity for glucocorticoids have been found in bone (251).

Estrogens and Androgens

Estrogens and androgens are important in skeletal maturation. Both the growth spurt and epiphysial closure at puberty are dependent upon these hormones, but the cellular mechanisms have not been determined. It is commonly held that the bone loss which accompanies aging is related to the loss of gonadal hormones. One concept is that estrogens and androgens inhibit bone resorption. Although there is evidence to support this both in vivo and in vitro (252–253), the in vitro studies have employed concentrations far in excess of those encountered physiologically. Hence, it seems premature to accept the hypothesis that sex hormones act as direct inhibitors of bone resorption, and worthwhile to seek other explanations for their in vivo effects, such as inhibition of PTH secretion (92).

Thyroid Hormones

It has long been known that the thyroid hormones, thyroxine (T_4) and triiodo-thyronine (T_3), are important in maintaining normal bone turnover. Addition of both thyroid and parathyroid hormones is required to restore bone turnover in thyroparathyroidectomized animals, and bone turnover is increased in animals and in humans in states of thyroid hormone excess (254). Recent evidence from our own laboratory suggests that T_4 and T_3 stimulate bone resorption directly at concentrations as low as 10^{-8} M (G. R. Mundy, J. L. Shapiro, E. M. Canalis, and L. G. Raisz, unpublished observations). It has been recently reported (225) that thyroid hormones and their analogs inhibit bone phosphodiesterase, but this effect is probably not the mechanism by which thyroid hormones stimulate bone resorption. The effects on bone resorption are observed with low concentrations of T_4 and T_3 and not with other thyronines, whereas when phosphodi-esterase inhibition occurs it is greatest with thyroid hormones which have much less calorigenic potency and bone-resorbing activity than T_4 or T_3. Moreover, the concentrations required to inhibit phosphodiesterase are much higher (10^{-4}–10^{-5} M) than those required to stimulate bone resorption.

Insulin and Glucagon

Insulin is required for normal skeletal growth and has been shown to stimulate bone formation and mineralization in vitro (256, 257). The reported effects were small, and the concentrations required were high. However, workers have recently observed that insulin can increase the rate of collagen synthesis more than 2-fold in fetal rat calvaria at concentrations as low as 10^{-9} M (E. M. Canalis, J. W. Dietrich, and L. G. Raisz, unpublished observations). There are conflicting reports on the effects of insulin on bone resorption. Stimulation has been reported in one study (258), but not in another (259).

Glucagon can inhibit bone resorption both directly (259) and indirectly by stimulating calcitonin secretion (260). Glucagon was also found to decrease proline incorporation into collagen in rats (261). In all of these studies large doses were used, and there is no evidence that glucagon has an important physiological role in mineral metabolism.

Growth Hormone and Somatomedins

A number of growth factors have now been identified in serum. Those factors which are growth hormone-dependent and which increase cartilage sulfation (sulfation factors) have been designated as somatomedins (262, 263). It is assumed that the pituitary regulation of skeletal growth is mediated by these factors. Somatomedin C has been shown to stimulate not only sulfate uptake in cartilage, but collagen synthesis in bone (264). Neither the regulation of the synthesis of somatomedin nor its importance in physiological growth has been established. Other factors which might play a role in growth, such as fibroblast growth factor (265), have been identified in pituitary extracts.

PROSTAGLANDINS

There is probably no other area of biomedical research in which there is more information than the study of prostaglandins. Most of this relates to metabolism and effects on smooth muscle or nerve. A role in bone metabolism was suggested by the findings that prostaglandins increased cAMP concentrations (266) and stimulated bone resorption in vitro (267). No physiological role for prosta-glandins in bone has been identified, but there is considerable evidence that prostaglandins can mediate pathological bone destruction in malignancy and inflammation.

In animal tumors, the development of hypercalcemia has been associated with increased prostaglandin production (268–270), and evidence for a role in the hypercalcemia of cancer has been obtained in a few human subjects (271).

Prostaglandins have also been implicated as mediators of bone destruction in arthritis (272), in dental cysts (273), and in periodontal disease (274, 275).

The major mechanism for these effects is presumably the stimulation of bone resorption. This stimulation occurs with a wide variety of prostaglandins, although PGE_2 is the most potent (276). Bone resorption can occur with local injections in vivo (277), and intravenous infusions of PGE_2 can raise serum calcium in the rat (278). Nevertheless, high doses are required which would have many other systemic effects. Hence, it is likely that, except in malignancy, the major role of prostaglandins in bone is as a local rather than a systemic hormone. The effects of prostaglandins on bone formation are not established. The labeling of collagen in chick tibiae was increased in acute studies in vitro (279); however, after 24-hr treatment with PGE at 10^{-6} M, bone collagen synthesis in fetal rat calvaria was substantially inhibited (280).

Bone tissue itself can produce prostaglandins, and this can be stimulated by complement activation (281). This probably requires an antibody to some cell surface component and could represent a mechanism for prostaglandin production in autoimmune disease. The interactions between prostaglandins and other hormones regulating mineral metabolism have received little attention. In the kidney, PGE_1 has been shown to inhibit the cAMP and phosphaturic responses to PTH, but not to dibutyryl cAMP, suggesting an interaction involving adenylate cyclase (282).

OSTEOCLAST-ACTIVATING FACTOR

Recently, a potent stimulator of bone resorption in supernatant fluid from cultures of normal human peripheral blood leukocytes activated by plant mitogen or an antigen to which the donor has been previously exposed was found (283). It has been named "osteoclast-activating factor" (OAF). OAF was first discovered during a search for the cause of alveolar bone loss which occurs adjacent to chronic inflammatory cells in periodontal disease. Although it could be the mediator responsible for producing osteolysis in chronic inflammation, there is now stronger evidence for a role in the bone lesions of lymphoproliferative disorders and particularly in myeloma. Its physiological function is unknown.

Bone-resorbing activity can be found in supernatant fluid of cultures of human peripheral blood leukocytes within 6 hr after activation with a mitogen and reaches a peak at 12–24 hr. OAF release appears to parallel the increase in RNA and protein synthesis and occurs before DNA synthesis has increased (284). The cell source has not yet been fully identified, but OAF secretion appears to depend upon macrophage-lymphocyte synergy. OAF-like resorbing activity has been found in the supernatant fluid of lymphoid cell lines and of short-term cultures of neoplastic cells from patients with myeloma (285, 286).

OAF is macromolecular and is inactivated by proteolytic enzymes (287). OAF does not cross-react with antibodies to PTH or prostaglandins, and its bone-resorbing activity cannot be extracted with lipid solvents which extract vitamin D metabolites and prostaglandins. The effects of OAF on bone resorption are similar to those of PTH. These effects include a steep dose-response curve, rapid onset of action, and the ability to induce prolonged resorption after brief exposure (288). As with PTH, OAF is inhibited by calcitonin, and this inhibition is followed by escape. OAF effects are also partially inhibited by increased medium phosphate concentration. Unlike PTH, which is relatively insensitive to glucocorticoids, the effect of OAF is inhibited by low concentrations (10^{-7} M) of cortisol. Both OAF and PTH inhibit collagen synthesis in cultured fetal rat bones (288). Since OAF has not been purified, it is not certain that stimulation of bone resorption and inhibition of collagen synthesis are a function of the same molecule. Its effects in vivo have been studied only briefly. When amounts of OAF and PTH which produced similar effects in vitro were injected into rats, the PTH-treated animals developed hypercalcemia and the OAF-treated animals did not. This suggests that OAF may function largely as a local hormone.

One possibility is that OAF is important in the initial stimulation of resorption which is required for the formation of the marrow cavity. Active lymphoid cells are present at this time, and bone resorption could be stimulated locally. Animal models with defective endosteal bone resorption and resultant osteopetrosis have been described, and there is some evidence that such animals have a deficiency in their lymphoid cells (289).

REFERENCES

1. Brewer, H. B., Jr., Fairwell, T., Rittel, W., Littledike, T., and Arnaud, C. D. (1974). Recent studies in the chemistry of human, bovine and porcine parathyroid hormone. Am. J. Med. 56:759.
2. Sauer, R. T., Niall, H. D., Hogan, M. L., Keutmann, H. T., O'Riordan, J. L. H., and Potts, J. T., Jr. (1974). The amino acid sequence of porcine parathyroid hormone. Biochemistry 13:1994.
3. MacGregor, R. R., Chu, L. L. H., Hamilton, J. W., and Cohn, D. V. (1973). Partial purification of parathyroid hormone from chicken parathyroid glands. Endocrinology 92:1312.
4. Niall, H. D., Sauer, R. T., Jacobs, J. W., Keutmann, H. T., Segre, G. V., O'Riordan, J. L. H., Aurbach, G. D., and Potts, J. T. (1974). The amino-acid sequence of the amino-terminal 37 residues of human parathyroid hormone. Proc. Nat. Acad. Sci. U. S. A. 71:384.
5. Keutmann, H. T., Niall, H. D., O'Riordan, J. L. H., and Potts, J. T., Jr. (1975). A reinvestigation of the amino-terminal sequence of human parathyroid hormone. Biochemistry 14:1842.
6. Hendy, G. N., Barling, P. M., and O'Riordan, J. L. H. (1974). Human parathyroid hormone: immunological properties of the amino terminus and of synthetic fragments. Clin. Sci. Mol. Med. 47:567.
7. Milhaud, G., Rivalle, P., Staub, J. F., and Jullienne, A. (1974). Synthesis and biological activity of 1-34 fragment of human parathyroid hormone. C. R. Soc. Biol. (Paris) 279:1015.
8. Murray, T. M., Muzaffar, S. A., Parsons, J. A., and Keutmann, H. T. (1975). A biologically active hormonal fragment isolated from bovine parathyroid glands (BPTH 1—65). Biochemistry 14:2705.

9. Tregear, G. W., van Rietschoten, J., Greene, E., Keutmann, H. T., Niall, H. D., Reit, B., Parsons, J. A., and Potts, J. T., Jr. (1973). Bovine parathyroid hormone: minimum chain length of synthetic peptide required for biological activity. Endocrinology 93:1349.

10. Segre, G. V., Niall, H. D., Habener, J. F., and Potts, J. T., Jr. (1974). Metabolism of parathyroid hormone: physiologic and clinical significance. Am. J. Med. 56:774.

11. Canterbury, J. M., Bricker, L. A., Levey, G. S., Kozlovskis, P. L., Ruiz, E., Zull, J. E., and Reiss, E. (1975). Metabolism of bovine parathyroid hormone: immunological and biological characteristics of fragments generated by liver perfusion. J. Clin. Invest. 55:1245.

12. Jacobs, J. W., Kemper, B., Niall, H. D., Habener, J. F., and Potts, J. T., Jr. (1974). Structural analysis of human proparathyroid hormone by a new microsequencing approach. Nature (Lond.) 249:155.

13. Hamilton, J. W., Niall, H. D., Jacobs, J. W., Keutmann, H. T., Potts, J. T., Jr., and Cohn, D. V. (1974). The N-terminal amino-acid sequence of bovine proparathyroid hormone. Proc. Nat. Acad. Sci. U. S. A. 71:653.

14. Kemper, B., Habener, J. F., Mulligan, R. C., Potts, J. T., Jr., and Rich, A. (1974). Pre-proparathyroid hormone: a direct translation product of parathyroid messenger RNA. Proc. Nat. Acad. Sci. U. S. A. 71:3731.

15. Chu, L. L. H., MacGregor, R. R., Liu, P. I., Hamilton, J. W., and Cohn, D. V. (1973). Biosynthesis of proparathyroid hormone and parathyroid hormone by human parathyroid glands. J. Clin. Invest. 52:3089.

16. Chu, L. L. H., MacGregor, R. R., Anast, C. S., Hamilton, J. W., and Cohn, D. V. (1973). Studies on the biosynthesis of rat parathyroid hormone and proparathyroid hormone: adaptation of the parathyroid gland to dietary restriction of calcium. Endocrinology 93:915.

17. Cohn, D. V., MacGregor, R. R., Chu, L. L. H., Huang, D. W. Y., Anast, C. S., and Hamilton, J. W. (1974). Biosynthesis of proparathyroid hormone: chemistry physiology and role in regulation. Am. J. Med. 56:767.

18. Habener, J. F., Kemper, B. W., Potts, J. T., Jr., and Rich, A. (1974). Calcium-dependent intracellular conversion of proparathyroid hormone to parathyroid hormone. Endocrinol. Res. Comm. 1:239.

19. Kemper, B. W., Habener, J. F., Rich, A., and Potts, J. T., Jr. (1975). Microtubules and the intracellular conversion of proparathyroid hormone to parathyroid hormone. Endocrinology 96:903.

20. Martin, T. J., Greenberg, P. B., and Michelangeli, V. (1973). Synthesis of human parathyroid hormone by cultured cells: evidence for release of prohormone by some adenomata. Clin. Sci. 44:1.

21. Benson, R. C., Jr., Riggs, B. L., Pickard, B. M., and Arnaud, C. D. (1974). Radioimmunoassay of parathyroid hormone in hypercalcemic patients with malignant disease. Am. J. Med. 56:821.

22. Licata, A. A., and Raisz, L. G. (1974). The release of glycoconjugates by rat parathyroid glands in tissue culture. II. Studies on uptake and incorporation of isotopically labeled glucosamine and characterization of secreted material. Biochim. Biophys. Acta 343:17.

23. Kemper, B., Habener, J. F., Rich, A., and Potts, J. T., Jr. (1974). Parathyroid secretion: discovery of a major calcium-dependent protein. Science 184:167.

24. Segre, G. V., Habener, J. F., Powell, D., Tregear, G. W., and Potts, J. T., Jr. (1972). Parathyroid hormone in human plasma: immunochemical characterization and biological implications. J. Clin. Invest. 51:3163.

25. Silverman, R., and Yalow, R. S. (1973). Heterogeneity of parathyroid hormone: clinical and physiologic implications. J. Clin. Invest. 52:1958.
26. Lindall, A. W., and Wong, E. T. (1975). Column chromatography of human serum parathyroid immunoreactive peptides. Proc. Soc. Exp. Bio. Med. 148:799.
27. Canterbury, J. M., and Reiss, E. (1972). Multiple immunoreactive molecular forms of parathyroid hormone in human serum. Proc. Soc. Exp. Biol. Med. 140:1393.
28. Arnaud, C. D., Goldsmith, R. S., Bordier, P. J., and Sizemore, G. W. (1974). Influence of immunoheterogeneity of circulating parathyroid hormone on results of radioimmunoassays of serum in man. Am. J. Med. 56:785.
29. Canterbury, J. M., Levey, G. S., and Reiss, E. (1973). Activation of renal cortical adenylate cyclase by circulating immunoreactive parathyroid hormone fragments. J. Clin. Invest. 52:524.
30. Parsons, J. A., Reit, B., and Robinson, C. J. (1973). A bioassay for parathyroid hormone using chicks. Endocrinology 92:454.
31. Dacke, C. G., and Kenny, A. D. (1973). Avian bioassay method for parathyroid hormone. Endocrinology 92:463.
32. Goltzmann, D., Peytremann, A., Callahan, E., Tregear, G. W., and Potts, J. T., Jr. (1975). Analysis of requirements for parathyroid hormone action in renal membranes with use of inhibiting analogues. J. Biol. Chem. 250:3199.
33. Chu, L. L. H., MacGregor, R. R., Hamilton, J. W., and Cohn, D. V. (1971). A bioassay for parathyroid hormone based on hormonal inhibition of CO_2 production from citrate in mouse calvarium. Endocrinology 89: 1425.
34. Webster, L. A., Atkins, D., and Peacock, M. A. (1974). A bioassay for parathyroid hormone using whole mouse calvaria in tissue culture. J. Endocrinol. 62:631.
35. O'Riordan, J. L. H., Woodhead, J. S., Hendy, G. N., Parsons, J. A., Robinson, C. J., Keutmann, H. T., Dawson, B. F., and Potts, J. T., Jr. (1974). Effect of oxidation on biological and immunological activity of porcine parathyroid hormone. J. Endocrinol. 63:117.
36. Goldsmith, R. S., Furszyfer, J., Johnson, W. J., Fournier, A. E., Sizemore, G. W., and Arnaud, C. D. (1973). Etiology of hyperparathyroidism and bone disease during chronic hemodialysis. III. Evaluation of parathyroid suppressibility. J. Clin. Invest. 52:173.
37. Sammon, P. J., Brand, J. S., Neuman, W. F., and Raisz, L. G. (1973). Metabolism of labeled parathyroid hormone. I. Preparation of biologically active ^{125}I-labeled parathyroid hormone. Endocrinology 92:1596.
38. McIntosh, C. H. S., and Hesch, R. D. (1975). Labelled antibody membrane assay for parathyroid hormone: a new approach to the measurement of receptor bound hormone. Biochem. Biophys. Res. Commun. 64:376.
39. Reiss, E., and Canterbury, J. M. (1973). Blood levels of parathyroid hormone in disorders of calcium metabolism. Ann. Rev. Med. 24:217.
40. Severson, A. R., Rothberg, P. F., Pratt, R. M., and Goggins, J. F. (1973). Effect of parathyroid hormone on the incorporation of ^{3}H-glucosamine into hyaluronic acid in bone organ culture. Endocrinology 92:1282.
41. Luben, R. A., Goggins, J. F., and Raisz, L. G. (1974). Stimulation by parathyroid hormone of bone hyaluronate synthesis in organ culture. Endocrinology 94:737.

42. Dietrich, J. W., Canalis, E. M., Maina, D., and Raisz, L. G. (1975). Inhibition of bone collagen synthesis in tissue culture by parathyroid hormone. Fed. Proc. 34:337.
43. Rasmussen, H., and Bordier, P. (eds.), The Physiological and Cellular Basis of Metabolic Bone Disease. Williams & Wilkins, Baltimore.
44. Herrmann-Erlee, M. P. M., and van der Meer, J. M. (1974). The effects of dibutyryl cyclic AMP, aminophylline and propranolol on PTE-induced bone resorption in vitro. Endocrinology 94:424.
45. Wong, G., and Cohn, D. C. (1974). Separation of parathyroid hormone and calcitonin-sensitive cells from non-responsive bone cells. Nature (Lond.) 252:713.
46. Rodan, S. B., and Rodan, G. A. (1974). The effect of parathyroid hormone and thyrocalcitonin on the accumulation of cyclic adenosine $3':5'$-monophosphate in freshly isolated bone cells. J. Biol. Chem. 249:3068.
47. Peck, W. A., Carpenter, J., Messinger, K., and DeBra, D. (1973). Cyclic $3'5'$-adenosine monophosphate in isolated bone cells: response to low concentrations of parathyroid hormone. Endocrinology 92:692.
48. Peck, W. A., Carpenter, J., and Messinger, K. (1974). Cyclic $3',5'$-adenosine monophosphate in isolated bone cells. II. Responses to adenosine and parathyroid hormone. Endocrinology 94:148.
49. Jande, S. S. (1972). Effects of parathormone on osteocytes and their surrounding bone matrix: an electron microscopic study. Z. Zellforsch. Anat. Mikrosk. Anat. 130:463.
50. Liu, C. C., Baylink, D. J., and Wergdahl, J. (1974). Vitamin D-enhanced osteoclastic bone resorption at vascular canals. Endocrinology 95:1011.
51. Agus, Z. S., Gardner, L. B., Beck, L. H., and Goldberg, M. (1973). Effects of parathyroid hormone on renal tubular reabsorption of calcium, sodium, and phosphate. Am. J. Physiol. 224:1143.
52. Vainsel, M. (1973). Effects of parathyroid hormone and calcium on renal reabsorption of bicarbonate in children. Biomedicine 18:112.
53. Beck, N., Kim, K. S., Wolak, M., and Davis, B. B. (1975). Inhibition of carbonic anhydrase by parathyroid hormone and cyclic AMP in rat renal cortex in vitro. J. Clin. Invest. 55:149.
54. Garg, L. C. (1975). Effect of parathyroid hormone and adenosine $3',5'$-monophosphate on renal carbonic anhydrase. Biochem. Pharmacol. 24:437.
55. Wen, S. F. (1974). Micropuncture studies of phosphate transport in the proximal tubule of the dog: the relationship to sodium reabsorption. J. Clin. Invest. 53:143.
56. Brunette, M. G., Taleb, L., and Carriere, S. (1973). Effect of parathyroid hormone on phosphate reabsorption along the nephron of the rat. Am. J. Physiol. 225:1076.
57. Kalu, D. N., Hadji-Georgopolous, A., Sarr, M. G., Solomon, B. A., and Foster, G. V. (1974). The role of parathyroid hormone in the maintenance of plasma calcium levels in rats. Endocrinology 95:1156.
58. Kalu, D. N., Hadji-Georgopolous, A., and Foster, G. V. (1975). Effect of calcium deprivation on parathyroid hormone-mediated bone and kidney contributions to the maintenance of plasma calcium in rats. J. Endocrinol. 64:299.
59. Biddulph, D. M., and Gallimore, L. B., Jr. (1974). Sensitivity of the kidney

to parathyroid hormone and its relationship to serum calcium in the hamster. Endocrinology 94:1241.

60. Birge, S. J., Switzer, S. C., and Leonard, D. R. (1974). Influence of sodium and parathyroid hormone on calcium release from intestinal mucosal cells. J. Clin. Invest. 54:702.

61. Birge, S. J., and Gilbert, H. R. (1974). Identification of an intestinal sodium and calcium-dependent phosphatase stimulated by parathyroid hormone. J. Clin. Invest. 54:710.

62. Fraser, D. R., and Kodicek, E. (1973). Regulation of 25-hydroxy cholecalciferol-1-hydroxylase activity in kidney by parathyroid hormone. Nature (New Biol.) 241:163.

63. Clark, I., and Rivera-Cordero, F. (1973). Effects of endogenous parathyroid hormone on calcium, magnesium and phosphate metabolism in rats. Endocrinology 92:62.

64. Barreras, R. F. (1973). Calcium and gastric secretion. Gastroenterology 64:1168.

65. Canterbury, J. M., Levy, G. S., Ruiz, E., and Reiss, E. (1974). Parathyroid hormone activation of adenylate cyclase in liver. Proc. Soc. Exp. Bio. Med. 147:366.

66. Moxley, M. A., Bell, N. H., Wagle, S. R., Allen, D. O., and Ashmore, J. (1974). Parathyroid hormone stimulation of glucose and urea production in isolated liver cells. Am. J. Physiol. 227:1058.

67. Rixon, R. H., and Whitfield, J. F. (1974). Parathyroid hormone and liver regeneration. Proc. Soc. Exp. Biol. Med. 146:926.

68. Whitfield, J. F., Rixon, R. H., MacManus, J. P., and Balk, S. D. (1973). Calcium, cyclic adenosine $3',5'$-monophosphate, and the control of cell proliferation: a review. In Vitro 8:257.

69. Werner, S., and Low, H. (1973). Stimulation of lipolysis and calcium accumulation by parathyroid hormone in rat adipose tissue in vitro after adrenalectomy and administration of high doses of cortisone acetate. Horm. Metab. Res. 5:292.

70. Gozariu, L., Forster, K., Faulhaber, J. D., Minne, H., and Ziegler, R. (1974). Parathyroid hormone and calcitonin: influences upon lipolysis of human adipose tissue. Horm. Metab. Res. 6:243.

71. Yasuda, K., Hurukawa, Y., Okuyama, M., Kikuchi, M., and Yoshinaga, K. (1975). Glucose tolerance and insulin secretion in patients with parathyroid disorders. N. Engl. J. Med. 292:501.

72. Guisado, R., Arieff, A. I., and Massry, S. G. (1975). Changes in electroencephalogram in acute uremia: effects of parathyroid hormone and brain electrolytes. J. Clin. Invest. 55:738.

73. Patten, B. M., Bilezikian, J. P., Mallette, L. E., Prince, A., Engel, W. K., and Aurbach, G. D. (1974). Neuromuscular disease in primary hyperparathyroidism. Ann. Intern. Med. 80:182.

74. Malbon, C. G., and Zull, J. E. (1974). Interactions of parathyroid hormone and plasma membranes from rat kidney. Biochem. Biophys. Res. Commun. 56:952.

75. Chase, L. R. (1975). Selective proteolysis of the receptor for parathyroid hormone in renal cortex. Endocrinology 96:70.

76. Blum, J. W., Fischer, J. A., Schwoerer, O., and Hunziker, W. (1974). Acute parathyroid hormone response: sensitivity, relationship to hypocalcemia and rapidity. Endocrinology 95:753.

77. MacGregor, R. R., Hamilton, J. W., and Cohn, D. V. (1975). The bypass of tissue hormone stores during the secretion of newly synthesized parathyroid hormone. Endocrinology 95:753.
78. Habener, J. F., Kemper, B., and Potts, J. T., Jr. (1975). Calcium-dependent intracellular degradation of parathyroid hormone: a possible mechanism for the regulation of hormone stores. Endocrinology 97:431.
79. Reaven, E. P. .and Reaven, G. M. (1975). A quantitative ultrastructural study of microtubule content and secretory granule accumulation in parathyroid glands of phosphate- and colchicine-treated rats. J. Clin. Invest. 56:49.
80. Chertow, B. S., Buschman, R. J., and Henderson, W. J. (1975). Subcellular mechanisms of parathyroid hormone secretion: ultrastructural changes in response to calcium, vitamin A, vinblastine and cytochalasin B. Lab. Invest. 32:190.
81. Williams, G. A., Hargis, G. K., Bowser, E. N., Henderson, W. J., and Martinex, N. J. (1973). Evidence for a role of adenosine $3',5'$-monophosphate in parathyroid hormone release. Endocrinology 92:687.
82. Mayer, G. P. (1974). Relative importance of calcium and magnesium in the control of parathyroid secretion. Endocrinol. Soc. 94:A-181.
83. Anast, C. S., Mohs, J. M., Kaplan, S. L., and Burns, T. W. (1972). Evidence for parathyroid failure in magnesium deficiency. Science 177:606.
84. Suh, S. M., Tashjian, A. H., Jr., Matsuo, N., Parkinson, D. K., and Fraser, D. (1973). Pathogenesis of hypocalcemia in primary hypomagnesemia: normal end-organ repressiveness to parathyroid hormone, impaired parathyroid gland function. J. Clin. Invest. 52:153.
85. Levi, J., Massry, S. G., Coburn, J. W., Llach, F., and Kleeman, L. R. (1974). Hypocalcemia in magnesium-depleted dogs: evidence for reduced responsiveness to parathyroid hormone and relative failure of parathyroid gland function. Metabolism 23:323.
86. Fischer, J. A., Blum, J. W., and Binswanger, U. (1973). Acute parathyroid hormone response to epinephrine in vivo. J. Clin. Invest. 52:2430.
87. Kukreja, S. C., Hargis, G. K., Bowser, E. N., Henderson, W. J., Fisherman, E. W., and Williams, G. A. (1975). Role of adrenergic stimuli in parathyroid hormone secretion in man. J. Clin. Endocrinol. Metab. 40:478.
88. Kukreja, S. C., Hargis, G. K., Rosenthal, I. M., and Williams, G. A. (1973). Pheochromocytoma causing excessive parathyroid hormone production and hypercalcemia. Ann. Intern. Med. 79:838.
89. Shimbo, S., and Nakano, Y. (1974). A case of malignant pheochromocytoma producing parathyroid hormone-like substance. Calcif. Tissue Res. 15:155.
90. Fucik, R. F., Kukreja, S. C., Hargis, G. K., Bowser, E. N., Henderson, W. J., and Williams, G. A. (1975). Effect of glucocorticoids on function of the parathyroid glands in man. J. Clin. Endocrinol. Metab. 40:152.
91. Williams, G. A., Peterson, W. C., Bowser, E. N., Henderson, W. J., Hargis, G. K., and Martinez, N. J. (1974). Interrelationship of parathyroid and adrenocortical function in calcium homeostasis in the rat. Endocrinology 95:707.
92. Au, W. Y. W. (1975). Effect of cortisol, β-estradiol, and testosterone on parathyroid hormone secretion by rat parathyroid glands in vitro. Fed. Proc. 34:336 (Abstr.).
93. Fischer, J. A., Binswanger, U., Fanconi, A., Illig, R. Baerlocher, K., and Prader, A. (1973). Serum parathyroid hormone concentrations in vitamin

D deficiency rickets of infancy: effects of intravenous calcium and vitamin D. Horm. Metab. Res. 5:381.

94. Henry, H. L., and Norman, A. W. (1975). Studies on the mechanisms of action of calciferol. VII. Localization of 1,25-dihydroxy-vitamin D_3 in chick parathyroid glands. Biochem. Biophys. Res. Commun. 62:781.

95. Oldham, S. B., Fischer, J. A., Shen, L. H., and Arnaud, C. D. (1974). Isolation and properties of a calcium-binding protein from porcine parathyroid glands. Biochemistry 13:4790.

96. Chertow, B. S., Baylink, D. J., Wergedal, J. E., Su, M. H. H., and Norman, A. W. (1975). Decrease in serum immunoreactive parathyroid hormone in rats and in parathyroid hormone secretion in vitro by 1,25-dihydroxycholecalciferol. J. Clin. Invest. 56:668.

97. Chertow, B. S., Williams, G. A., Kiuni, R., Stewart, K. L., Hargis, G. K., and Flayter, R. L. (1974). The interactions between vitamin A, vinblastine and cytocholism B in parathyroid hormone secretion. Proc. Soc. Exp. Biol. Med. 147:16.

98. Fujita, T., Orimo, H., Ohata, M., Okano, K., and Yoshikawa, M. (1973). Loss of immunoreactivity of human serum parathyroid hormone by the action of rat kidney enzyme, preferentially hydrolyzing parathyroid hormone. Horm. Res. 4:213.

99. Sutcliffe, H. S., Martin, T. J., Eisman, J. A., and Pilczk, R. (1973). Binding of parathyroid hormone to bovine kidney-cortex plasma membranes. Biochem. J. 134:913.

100. Singer, F. R., Segre, G. V., Habener, J. F., and Potts, J. T., Jr. (1975). Peripheral metabolism of bovine parathyroid hormone in the dog. Metabolism 24:139.

101. Kruska, K. A., Kopelman, R., Rutherford, W. E., Klahr, S., and Slatopolsky, E. (1975). Metabolism of immunoreactive parathyroid hormone in the dog: the role of the kidney and the effects of chronic renal disease. J. Clin. Invest. 56:39.

102. Catherwood, B., and Singer, R. R. (1974). Generation of a carboxyl-terminal fragment of bovine parathyroid hormone by canine renal plasma membranes. Biochem. Biophys. Res. Commun. 57:469.

103. Pearse, A. G. E. (1969). The cytochemistry and ultrastructure of polypeptide hormone-producing cells of the APUD series and the embryologic, physiologic and pathologic implications of the concept. J. Histochem. Cytochem. 17:303.

104. Polak, J. M., Pearse, A. G. E., LeLivre, C., Fountaine, J., and Douarin, N. M. (1974). Immunocytochemical confirmation of the neural crest origin of avian calcitonin producing cells. Histochemistry 40:209.

105. Voelkel, E. F., Tashjian, A. H., Jr., Davidoff, F. F., Cohen, R. B., Perlia, C. P., and Wurtman, R. J. (1974). Concentration of calcitonin and catecholamines in pheochromocytomas, a mucosal neuroma and medullary thyroid carcinoma. J. Clin. Endocrinol. Metab. 37:297.

106. Heynen, G., and Franchimont, P. (1974). Human calcitonin radioimmunoassay in normal and pathological conditions. Eur. J. Clin. Invest. 4:218.

107. Silva, O. L., Becker, K. L., Primack, A., Doppman, J., and Snider, R. H. (1974). Ectopic secretion of calcitonin by OAT-cell carcinoma. N. Engl. J. Med. 290:1122.

108. Coombes, R. C., Hillyard, C., Greenberg, P. B., and MacIntyre, I. (1974). Plasma-immunoreactive-calcitonin in patients with non-thyroid tumours. Lancet i:1080.

109. Feinblatt, J. D., Tai, L. R., and Kenney, A. D. (1974). Avian parathyroid glands in organ culture: secretion of parathyroid hormone and calcitonin. Endocrinology 96:282.
110. Burford, H. J., Ontjes, D. A., Cooper, C. W., Parlow, A. F., and Hirsch, P. F. (1975). Purification, characterization and radioimmunoassay of thyrocalcitonin from rat thyroid glands. Endocrinology 96:340.
111. Maier, R., Riniker, B., and Rittel, W. (1974). Analogs of human calcitonin. I. Influence of modifications in amino acid positions 29 and 31 on hypocalcemic activity in the rat. FEBS Lett. 48:69.
112. Marx, S. J., Woodard, C. J., and Aurbach, G. D. (1972). Calcitonin receptors of kidney and bone. Science 178:999.
113. Marx, S. J., Woodward, C., Aurbach, G. D., Glossman, H., and Keutmann, H. T. (1973). Renal receptors of calcitonin: binding and degradation of hormone. J. Biol. Chem. 248:4797.
114. Marx, S. J., and Aurbach, G. D. (1975). Renal receptors for calcitonin: coordinate occurrence with calcitonin-activated adenylate cyclase. Endocrinology 97:448.
115. Marx, S. J., Gavin, J. R., Aurbach, G. D., and Buell, D. N. (1974). Calcitonin receptors on cultured human lymphocytes. J. Biol. Chem. 249:6812.
116. McManus, J. P., and Whitfield, J. F. (1970). Inhibition by thyrocalcitonin of the mitogenic actions of parathyroid hormone and cyclic adenosine-$3',5'$-monophosphate by rat thymocytes. Endocrinology 86:934.
117. Whitfield, J. F., McManus, J. P., and Gillan, D. J. (1974). Inhibition by thyrocalcitonin (calcitonin) of the cyclic AMP-mediated stimulation of thymocyte proliferation by epinephrine. Horm. Metab. Res. 3:348.
118. Whitfield, J. F., McManus, J. D., Franks, D. J., Braceland, D. M., and Cullan, D. J. (1972). Calcium-mediated effects of calcitonin on cyclic AMP formation and lymphoblast proliferation in thymocyte populations exposed to prostaglandin E_1. J. Cell. Physiol. 80:315.
119. Smith, D. M., and Johnston, C. C., Jr. (1975). Cyclic $3',5'$-adenosine monophosphate levels in separated bone cells. Endocrinology 96:1261.
120. Raisz, L. G., Au, W. Y. W., Simmons, H., and Mandelstam, P. (1972). Calcitonin in human serum: detection by tissue culture bioassay in medullary carcinoma of the thyroid and other disorders. Arch. Intern. Med. 129:889.
121. Singer, F. R., and Habener, J. F. (1974). Multiple immunoreactive forms of calcitonin in human plasma. Biochem. Biophys. Res. Commun. 61: 710.
122. Deftos, L. J., Roos, B. A., Bronzert, D., and Parthemore, J. G. (1975). Immunochemical heterogeneity of calcitonin in plasma. J. Clin. Endocrinol. Metab. 40:409.
123. Sizemore, G. W., Heath, H., and Larson, J. M. (1975). Immunochemical heterogeneity of calcitonin in plasma of patients with medullary thyroid carcinoma. J. Clin. Invest. 55:1111.
124. Deftos, L. J., Powell, D., Parthemore, J. G., and Potts, J. D., Jr. (1973). Secretion of calcitonin in hypocalcemic states in man. J. Clin. Invest. 52:3109.
125. Silva, O. L., Snider, R. H., and Becker, K. L. (1974). Radioimmunoassay of calcitonin in human plasma. Clin. Chem. 20:337.
126. Borle, A. B. (1975). Regulation of cellular calcium metabolism and calcium transport by calcitonin. J. Membr. Biol. 21:125.

127. Meyer, R. A., and Meyer, M. H. (1975). Thyrocalcitonin injection to rats increases the liver inorganic phosphate. Endocrinology 96:1048.
128. Talmage, R. V., Whitehurst, L. A., and Anderson, J. J. B. (1973). Effect of calcitonin and calcium infusion on plasma phosphate. Endocrinology 92:792.
129. Kallio, D. M., Garant, P. R., and Minkin, C. (1972). Ultrastructural effects of calcitonin on osteoclasts in tissue culture. J. Ultrastruct. Res. 39:205.
130. Lucht, U. (1973). Effects of calcitonin on osteoclasts in vivo: an ultra-structural and histochemical study. Z. Zellforsch. Mikrosk. Anat. 145:75.
131. Holtrop, M. E., Raisz, L. G., and Simmons, H. A. (1974). The effects of parathyroid hormone, colchicine and calcitonin on the ultrastructure and the activity of osteoclasts. J. Cell. Biol. 60:346.
132. Mundy, G. R., and Raisz, L. G. (1974). Drugs for disorders of bone: pharmacological and clinical considerations. Drugs 8:250.
133. Au, W. Y. W. (1977). Synergistic effect of prednisone on calcitonin treat-ment of hypercalcemia due to recurrent parathyroid carcinoma. Arch. Intern. Med. 35:1594.
134. Haddad, J. A., Jr., and Caldwell, J. A. (1972). Calcitonin resistance: clinical and immunologic studies in subjects with Paget's disease of bone treated with porcine and salmon calcitonins. J. Clin. Invest. 51:3133.
135. Hirsch, P. F., and Munson, P. L. (1969). Thyrocalcitonin. Physiol. Rev. 49:548.
136. Krane, S. M., Harris, E. D., Jr., Singer, F. R., and Potts, J. T., Jr. (1973). Acute effects of calcitonin on bone formation in man. Metabolism 22:51.
137. Heersche, J. N. M., Marcus, R., and Aurbach, G. D. (1974). Calcitonin and the formation of $3',5'$-AMP in bone and kidney. Endocrinology 94:241.
138. Nielsen, P. S., Buchanan-Lee, B., Matthews, E. W., Moseley, J. M., and Williams, C. C. (1971). Acute effects of synthetic porcine calcitonins on the renal excretion of magnesium, inorganic phosphate, sodium and potassium. J. Endocrinol. 51:455.
139. Bijvoet, L. L. M., and Foreling, P. G. A. M. (1972). Calcitonin, parathyroid hormone, and the kidney. Clinical Aspects of Metabolic Bone Disease, Henry Ford Hospital Symposium. Excerpta Med. Int. Cong. Series 270.
140. Aurbach, G. D., and Heath, D. A. (1974). Parathyroid hormone and calcitonin regulation of renal function. Kidney Int. 6:331.
141. Hotz, J., Goebell, H., Minne, H., and Ziegler, R. (1974). Persistent inhibi-tion of gastric secretion by an intravenous 12-hour infusion of calcitonin in normals, peptic ulcer and high risk patients. Digestion 11:311.
142. Bartlett, J. P., and Bates, R. F. L. (1974). Calcitonin given intragastrically and resistance to histamine-induced peptic ulcer in guinea-pigs. J. Endo-crinol. 63:407.
143. Becker, H. D., Reeder, D. D., Scurry, M. T., and Thompson, J. C. (1974). Inhibition of gastrin release and gastric secretion by calcitonin in patients with peptic ulcer. Am. J. Surg. 127:71.
144. Bieberdorf, F. A., Gray, T. K., Walsh, J. H., and Fordtran, J. S. (1974). Effect of calcitonin on meal-stimulated gastric acid secretion and serum gastrin concentration. Gastroenterology 66:343.
145. Gray, T. K., Bieberdorf, F. A., and Fordtran, J. S. (1973). Thyrocalcitonin and the jejunal absorption of calcium, water and electrolytes in normal subjects. J. Clin. Invest. 52:3084.

146. Tanzer, F. S., and Navia, J. M. (1973). Calcitonin inhibition of intestinal phosphate absorption. Nature (New Biol.) 242:221.
147. Swaminathan, R., Ker, J., and Care, A. D. (1974). Calcitonin and intestinal calcium absorption. J. Endocrinol. 61:83.
148. Kurokawa, K., Nagata, N., Sasaki, M., and Nakane, K. (1974). Effects of calcitonin on the concentration of cyclic adenosine $3',5'$-monophosphate in rat kidney in vivo and in vitro. Endocrinology 94:1514.
149. Harrell, A., Binderman, I., and Rodan, G. A. (1973). The effect of calcium concentration on calcium uptake by bone cells treated with thyrocalcitonin (TCT) hormone. Endocrinology 92:550.
150. Yamaguchi, M., Takei, Y., and Yamamoto, T. (1975). Effect of thyrocalcitonin on calcium concentration in liver of intact and thyroparathyroidectomized rats. Endocrinology 96:1004.
151. Raisz, L. G., Trummel, C. L., and Simmons, H. (1972). Induction of bone resorption in tissue culture: prolonged response after brief exposure to parathyroid hormone or 25-hydroxychole calciferol. Endocrinology 90:744.
152. Pento, J. T., Glick, S. M., Kagan, A., and Gorgein, P. C. (1974). The relative influence of calcium, strontium, and magnesium on calcitonin secretion in the pig. Endocrinology 94:1176.
153. Swaminathan, R., Bates, R. F. L., Bloom, S. R., Ganguli, P. C., and Care, A. D. (1973). The relationship between food, gastro-intestinal hormones and calcitonin secretion. J. Endocrinol. 59:217.
154. Talmage, R. V., Roycroft, J. H., and Anderson, J. J. B. (1975). Daily fluctuations in plasma calcium, phosphate and their radionucleotide concentrations in the rat. Calcif. Tissue Res. 17:91.
155. Perault-Staub, A. M., Staub, J. F., and Milhaud, G. (1974). A new concept of plasma calcium homeostasis in the rat. Endocrinology 95:480.
156. Bell, N. H., and Queener, S. (1974). Stimulation of calcitonin synthesis and release in vitro by calcium and dibutyryl cyclic AMP. Nature (London) 248:343.
157. Roos, B., Bundy, L. L., Bailey, R., and Deftos, L. J. (1974). Calcitonin secretion *in vitro*. I. Endocrinology 95:1142.
158. Bell, N. H. (1975). Further studies on the regulation of calcitonin release *in vitro*. Horm. Metab. Res. 7:77.
159. Roos, B. A., Bundy, L. L., Miller, E. A., and Deftos, L. J. (1975). Calcitonin secretion by monolayer cultures of human c-cells derived from medullary thyroid carcinoma. Endocrinology 97:39.
160. Hsu, H. H. T., and Haymovtis, A. (1974). On the nature of degradation of calcitonin by mammalian cells. Proc. Soc. Exp. Biol. Med. 146:1044.
161. Clark, M. B., Williams, C. C., Nathanson, B. M., Horton, R. E., Glass, H. I., and Foster, G. V. (1974). Metabolic fate of human calcitonin in the dog. J. Endocrinol. 61:199.
162. Hirsch, P. F., Sliwowski, A., Orimo, H., Darago, L. S., and Mewborn, Q. A. (1973). On the mode of the hypocalcemic action of thyrocalcitonin and its enhancement by phosphate in rats. Endocrinology 93:12.
163. Kalu, D. N., Hadkigeorgopoulos, A., and Foster, G. V. (1975). Evidence for physiological importance of calcitonin in regulation of plasma calcium in rats. J. Clin. Invest. 55:722.
164. Deftos, L. J., Watts, E. G., Copp, D. H., and Potts, J. T., Jr. (1974). A radioimmunoassay for salmon calcitonin. Endocrinology 94:155.
165. Gariel, J. M., Care, A. D., and Bartlett, J. P. (1974). A radioimmunoassay

for ovine calcitonin: an evaluation of calcitonin secretion during gestation, lactation and foetal life. J. Endocrinol. 62:497.

166. Culter, G. B., Jr., Habener, J. F., Dee, P. C., and Potts, J. T., Jr. (1974). Radioimmunoassay for chicken calcitonin. FEBS Lett. 28:209.

167. Watts, E. G., Copp, D. H., and Deftos, L. J. (1975). Changes in plasma calcitonin and calcium during the migration of the salmon. Endocrinology 96:214.

168. Omdahl, J. L., and DeLuca, H. F. (1973). Regulation of vitamin D metabolism and function. Physiol. Rev. 53:327.

169. Avioli, L. V., and Haddad, J. G. (1973). Vitamin D: current concepts. Metabolism 22:507.

170. Kodicek, E. (1974). The story of vitamin D. Lancet i:325.

171. DeLuca, H. F. (1974). Vitamin D: the vitamin and the hormone. Fed. Proc. 33:2211.

172. DeLuca, H. F. (1975). The kidney as an endocrine organ involved in the function of vitamin D. Am. J. Med. 58:39.

173. Kleiner-Bossaller, A., and DeLuca, H. F. (1974). Formation of 1,24,25-trihydroxyvitamin D_3 from 1,25-dihydroxyvitamin D_3. Biochim. Biophys. Acta 338:489.

174. Holick, M. F., Semmler, E. J., Schnoes, H. K., and DeLuca, H. F. (1973). Hydroxyderivative of vitamin D_3: a highly potent analog of 1-α-25-dihydroxyvitamin D_3. Science 180:190.

175. Norman, A. W., Mitra, M. N., Okamura, W. H., and Wing, R. M. (1975). Vitamin D: 3-deoxy-1α-hydroxyvitamin D_3, biologically active analog of 1α,25-dihydroxyvitamin D_3. Science 188:1013.

176. Zerwekh, J. E., Brambaugh, P. F., Haussler, D. H., Cork, D. J., and Haussler, M. R. (1974). 1α-hydroxyvitamin D_3: an analog of vitamin D_3 which apparently acts by metabolism to 1α,25-dihydroxyvitamin D_3. Biochemistry 13:4097.

177. Haddad, J. G., and Hahn, T. J. (1973). Natural and synthetic sources of circulating 25-hydroxyvitamin D in man. Nature (London) 244:515.

178. Neer, R. M., Davis, T. R. A., Walcott, A., Koski, S., Schepis, P., Taylor, J., Thorington, C., and Wurtman, R. J. (1971). Stimulation by artificial lighting of calcium absorption in elderly human subjects. Nature (London) 229:255.

179. Stamp, T. C. B., and Round, J. M. (1974). Seasonal changes in human plasma levels of 25-hydroxyvitamin D. Nature (London) 247:563.

180. Bhattacharyya, M. N., and DeLuca, H. F. (1974). Subcellular location of rat liver calciferol-25-hydroxylase. Arch. Biochem. Biophys. 160:58.

181. Bhattacharyya, M. H., and DeLuca, H. F. (1973). The regulation of rat liver calciferol-25-hydroxylase. J. Biol. Chem. 248:2969.

182. Ghazarian, J. G., Jefcoste, C. R., Knutson, J. C., Orma-Johnson, W. H., and DeLuca, H. F. (1974). Mitochondrial cytochrome P_{450}. A component of chick kidney 25-hydroxycholecalciferol-1α-hydroxylase. J. Biol. Chem. 249:3026.

183. Ghazarian, J. G., and De Luca, H. F. (1974). 25-hydroxycholecalciferol-1-hydroxylase: a specific requirement for NADPH and a hemoprotein component in chick kidney mitochondria. Arch. Biochem. Biophys. 160:63.

184. Larkins, R. G., MacAvley, S. J., Rapaport, D., and Martin, T. J. (1974). Effects of nucleotides, hormones, ions and 1,25-dihydroxycholecalciferol on 1,25-dihydroxycholecalciferol production in isolated chick renal tubules. Clin. Sci. Mol. Med. 46:569.

185. Bikle, D. D., and Rasmussen, H. (1975). The ionic control of 1,25-dihydroxyvitamin D_3 production in isolated chick renal tubules. J. Clin. Invest. 55:292.
186. Bikle, D. D., Murphy, E. W., and Rasmussen, H. (1975). The ionic control of 1,25-dihydroxyvitamin D_3 synthesis in isolated chick renal mitochondria: the role of calcium as influenced by inorganic phosphate and hydrogen ion. J. Clin. Invest. 55:299.
187. Bishop, J. E., and Norman, A. W. (1975). Studies on calciferol metabolism: metabolism of 25-hydroxy-vitamin D_3 by the chicken embryo. Arch. Biochem. Biophys. 167:769.
188. Edelstein, S., Lawson, D. E. M., and Kodicek, E. (1973). The transporting proteins of cholecalciferol and 25-hydroxycholecalciferol in serum of chicks and other species: partial purification and characterization of the chick proteins. Biochem. J. 135:417.
189. Belsey, R. E., DeLuca, H. F., and Potts, J. T., Jr. (1974). Selective binding properties of vitamin D transport protein in chick plasma in vitro. Nature (Lond.) 247:208.
190. Rojanasathit, S., and Haddad, J. G. (1975). Ontogeny and effect of vitamin D depletion on specific serum binding of 25-hydroxycholecalciferol in the rat. Proceedings of the 57th Meeting of the Endocrine Society.
191. Mawer, E. B., Backhouse, J., Hill, L. F., Lumb, G. A., deSilva, P., Taylor, C. M., and Stanbury, S. W. (1975). Vitamin D metabolism and parathyroid function in man. Clin. Sci. Mol. Med. 48:349.
192. Henry, H. L., Midgett, R. J., and Norman, A. W. (1974). Regulation of 25-hydroxyvitamin D_3-1-hydroxylase in vivo. J. Biol. Chem. 249:7584.
193. Garabedian, M., Holich, M. F., DeLuca, H. F., and Boyle, I. B. (1972). Control of 25-hydroxycholecalciferol metabolism by parathyroid glands. Proc. Natl. Acad. Sci. U. S. A. 69:1673.
194. Fraser, D. R., and Kodicek, E. (1973). Regulation of 25-hydroxycholecalciferol-1-hydroxylase activity in kidney by parathyroid hormone. Nature (New Biol.) 241:163.
195. Tanaka, Y., and DeLuca, H. F. (1973). The control of 25-hydroxyvitamin D metabolism by inorganic phosphorus. Arch. Biochem. Biophys. 154:566.
196. Gray, R. W., Weber, H. P., Dominguez, J. H., and Lemann, J. (1974). The metabolism of vitamin D_3 and 25-hydroxyvitamin D_3 in normal and anephric humans. J. Clin. Endocrinol. Metab. 39:1045.
197. Hahn, T. J., Hendin, B. A., Scharp, C., and Haddad, J. G. (1972). Effect of chronic anticonvulsant therapy on serum 25-hydroxycholecalciferol levels in adults. N. Engl. J. Med. 287:900.
198. Arnaud, S. B., Goldsmith, R. S., Lamber, P. W., and Go, V. L. W. (1975). 25-hydroxyvitamin D_3: evidence of an enterohepatic circulation in man. Proc. Soc. Exp. Biol. Med. 149:570.
199. Carre, M., Ayigbede, O., Miravet, L., and Rasmussen, H. (1974). The effect of prednisolone upon the metabolism and action of 25-hydroxy- and 1,25-dihydroxyvitamin D_3. Proc. Natl. Acad. Sci. U. S. A. 71:2996.
200. Brumbaugh, P. F., and Haussler, M. R. (1974). 1α,25-dihydroxycholecalciferol receptors in intestine. I. Association of 1α,25-dihydroxycholecalciferol with intestinal mucosa chromatin. J. Biol. Chem. 249:1251.
201. Brumbaugh, P. F., and Haussler, M. R. (1974). 1α,25-dihydroxycholecalciferol receptors in intestine. II. Temperature-dependent transfer of

the hormone to chromatin via a specific cytosol receptor. J. Biol. Chem. 249:1158.

202. Brumbaugh, P. F., and Haussler, M. R. (1975). Specific binding of 1-α 25 dihydroxycholecalciferol to nuclear components of chick intestine. J. Biol. Chem. 250:1588.

203. Haddad, J. G., Hahn, T. J., and Birge, S. F. (1973). Vitamin D metabolites: specific binding by rat intestinal cytosol. Biochim. Biophys. Acta 329:93.

204. Corradino, R. A. (1973). Embryonic chick intestine in organ culture: response to vitamin D_3 and its metabolites. Science 179:402.

205. Weber, J. C., Pons, V., and Kodicek, E. (1971). The localization of 1,25-dihydroxycholecalciferol in bone cell nuclei of rachitic chicks. Biochem. J. 125:147.

206. Emtage, J. S., Lawson, D. E. M., and Kodicek, E. (1974). The response of the small intestine to vitamin D: isolation and properties of chick intestinal polyribosomes. Biochem. J. 140:239.

207. Wong, R. G., and Norman, A. W. (1975). Studies on the mechanism of action of calciferol. VIII. Effects of dietary vitamin D and the polyene antibiotic, filipin, in vitro, on the intestinal cellular uptake of calcium. J. Biol. Chem. 250:2411.

208. Corradino, R. A. (1974). Embryonic chick intestine in organ culture: interaction of adenylate cyclase system and vitamin D_3-mediated calcium absorptive mechanism. Endocrinology 94:1607.

209. Mahgoub, A., and Sheppard, H. (1975). Early effect of 25-hydroxychole-calciferol (25-OHD$_3$) and 1,25-dihydroxycholecalciferol (1,25-(OH)$_2$-D$_3$) on the ability of parathyroid hormone to elevate cyclic AMP of intact bone cells. Biochem. Biophys. Res. Commun. 62:901.

210. Fullmer, C. S., and Wasserman, R. H. (1975). Isolation and partial charac-terization of intestinal calcium-binding proteins from the cow, pig, horse, guinea pig and chick. Biochim. Biophys. Acta 393:134.

211. Morrissey, R. L., Bucci, T. J., Empson, R. N., Jr., and Lufkin, E. G. (1975). Calcium-binding protein: its cellular localization in jejunum, kidney and pancreas. Proc. Soc. Exp. Biol. Med. 149:56.

212. Warner, R. R., and Coleman, J. R. (1975). Electron probe analysis of calcium transport by small intestine. J. Cell. Biol. 64:54.

213. Borle, A. B. (1974). Kinetic studies of calcium movements in intestinal cells: effects of vitamin D deficiency and treatment. J. Membr. Biol. 16:207.

214. Kowarski, S., and Schachter, D. (1973). Vitamin D and adenosine tri-phosphatase dependent on divalent cations in rat intestinal mucosa. J. Clin. Invest. 52:2765.

215. Wasserman, R. H., and Taylor, A. N. (1973). Intestinal absorption of phosphate in the chick: effect of vitamin D_3 and other parameters. J. Nutr. 103:586.

216. Chen, T. C., Castillo, L., Korycka-Dahl, M., and DeLuca, H. F. (174). Role of vitamin D metabolites in phosphate transport of rat intestine. J. Nutr. 104:1056.

217. Taylor, A. N. (1974). In vitro phosphate transport in chick ileum: effect of cholecalciferol, calcium, sodium and metabolic inhibitors. J. Nutr. 104:489.

218. Spielvogel, A. M., Farley, R. D., and Norman, A. W. (1972). Studies on the mechanism of action of calciferol. V. Turnover time of chick intestinal

epithelial cells in relation to the intestinal action of vitamin D. Exp. Cell. Res. 74:359.

219. Birge, S. J., and Alpers, D. H. (1973). Stimulation of intestinal mucosal proliferation by vitamin D. Gastroenterology 64:977.

220. Trummel, C. L., Raisz, L. G., Blunt, J. W., and DeLuca, H. F. (1969). 25 Hydroxycholecalciferol: metabolite of vitamin D_3 which stimulates bone resorption in tissue culture. Science 163:1450.

221. Raisz, L. G., Trummel, C. L., Holick, M. F., and DeLuca, H. F. (1972). 1,25-Dihydroxycholecalciferol: a potent stimulator of bone resorption in tissue culture. Science 175:768.

222. Reynolds, J. J., Holick, M. F., and DeLuca, H. F. (1974). The effects of vitamin D analogs on bone resorption. Calcif. Tissue Res. 15:333.

223. Trummel, C. L., Raisz, L. G., Hallick, R. B., and DeLuca, H. F. (1971). 25 Hydroxy-dihydroxytachysterol; stimulation of bone resorption in tissue culture. Biochem. Biophys. Res. Commun. 44:1096.

224. Garabedian, M., Tanaka, Y., Holick, M. F., and DeLuca, H. F. (1974). Response of intestinal calcium transport and bone calcium mobilization to 1,25-dihydroxyvitamin D_3 in thyroparathyroidectomized rats. Endocrinology 94:1022.

225. Avioli, V. (1972). Vitamin D, the kidney and calcium homeostasis. Kidney Int. 2:241.

226. Popovtzer, M. M., Robinette, J. B., DeLuca, H. F., and Holick, M. F. (1974). The acute effect of 25-hydroxycholecalciferol on renal handling of phosphorus: evidence for a parathyroid hormone-dependent mechanism. J. Clin. Invest. 53:913.

227. Puschett, J. B., Fernandez, P. C., Boyle, I. T., Gray, R. W., Omdahl, J. L., and DeLuca, H. F. (1972). The acute renal tubular effects of 1,25-dihydroxycholecalciferol. Proc. Soc. Exp. Biol. Med. 141:379.

228. Puschett, J. B., Moranz, J., and Kurnick, W. S. (1972). Evidence for a direct action of cholecalciferol and 25-hydroxycholecalciferol on the renal transport of phosphate, sodium and calcium. J. Clin. Invest. 51:373.

229. Puschett, J. B., Beck, N. S., Jelonik, A., and Fernandez, P. (1974). Study of the renal tubular interactions of thyrocalcitonin, cyclic adenosine 3',5'-monophosphate, 25-hydroxycholecalciferol, and calcium ion. J. Clin. Invest. 53:756.

230. Rasmussen, H., Jensen, P., Lake, W., Friedmann, N., and Goodman, D. B. P. (1975). Cyclic nucleotides and cellular metabolism. Advances in Cyclic Nucleotide Research, Vol. 5, p. 375. Raven Press, New York.

231. Beck, N., Singh, H., Reed, S. W., and Davis, B. B. (1974). Direct inhibitory effect of hypercalcemia on renal actions of parathyroid hormone. J. Clin. Invest. 53:717.

232. Bingham, P. J., and Raisz, L. G. (1974). Bone growth in organ culture: effects of phosphate and other nutrients on bone and cartilage. Calcif. Tissue Res. 14:31.

233. Wergedal, J., Stauffer, M., Baylink, D., and Rich, C. (1973). Inhibition of bone matrix formation, mineralization and resorption in thyroparathyroidectomized rats. J. Clin. Invest. 52:1052.

234. Stauffer, M., Baylink, D. Wergeda, J., and Rich, C. (1973). Decreased bone formation, mineralization, and enhanced resorption in calcium-deficient rats. Am. J. Physiol. 225:269.

235. Asher, M. A., Sledge, C. B., and Glimcher, M. J. (1974). The effect of

238   Raisz, Mundy, Dietrich, and Canalis

inorganic orthophosphate on the rates of collagen formation and degradation in bone and cartilage in tissue culture. J. Clin. Endocrinol.
Metab. 38:376.

236. Raisz, L. G., and Niemann, I. (1969). Effect of phosphate, calcium and
magnesium on bone resorption and hormonal responses in tissue culture.
Endocrinology 85:446.

237. Jowsey, J., Reiss, E., and Canterbury, J. M. (1974). Long-term effects of
high phosphate intake on parathyroid hormone levels and bone metabolism. Acta Orthop. Scand. 45:801.

238. Barzel, U. S. (1975). The effect of chronic ammonium chloride ingestion
on parathyroid hormone function. Nephron 14:339.

239. Beck, N., Kim, H. P., and Kim, K. S. (1975). Effect of metabolic acidosis
on renal action of parathyroid hormone. Am. J. Physiol. 228:1483.

240. Russell, R. G. G., and Fleisch, H. (1975). Pyrophosphate and diphosphonates in skeletal metabolism: physiological, clinical and therapeutic
aspects. Clin. Orthop. 108:241.

241. Beck, N., and Davis, B. B. (1975). Impaired renal response to parathyroid
hormone in potassium depletion. Am. J. Physiol. 228:179.

242. Raisz, L. G., and Bingham, P. J. (1972). Effect of hormones on bone
development. Ann. Rev. Pharmacol. 12:337.

243. Philips, L. S. (1974). Advances in Human Growth Hormone Research, p.
50. Government Printing Office, Washington, D. C.

244. Frantz, A. G., and Rabkin, M. T. (1965). Human growth hormone: clinical
measurement, response to hypoglycemia and suppression by corticosteroids. N. Engl. J. Med. 271:1375.

245. Krawitt, E. L. (1972). The role of intestinal transport proteins in cor-
tisone-mediated suppression of Ca^{2+} absorption. Biochim. Biophys. Acta
274:179.

246. Favus, M. J., Walling, M. W., and Kimberg, D. V. (1973). Effects of
1,25-dihydroxycholecalciferol on intestinal calcium transport in
cortisone-treated rats. J. Clin. Invest. 52:1680.

247. Favus, M. J., Kimber, D. V., Miller, G. N., and Gershon, E. (1973). Effects
of cortisone administration on the metabolism and localization of
25-hydroxycholecalciferol in the rat. J. Clin. Invest. 52:1328.

248. Lukert, B. P., Stanbury, S. W., and Mawer, E. B. (1973). Vitamin D and
intestinal transport of calcium: effects of prednisone. Endocrinology
93:718.

249. Raisz, L. G., Trummel, C. L., Wener, J., and Simmons, H. (1972). Effect of
glucocorticoids on bone resorption in tissue culture. Endocrinology
90:961.

250. Peck, W. A., and Messinger, K. (1970). Nucleoside and ribonucleic acid
metabolism in isolated bone cells: effects of insulin and cortisol in vitro.
J. Biol. Chem. 245:2722.

251. Feldman, D., Dziak, R., Koehler, R., and Stern, P. (1975). Cytoplasmic
glucocorticoid bonding proteins in bone. Endocrinology 96:29.

252. Gallagher, J. C., and Wilkinson, R. (1973). The effect of ethinyloestradiol
on calcium and phosphorus metabolism of postmenopausal women with
primary hyperparathyroidism. Clin. Sci. Mol. Med. 45:785.

253. Atkins, D., Zanelli, J. M., Peacock, M., and Nordin, B. E. C. (1972). The
effect of oestrogens on the response of bone to parathyroid hormone in
vitro. J. Endocrinol. 54:107.

254. Krane, S. M. (1971). Thyroid Diseases, 598. Harper and Row, New York.

255. Marcus, R. (1975). Cyclic nucleotide phosphodiesterase from bone: characterization of the enzyme and studies of inhibition by thyroid hormones. Endocrinology 96:400.
256. Schwartz, P. L., Wettenhau, R. E. H., Troedel, M. A., and Bornstein, J. (1970). A long term effect of insulin on collagen synthesis by new born rat bone *in vitro*. Diabetes 19:465.
257. Perlish, J. S., Bashey, R. I., and Fleischmajer, R. (1973). The *in vitro* effect of insulin on collagen synthesis in embryonic chick tibia. Proc. Soc. Exp. Biol. Med. 142:1152.
258. Puche, R. C., Romano, M. C., Locatto, M. E., and Ferretti, J. L. (1973). The effect of insulin on bone resorption. Calcif. Tissue Res. 12:8.
259. Stern, P. H., and Bell, N. H. (1970). Effects of glucagon on serum calcium in the rat and on bone resorption in tissue culture. Endocrinology 87:111.
260. Bell, N. H., and Kimble, J. B. (1970). Effects of glucagon, dibutyryl cyclic 3',5-adenosine monophosphate and theophylline on calcitonin secretion *in vitro*. J. Clin. Invest. 49:1368.
261. Kalu, D. N., Hillyard, C., and Foster, G. V. (1972). Effect of glucagon on bone collagen metabolism in the rat. J. Endocrinol. 55:245.
262. Van Wyk, J. J., Underwood, L. E., Hintz, R. L., Clemmons, D. R., Voina, S. J., and Weaver, R. P. (1974). The somatomedins: a family of insulin-like hormones under growth hormone control. Recent Prog. Horm. Res. 30:259.
263. Bomboy, J. D., and Salmon, W. D. (1975). Somatomedin. Clin. Orthop. 108:228.
264. Canalis, E. M., Hintz, R., Dietrich, J. W., Maina, D. M., and Raisz, L. G. (1975). Clin. Res. 23:316A.
265. Gospodarowicz, D. (1975). Purification of a fibroblast growth factor from bovine pituitary. J. Biol. Chem. 250:2515.
266. Chase, L. R., and Aurbach, G. D. (1970). Effects of parathyroid hormone on the concentration of adenosine 3',5'-monophosphate in skeletal tissue in vitro. J. Biol. Chem. 245:1520.
267. Klein, D. C., and Raisz, L. G. (1970). Prostaglandins: stimulation of bone resorption in tissue culture. Endocrinology 86:1456.
268. Tashijian, A. H., Jr., Voelkel, E. F., Levine, L., and Goldhaber, P. (1972). Evidence that the bone resorption stimulating factor produced by mouse fibrosarcoma cells is prostaglandin E_2: a new model for the hypercalcemia of cancer. J. Exp. Med. 136:1329.
269. Powles, T. J., Clark, S. A., Easty, D. M., Easty, G. C., and Munro-Neville, A. (1973). The inhibition by aspirin and indomethacin of osteolytic tumour deposits and hypercalcaemia in rats with Walker tumours and in possible application to human breast cancer. Br. J. Cancer. 28:210.
270. Voelkel, E. F., Tashjian, A. H., Jr., Franklin, R., Wasserman, E., and Levine, L. (1975). Hypercalcemia and tumor-prostaglandins: the VX_2 carcinoma model in the rabbit. Metabolism 24:973
271. Seyberth, H. W., Morgan, J. L., Sweetman, B. J., and Oates, J. A. (1975). Inhibition of increased prostaglandin synthesis in patients with tumor associated hypercalcemia. Clin. Res. 23:423A.
272. Robinson, D. R., Tashjian, A. H., Jr., and Levine, L. (1975). Prostaglandin induced bone resorption by rheumatoid synovia. Clin. Res. 23:443A.
273. Harris, M., Jenkins, M. V., Bennett, A., and Wills, M. R. (1973). Prosta-

glandin production and bone resorption by dental cysts. Nature (Lond.) 245:213.

274. Goodson, J. M., Dewhirst, F. E., and Brunetti, A. (1974). Prostaglandin E_2 levels and human periodontal disease. Prostaglandins 6:81.

275. Goldhaber, P., Radadiija, L., Beyer, W. R., and Kornhauser, A. (1973). Bone resorption in tissue culture and its relevance to periodontal disease. J. Am. Dent. Assoc. 87:1027.

276. Dietrich, J. W., Goodson, J. M., and Raisz, L. G. Stimulation of bone resorption by various prostaglandins in organ culture. Prostaglandins, in press.

277. Goodson, J. M., McClatchy, K., and Revell, C. (1974). Prostaglandin-induced resorption of the adult rat calvarium. J. Dent. Res. 53:670.

278. Franklin, R. B., and Tashjian, A. H., Jr. (1975). Intravenous infusion of prostaglandin E_2 raises plasma calcium concentration in the rat. Endocrinology 97:240.

279. Blumenkrantz, N., and Sondergaard, J. (1972). Prostaglandin E_1 and F_1 alpha biosynthesis of collagen. Nature (New Biol.) 239:246.

280. Raisz, L. G., and Koolemans-Beynen, A. R. (1974). Inhibition of bone collagen synthesis by prostaglandin E_2 in organ culture. Prostaglandins 8:377.

281. Raisz, L. G., Sandberg, A., Goodson, J. M., Simmons, H. A., and Mergenhagen, S. E. (1974). Complement-dependent stimulation of bone resorption mediated by prostaglandins. Science 185:789.

282. Beck, N. P., DeRubertis, F. R., Michelis, M. F., Fusco, R. D., Field, J. B., and Davis, B. B. (1972). Effect of prostaglandin E_1 on renal actions of parathyroid hormone. J. Clin. Invest. 51:2352.

283. Horton, J. E., Raisz, L. G., Simmons, H. A., Oppenheim, J. J., and Mergenhagen, S. E. (1972). Bone resorbing activity in supernatant fluid from cultured human peripheral blood leukocytes. Science 177:793.

284. Horton, J. D., Oppenheim, J. J., Mergenhagen, S. E., and Raisz, L. G. (1974). Macrophage lymphocyte synergy in the production of osteoclast activating factor (OAF). J. Immunol. 113:1278.

285. Mundy, G. R., Luben, R. A., Raisz, L. G., Oppenheim, J. J., and Buell, D. N. (1974). Bone resorbing activity in supernatants from lymphoid cell lines. N. Engl. J. Med. 290:867.

286. Mundy, G. R., Raisz, L. G., Cooper, R. A., Schechter, G. P., and Salmon, S. E. (1974). Evidence for the secretion of an osteoclast stimulating factor in myeloma. N. Engl. J. Med. 291:1041.

287. Luben, R. A., Mundy, G. R., Trummel, C. L., and Raisz, L. G. (1974). Partial purification of osteoclast activating factor from phyto-hemagglutinin-stimulated human leukocytes. J. Clin. Invest. 53:1473.

288. Raisz, L. G., Luben, R. A., Mundy, G. R., Dietrich, J. W., Horton, J. E., and Trummel, C. L. (1975). Effect of osteoclast activating factor from human leukocytes on bone metabolism. J. Clin. Invest. 56:408.

289. Walker, D. G. (1972). Congenital osteopetrosis in mice cured by parabiotic union with normal siblings. Endocrinology 91:916.

International Review of Physiology
Endocrine Physiology II, Volume 16
Edited by S. M. McCann
Copyright 1977   University Park Press   Baltimore

7
Cyclic Nucleotides in Mode of Hormone Action

J. N. FAIN and F. R. BUTCHER

Brown University,
Providence, Rhode Island

It is impossible in one article to review adequately all the recent advances in a rapidly growing area such as cyclic nucleotides. During the 3 years preceding the preparation of this article (October, 1975), 3,901 articles which listed cyclic AMP as an index term and 515 articles mentioning cyclic GMP appeared on journals covered by *Index Medicus* (based on Medline citations). There is even a journal devoted exclusively to cyclic nucleotide research. The proceedings have been published of the Second International Conference on Cyclic AMP (1) and of a conference on cyclic nucleotides in disease (2). A memorial issue was also published on cyclic nucleotides and mammalian cells in honor of Earl W. Sutherland, who died in 1974 (3).

The increase in number of articles on cyclic nucleotides during the past 4 years has been so rapid that it is impossible for any one individual to keep up with all areas. However, the literature on cyclic nucleotides which appeared during the first 12 years after the discovery of cyclic AMP in 1957 was reviewed in a single volume by Robison et al. (4). The monograph is still the best introduction to the field and is well on its way to becoming a classic. Most reviews written since that time have been limited to special aspects of cyclic nucleotides.

Table 1 is a compilation of some recent reviews. This review is devoted to selected aspects of progress during the past 2–3 years which appear particularly significant. Some areas have been neglected because excellent reviews have recently appeared (Table 1) or because they are not particularly relevant to the role of cyclic nucleotides in mode of hormone action.

The discovery of cyclic GMP and AMP has probably contributed more than anything else to the amazing progress made during the past 10 years in understanding how hormones regulate metabolism in mammalian cells. One sometimes feels when reading the current literature that every known hormone affects either the level of cyclic AMP or GMP or both. The real problem is which of the hormone-induced changes in intracellular cyclic nucleotides directly reflect the action of the hormone and which are secondary results of some more fundamental change.

The history of cyclic AMP research dates from 1957 when Sutherland and Rall (34,35) discovered that the heat-stable compound formed by particulate fractions from liver homogenates after incubation with ATP, magnesium ions, and glucagon or epinephrine, which activated hepatic phosphorylase, was cyclic AMP. Cyclic GMP was discovered 6 years later in rat urine by Price and his colleagues (36). However, the significance of cyclic GMP has been difficult to demonstrate. There is no established activation of guanylate cyclase by hormones in cell-free systems. Furthermore, there is no protein with a known function which is phosphorylated by a cyclic GMP-sensitive protein kinase. In contrast, many hormones readily activate adenylate cyclase in broken cell preparations, and the cyclic AMP which is formed activates a protein kinase which phosphorylates regulatory enzymes.

Table 1. Recent review articles on cyclic nucleotides

Area of review	Author	Date published	Reference
General reviews			
Adenyl cyclase	Perkins	1973	5
Hormone binding and	Birnbaumer et al.	1974	6
cyclase activation	Helmreich et al.	1976	7
Cyclic nucleotide phospho-diesterases	Appleman et al.	1973	8
Protain kinase and protein	Langan	1973	9
phosphorylation	Rubin and Rosen	1975	10
	Cohen et al.	1976	11
	Krebs and Stull	1975	12
	Corbin et al.	1975	13
Cyclic GMP	Goldberg et al.	1973, 1975	14,15
	Goldberg	1974	16
Growth regulation	Pastan et al.	1975	17
Glycogen metabolism	Soderling and Park	1974	18
Protein synthesis	Wicks	1974	19
Analogs of cyclic AMP and cyclic GMP	Simon et al.	1973	20
Calcium and cyclic nucleotide interactions	Rasmussen et al.	1972,1974	21,22
	Berridge	1975	23
Immune response	Parker et al.	1974	24
Reviews of particular tissues			
Smooth muscle	Bär	1974	25
Adrenal cortex	Halkerston	1975	26
Gonads	Marsh	1975	27
Cardiac muscle	Entman	1974	28
Insulin secretion by islets of Langerhans	Montague and Howell	1975	29
Normal and proliferating epidermis	Voorhees et al.	1974	30
Cultured mammalian cells	Chlapowski et al.	1975	31
Nervous system	Daly	1975	32
Fat cells	Fain	In press	33

The current dogma is that all effects of cyclic AMP in mammalian cells are secondary to increased phosphorylation of target proteins. Whether or not this is actually the case is unclear at the moment. Probably cyclic AMP has other effects besides activation of protein kinase in mammalian systems. There is also increasing evidence that many hormones which elevate cyclic AMP have other effects which are not secondary to cyclic AMP elevation but act synergistically with cyclic AMP.

A major problem today is the uncritical attempt to involve cyclic nucleotides in the action of every hormone, in growth regulation, and even in cancer. Like all great discoveries, that of cyclic nucleotides first went through a period of initial opposition, followed by a period of increasing acceptance which culminated with the awarding of the Nobel Prize to Earl Sutherland in 1971. For the past 4 years we have been literally inundated with reports of cyclic nucleotide involvement in virtually every biological process. Many of these reports adopted a rather uncritical approach to cyclic nucleotides.

Pharmaceutical firms embarked on large programs of research on cyclic nucleotides. Virtually every known drug has been tested for effects on cyclic AMP formation, degradation, or action. These research efforts did not produce a new wonder drug within 36–48 months so many firms dropped their research programs on cyclic nucleotides. This is unfortunate as there is substantial evidence that methylxanthines (the active ingredients in cola beverages, tea, and coffee) and opiates affect cyclic nucleotide metabolism. The opiate story is the most recent link between drug action and cyclic nucleotides and is discussed later in this chapter.

CYCLIC NUCLEOTIDES, YIN-YANG, AND Ca^{2+}

Probably the most important hypothesis to explain the interactions of cyclic AMP, cyclic GMP, and Ca^{2+} is that of Berridge (23). Much of the information about the relative roles and importance of cyclic AMP, cyclic GMP, and Ca^{2+} has been more confusing than enlightening. Goldberg et al. (14) originally emphasized that in many systems the level of cyclic AMP went down when cyclic GMP was elevated and vice versa. Goldberg called this a Yin-Yang relationship, based on the Oriental concept of two major opposing forces in the universe. However, it was soon realized that in many cells both cyclic AMP and cyclic GMP are simultaneously elevated, which is incompatible with the Yin-Yang hypothesis. Goldberg et al. in their most recent formulation of this hypothesis divided cyclic

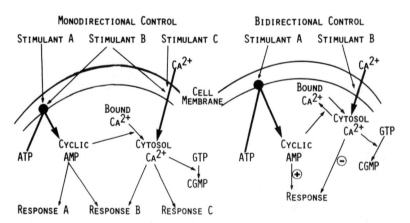

Figure 1. A model for mono- and bidirectional control of metabolism by Ca^{2+} and cyclic nucleotides based on the hypothesis of Berridge (23).

nucleotide interactions into those which fit the Yin-Yang hypothesis and those which do not (15).

It remained for Berridge (23) to place more emphasis on the role of Ca^{2+} in monodirectional and bidirectional control. Bidirectional control is in essence another name for Yin-Yang control since both terms describe situations in which cyclic AMP and cyclic GMP are related in a reciprocal fashion. The difference is that the Yin-Yang hypothesis suggests that there is antagonism between the actions of cyclic AMP or cyclic GMP. In contrast, Berridge (23) postulated that the antagonism is primarily between cyclic AMP and Ca^{2+}. Berridge (23) suggested that the level of cyclic GMP is regulated by and reflects change in the free intracellular Ca^{2+} concentration.

Figure 1 summarizes monodirectional and bidirectional control. The five major differences between the two types of control are as follows.

Monodirectional control	Bidirectional control
1. Stimulants may increase both intracellular cyclic AMP and cytosol Ca^{2+}.	1. One group of stimulants increases cyclic AMP and a different group increases Ca^{2+}.
2. Cyclic AMP increases cytosol Ca^{2+}.	2. Cyclic AMP lowers cytosol Ca^{2+}.
3. Ca^{2+} action is enhanced by cyclic AMP.	3. Ca^{2+} action is opposed by cyclic AMP.
4. Cyclic AMP and cyclic GMP may both be elevated at the same time.	4. Cyclic GMP elevation is associated with drop in cyclic AMP.
5. Elevated cytosol Ca^{2+} has little influence on cyclic AMP level.	5. Elevated cytosol Ca^{2+} lowers cyclic AMP.

One type of monodirectional control involves activation of membrane-bound adenylate cyclase by stimulants of the A type (Figure 1). Another type of response occurs when stimulant C elevates intracellular calcium. The increase in intracellular free Ca^{2+} concentration (cytosol Ca^{2+}) could result from either decreased efflux, increased influx of extracellular Ca^{2+}, or release of bound calcium sequestered in mitochondria, sarcoplasmic reticulum, endoplasmic reticulum and other cellular structures. The third type of monodirectional control results from stimulants which increase both intracellular cyclic AMP and Ca^{2+}. This results in a response in which Ca^{2+} and cyclic AMP act synergistically (*response B* in Figure 1).

Bidirectional control is relatively simple in that there is usually a single response for a particular differentiated cell type which is reciprocally controlled by the level of cyclic AMP and Ca^{2+}. Stimulants of the A type elevate cyclic AMP, which lowers cytosol Ca^{2+} by increasing either its efflux from the cell or uptake into cytoplasmic organelles where it is bound (Figure 1). Stimulants of the B type elevate cytosol Ca^{2+}, which in turn increases guanylate cyclase activity. In bidirectional cells, an elevated cytosol Ca^{2+} lowers cyclic AMP through either activation of cyclic AMP phosphodiesterase or inhibition of adenylate cyclase.

Table 2. Examples of two types of interaction between cyclic AMP, cyclic GMP, and Ca[2+]

Monodirectional control[a]	Bidirectional control (Yin-Yang)
1. Release of hormones by pituitary, adrenal medulla, and endocrine pancreas	1. Contraction and relaxation of muscle
2. Release of enzymes by exocrine pancreas and parotid	2. Aggregation and dispersion of melanin in melanophores
3. Water transport in toad bladder	3. Platelet aggregation
4. Steroid hormone formation and release	4. Histamine release by mast cells
5. Photoreception in eye	

Modified from Berridge (23).

[a]Hepatic gluconeogenesis and glycogenolysis and triglyceride lipolysis in fat cells appear to be monodirectional with respect to Ca[2+] and cyclic AMP interactions. They are bidirectional in that insulin can oppose the action of hormones which elevate cyclic AMP in these cells.

Examples of hormonal responses of each type are shown in Table 2. This list follows the classification of responses used by Berridge (23). Lipolysis in fat cells and hepatic glucose release are not easily classified. They are bidirectional in the broader sense of the term since the action of hormones which stimulate cyclic AMP is opposed by insulin. Insulin is able to elevate cyclic GMP and lower cyclic AMP in fat cells and liver, which are monodirectional in the sense that an elevation of cytosol Ca[2+] either mimics the action of cyclic AMP (hepatic glycogenolysis) or has no effect (fat cell lipolysis). Insulin is thought to elevate intracellular Ca[2+] which should result in antagonism to cyclic AMP if control is bidirectional. The inconsistency can be resolved by postulating that in fat cells and hepatic cells regulation is monodirectional with respect to Ca[2+] and cyclic GMP interactions. The bidirectional control results from insulin action through an unknown second messenger. This problem is discussed in more detail in the section of this chapter devoted to the regulation of hepatic glucose production.

The role of cyclic nucleotides in cell division can be either bidirectional or monodirectional. We postulate that much of the confusion generated in this area could be clarified by postulating that bidirectional control exists where cell division is associated with a rise in Ca[2+] and cyclic GMP but a fall in cyclic AMP. However, monodirectional control exists when cell division is associated with rises in both cyclic AMP and cyclic GMP.

METHODOLOGY

An entire volume with 57 articles on cyclic nucleotide methodology appeared in 1974 (37). Two earlier works on the same subject were published in 1972 (38,39). These volumes can be consulted for methodology in this area, but advances have come so rapidly that many of the published procedures are now obsolete. Good examples of obsolete procedures are assays for cyclic nucleotides based on protein kinase activation, enzymatic cycling, luminescence assays, or high pressure ion exchange chromatography.

The rapid advances in recent years have resulted in part from the development of techniques which have made it relatively easy to assay cyclic nucleotides. The original assay for cyclic AMP used by Sutherland and his colleagues was based on the ability of the nucleotide to enhance the rate of activation of dog liver phosphorylase. The assay was difficult to perform and even led to some doubt about the importance of cyclic AMP since for quite a few years Sutherland's laboratory was virtually the only one to get consistent data. There are a multitude of factors which can interfere with this assay, but nearly all the results obtained with this assay have been confirmed by newer procedures. An entire chapter in the monograph on cyclic AMP by Robison et al. (4) was devoted to the phosphorylase assay for cyclic AMP, which is now only of historical importance.

Radioligand binding assays for the determination of cyclic AMP and GMP are so superior to other assays that they are now universally accepted as the methods of choice. Cyclic AMP can be readily determined by using various modifications of the protein kinase binding assay of Gilman (40). We prefer for reasons of convenience and economy to separate bound from unbound cyclic AMP by charcoal precipitation according to the procedure of Brown et al. (41) rather than with the use of Millipore filters as originally described by Gilman (40). Binding protein fraction from either rabbit muscle protein kinase preparations (40) or more conveniently a $10,000 \times g$ supernatant fraction from bovine adrenals (41) can be used.

Steiner et al. (42) developed radioimmunoassays for both cyclic AMP and cyclic GMP. It is generally very difficult to measure cyclic GMP with protein kinase binding assays because of the low specific radioactivity of tritiated cyclic GMP and the low level of cyclic GMP in tissues as compared to cyclic AMP. Even the radioimmunoassay for cyclic GMP was not sensitive enough to provide a convenient procedure for most samples. However, Cailla et al. (43) found that the sensitivity of the radioimmunoassay for cyclic nucleotides was greatly enhanced if the samples were succinylated prior to assay. Acetylation (44) also increased the sensitivity of the radioimmunoassay for cyclic nucleotides. The antigen is prepared with the use of cyclic nucleotides succinylated at the $O^{2'}$ position and linked to serum albumin, which results in antibodies which are much more sensitive to $O^{2'}$-acylated cyclic nucleotides. The radioimmunoassay with the use of succinylated or acetylated samples of cyclic AMP or cyclic GMP detects femtomole concentrations of the nucleotides and has revolutionized the assay of cyclic GMP. The routine $O^{2'}$ acylation of cyclic nucleotides with acetic or succinic anhydride occurs with virtually 100% yield in water.

The radioligand binding assays are much more sensitive and often much cheaper to use for analysis of cyclic GMP or cyclic AMP formed during assay of adenylate or guanylate cyclase activity than the use of the radioactive GTP or ATP. Tissue samples or those from cyclase assays can sometimes be analyzed for cyclic AMP or cyclic GMP without purification of the samples. However, when purification is required, particularly useful procedures use column chromatography over neutral alumina (45) or Dowex 1 (46) or a combination of both. The procedure of White and Zenser (45) was modified by Jakobs et al. (47) to allow absorption of the cyclic nucleotides in acid to neutral alumina and subsequent elution with ammonium formate.

To purify or not to purify samples is a question which investigators must answer experimentally for themselves. There are compounds which do interfere with the protein binding assay for cyclic AMP (48). In addition to sample purification, in many cases the problems caused by interfering compounds can be obviated by diluting the samples or by maintaining a constant amount of the interfering substances in each assay tube. These problems are discussed by Albano et al. (48). The above comments regarding sample purification before assaying cyclic AMP are also true for cyclic GMP.

With the advent of a multitude of commercial assay kits for cyclic AMP and cyclic GMP, we are concerned that the novice might be misled as to the necessity of sample purification. Regardless of what the literature accompanying these commercial kits might claim about the lack of need for sample purification we advise each user to these kits to establish for himself whether or not sample purification is essential for these particular experiments.

CYCLIC GMP

Control of Tissue Cyclic GMP Levels

Since the initial report of the natural occurrence of cyclic GMP, several agents have been found which elevate cyclic GMP. Some of these are summarized in Table 3. The first report of an elevation of cyclic GMP by a hormone appeared in June, 1970 (51). George et al. (51) found that acetylcholine elevated the level of cyclic GMP in the heart. Previously, there had been several unsuccessful attempts to demonstrate effects of hormones on tissue cyclic GMP levels (84,85). Although the list of hormones and other agents which modify tissue levels of cyclic GMP continues to grow, we still lack knowledge of any cause and effect relationship between changes in tissue cyclic GMP levels and the ultimate effect of hormones on their target tissues.

If the four criteria used by Sutherland to implicate a role for cyclic AMP in mediating the response to an agent are applied to cyclic GMP, the only criterion which is fulfilled is that the cyclic GMP levels change either before or coincident with the physiological response to the agent.

The effects of exogenous cyclic GMP may be extremely difficult to interpret. In many instances, the added cyclic GMP may mimic the effects of cyclic AMP or modify cyclic AMP levels through an effect on the cyclic AMP phospho-

Table 3. Agents that elevate cyclic GMP

Agent	Tissue	Reference	Agent	Tissue	Reference
Cholinergic	Lung	49, 50	ACTH	Adrenal	73, 74
	Heart	51, 52, 53	Prostaglandin $F_{2\alpha}$	Uterus	59
	Ductus deferens	54		Digital veins	59
	Submaxillary gland	54	Estrogens	Uterus	75
	Parotid	185	Methyl isobutyl xanthine	Ductus deferens	54
	Liver	55, 56, 57		Submaximallary parotid	54
	Adipose	55, 58	Ascorbic acid	Platelets	15
	Uterus	59	Histamine	Monocytes	76
	Neutrophils	60		Umbilical artery	77
	Ileum	53	Morphine	Neuroblastoma-glioma hybrid cell line	78
	Thyroid	57			
	Tracheal smooth muscle	61, 62	Serotonin	Monocytes	79
	Pancreas	63, 64			
	Brain	53	Secretin	Pancreas	64
α-Adrenergic	Ductus deferens	65	Pancreozymin	Pancreas	64
	Human plasma	66	Bradykinin	Lung	80
	Parotid	67	A-23187	Parotid	81
Insulin	Liver	55, 56		Thyroid	82
	Adipose	55, 58		Neutrophils	83
	Fibroblasts	59		Umbilical artery	77
Somatostatin	Anterior pituitary	68		Liver	56
Serum factors	Fibroblasts	69, 70		Adipose tissue	58
Phytohemagglutin	Lymphocytes	71			
High K^+	Cerebellum	72			
	Ductus deferens	65			

Table 4. Tissues responding to exogenous cyclic GMP or cyclic GMP analogs

Tissue	Response	Reference
Diaphragm muscle	Sugar transport	86
Polymorphonuclear neutrophils	Chemotaxis	87, 88, 89
Leukocytes	Lysosomal enzyme release	60, 90, 91
Mast cells	Histamine release	92
Fibroblasts	Transport of leucine, uridine, and glucose	93
Superior cervical ganglia	Polarization of postsynaptic membrane	94
Somatosensory cells of cortex	Neuronal firing	95
Isolated lymphocyte nuclei	[^{3}H] Uridine incorporation into RNA	59
Lymphocytes	[^{3}H] Uridine and [^{3}H] thymidine in RNA and DNA, respectively	96
	Proliferation	97
	Phosphorylation of nuclear acidic proteins	98
Parotid	K$^+$ efflux	67

diesterase. Only in cases in which the response of a given tissue to added cyclic AMP differs from that for added cyclic GMP are the results less ambiguous. Some examples of systems responding to exogenous cyclic GMP are listed in Table 4.

Ideas on how cyclic GMP might change cellular events in the various target cells have been based on analogies to cyclic AMP action. Just as there are cyclic AMP-dependent protein kinases which appear to control the activity of a number of intracellular enzymes, so too are there cyclic GMP-dependent protein kinases. However, unlike the case for cyclic AMP there are no identified physiological substrates for cyclic GMP-dependent protein kinases.

Guanylate Cyclase

Guanylate cyclase, the enzyme which catalyzes cyclic GMP formation from GTP, has several unique properties which distinguish it from adenylate cyclase. In contrast to adenylate cyclase, which is almost entirely localized in the plasma membrane, guanylate cyclase is found in both particulate and soluble fractions. The ratio of the amount of guanylate cyclase in the soluble fraction to that in the particulate fraction varies from one tissue to another. Kimura and Murad have recently summarized the subcellular distribution of guanylate cyclase in several tissues (99). In the lung, 80% of guanylate cyclase was in the soluble fraction (100), whereas in intestinal mucosa 90% of the activity was in the particulate fraction sedimented at 105,000 $\times$ g (100). Furthermore, the activity of guanylate cyclase in the particulate fraction was increased in regenerating liver, fetal liver, and a hepatoma, in contrast to normal liver (101). At the same time, the percentage of enzyme in the soluble fraction in the same three tissues decreased relative to normal liver (101).

The guanylate cyclase in the soluble and particulate fractions seems to be different on the basis of kinetic properties and molecular sieve chromatography (102, 103). The kinetic behavior of the particulate and soluble guanylate cyclase activities with respect to divalent cation effects is particularly striking. Guanylate cyclase from all sources has an absolute requirement for Mn^{2+}. The actual substrate is Mn-GTP, and some free Mn^{2+} is required (100, 103). At saturating concentrations of Mn-GTP, the K_m for Mn^{2+} of the soluble cyclase was 2×10^{-4} M, whereas that of the particulate enzyme approached zero (103). The soluble guanylate cyclase fractions from liver (102), heart (100), and lung (103) were stimulated by Ca^{2+}. Stimulation of soluble guanylate cyclase activity by Ca^{2+} was related to the Mn^{2+} to GTP ratio. The effect of Ca^{2+} was greatest when GTP was in excess of Mn^{2+} and was the smallest at near saturating amounts of Mn^{2+} and Mn-GTP. Chrisman et al. (103) found that 0.1–4 mM Ca^{2+} increased the concentration of free Mn^{2+} by displacing it from Mn-GTP to form Ca-GTP. Unlike its effect on the soluble enzyme, Ca^{2+} inhibits the particulate guanylate cyclase. This is true for the particulate enzyme from heart (100), lung (103), liver (102), and parotid (104).

Modulation of guanylate cyclase activity by hormones is poorly understood. There are only a few reports of direct effects of hormones on guanylate cyclase (105, 106). The failure to demonstrate direct effects of hormones on guanylate cyclase activity has led to the suggestion that hormones are indirect activators. Schultz et al. (54) have proposed that Ca^{2+} is required for hormones to increase cellular levels of cyclic GMP. Hormones might elevate cyclic GMP levels by increasing the concentration of free Ca^{2+} accessible to the soluble cyclase. Alternatively, Ca^{2+} could function as a cofactor which initiates the release or synthesis of some as yet unidentified activator of guanylate cyclase. Since the activity of particulate guanylate cyclase was increased by solubilization with Triton X-100, it is possible that hormones might affect the ratio of particulate to soluble enzyme. Thus far the only indications of a change in the ratio of particulate to soluble activity are in rapidly growing tissues such as fetal liver, regenerating liver, and a hepatoma (101). A mechanism involving redistribution of the enzyme activity would be hard to reconcile for those tissues in which nearly all of the guanylate cyclase activity was already in the soluble form.

It has been reported that guanylate cyclase undergoes autoactivation in the test tube (107, 108). This mechanism appears to involve an oxidation-reduction reaction of some component which results in increased guanylate cyclase activity. If the autoactivation process has a counterpart in the cell, it is possible that hormones could modulate the activity of guanylate cyclase by controlling the oxidation-reduction state of a component which regulates guanylate cyclase activity. It has been proposed that insulin regulates glucose transport in adipose tissue by altering the oxidation-reduction state of membrane sulfhydryl groups (109).

Kimura et al. (110) have demonstrated that sodium azide increased the activity of guanylate cyclase from a number of tissues independent of possible effects of azide on substrate depletion or cyclic GMP hydrolysis. With liver and kidney, the effect of azide was greater on the soluble enzyme than on the particulate, whereas just the opposite was true for enzyme preparations from several areas of the brain. Azide was without effect on the soluble enzyme from cerebral cortex and cerebellum but increased the activity of the particulate enzyme 60- and 20-fold, respectively. No effect of azide was observed with either the particulate or soluble guanylate cyclase from heart, spleen, or small intestinal smooth muscle or small intestinal mucosa. Azide should be a fruitful probe for studying guanylate cyclase.

Protein Phosphorylation

Kuo and Greengard (111) originally reported that only low levels of cyclic GMP-dependent protein kinase activity were present in mammalian tissues. Subsequently, Kuo (112) detected a protein kinase in mammalian tissues which was stimulated by low levels of cyclic GMP. The presence of a protein kinase modulator was essential. This was apparently the same modulator fraction described by Walsh et al. (113) that inhibited cyclic AMP-stimulated protein kinase activity. Kuo (112) also confirmed the report of Hofmann and Sold (114) that inorganic phosphate enhanced the stimulation of protein kinase by cyclic GMP and suppressed that by cyclic AMP. Kuo (112) separated the cyclic GMP-dependent protein kinase activity from the cyclic AMP-dependent protein kinase activity by chromatography on Sephadex G-200. The lung cyclic GMP-dependent protein kinase activity purified by Sephadex chromatography was half-maximally activated by 30 nM cyclic GMP. Kuo (115) has also reported that the level of the protein kinase modulator was lower in adipose tissue from diabetic rats than in controls. This suggests that variations in the level of protein kinase modulator might alter the ratio in intracellularly active cyclic AMP- and cyclic GMP-dependent protein kinase activities.

Takai et al. (116) have reported the purification of a cyclic GMP-dependent protein kinase from bovine cerebellum. The protein kinase was half-maximally activated by 1.7×10^{-8} M cyclic GMP or 1×10^{-6} M cyclic AMP. In addition, the purified cyclic GMP-dependent protein kinase could not activate muscle glycogen phosphorylase kinase further, suggesting that it was distinct from the cyclic AMP-dependent protein kinase.

Casnellie and Greengard (117) reported a cyclic GMP-dependent phosphorylation of an endogenous protein in a membrane fraction from mammalian smooth muscle by an endogenous protein kinase. A half-maximal increase in phosphorylation of the membrane protein was attained at 20–30 nM cyclic GMP, whereas approximately a 10-fold higher concentration of cyclic AMP was required. Since it has been suggested that the effects of cholinergic agonists on smooth muscle contractility are mediated by cyclic GMP, it is tempting to speculate about the functional significance of the cyclic GMP-dependent phosphorylation of the smooth muscle membrane protein. However, until the findings of Casnellie and Greengard (117) are corroborated and extended, such speculation would be premature. Johnson and Hadden (118) have reported that cyclic GMP added to suspensions of lymphocytes enhanced the phosphorylation of nuclear acidic proteins. Exogenous cyclic AMP or monobutyryl cyclic AMP was without effect. The differences in the effects of cyclic AMP and cyclic GMP were not due to alterations in the specific radioactivity of the ATP pool. Apparently, the effect of added cyclic GMP resulted from the activation of a cyclic GMP-dependent protein kinase. However, this was not demonstrated directly.

Gill and Kanstein (119) successfully separated a cyclic GMP receptor protein from a cyclic AMP receptor protein of bovine adrenal cortex. It was not determined whether the cyclic GMP binding activity was associated with a cyclic GMP-dependent protein kinase activity.

Even though there are reports of cyclic GMP-dependent protein kinases and altered phosphorylation patterns of specific proteins by added cyclic GMP, there is still no compelling evidence that changes in cellular responses associated with changes in cyclic GMP are caused by alterations in cyclic GMP-dependent phosphorylations. This by no means lessens the importance of these studies. The major problem in this area is the lack of a defined biochemical system analogous to the glycogen phosphorylase enzyme complex which is modulated by cyclic GMP. The systems described so far that are sensitive to cyclic GMP are complex multistep systems. The elucidation of these steps will be arduous but necessary if the role of cyclic GMP-mediated protein phosphorylation in these various systems is to be understood.

Regulation of Cell Proliferation

Many articles have appeared which suggest that cyclic AMP levels are lower in rapidly proliferating tissues (see refs. 17 and 31 for reviews). However, increased rates of proliferation are not always associated with lowered levels of cyclic AMP. It has been observed that cyclic GMP levels are elevated in some hepatomas (120, 121) as well as in psoriatic epidermis (122). Murad et al. (123) observed an elevation in the level of cyclic GMP in the urine of rats bearing Morris Hepatoma 3824A. The urinary level of cyclic GMP correlated well with increased tumor size, and the level of cyclic GMP in the urine fell after tumor removal or treatment with various antitumor agents such as 5-fluorouracil or irradiation.

Several mitogenic stimuli have been associated with elevated cyclic GMP levels. Hadden et al. (71) observed that concanavalin A and phytohemagglutinin caused a 10–50-fold increase in the level of cyclic GMP in lymphocytes. The effect was maximal by 20 min. Cyclic AMP was increased approximately 70% above control values during the same period. Seifert and Rudland (69, 70) reported that cyclic GMP levels in Balb/c 3T3 were increased maximally 10 min after addition of 20% serum and fresh medium to resting serum-starved cells. The serum-depleted cells were arrested in the G_1 phase of the cell cycle (94%) and behaved synchronously through subsequent phases of the cell cycle after the second addition of serum and fresh medium (70). Seifert and Rudland (70) reported that in synchronized cells the initial 10-min peak in cyclic GMP level was followed by a second peak 30–32 hr after the second addition of serum and fresh medium. Although fluctuations of cyclic GMP appeared restricted to G_0 and G_1, cyclic AMP levels fluctuated throughout the cell cycle. These data suggest that changes in cyclic GMP levels are restricted to a unique portion of the cell cycle. Moens et al. (124) also reported that serum addition to serum-starved fibroblasts resulted in elevated cyclic GMP.

Weinstein et al. (96) found that 8-bromocyclic GMP added to suspensions of splenic lymphocytes increased the incorporation of uridine and thymidine into RNA and DNA, respectively. However, the stimulation by cyclic GMP or cyclic GMP analogs was only 20% of that caused by concanavalin A. Dibutyryl cyclic AMP, which completely blocked the effects of concanavalin A on thymidine incorporation into DNA, had no effect on the stimulation caused by 8-bromo-cyclic GMP. Weinstein et al. (96) concluded that 8-bromocyclic GMP stimulated only a small subpopulation of the lymphocytes. Possibly the small stimulatory effect of cyclic GMP on nucleotide incorporation was unrelated to the action of concanavalin A. Kram and Tomkins (93) have reported that the inhibitory effect of dibutyryl cyclic AMP on uridine, leucine, and 2-deoxyglucose uptake by cultured 3T3 fibroblasts was prevented by cyclic GMP. Diamantstein and Ulmer (97) reported that cyclic GMP enhanced and cyclic AMP inhibited proliferation of B and T lymphocytes. It appears that cyclic GMP may very well be important in modulation of cell growth. However, far too few systems have been examined for any definitive statements. Future studies on the role of cyclic nucleotides in cell proliferation should also include studies on a possible role for calcium. It has been amply pointed out that calcium may be an important component of mitogenic signals (125–128).

It is difficult to assess the relative roles of cyclic AMP and cyclic GMP in the regulation of cell proliferation. The levels of both cyclic nucleotides appear to change under various growth conditions. It is not clear whether changes in one cyclic nucleotide are more important than changes in the other or whether the resulting changes in growth are a consequence of the coordinated change in the levels of both cyclic nucleotides. No doubt studies with synchronized cells are essential, but studies which simply measure cyclic nucleotide changes during the cell cycle or after changing the serum concentration are not enough. For example, agents which selectively modify the level of one cyclic nucleotide and not the other should be used.

CYCLIC AMP

Adenylate Cyclase Regulation

Activation by Cholera Toxin   Cholera is a dramatic and potentially fatal rise in intestinal fluid secretion due to an enterotoxin formed by *Vibrio cholerae*

(129). The molecular mechanism for this disease process involves activation of adenylate cyclase. The resulting rise in cyclic AMP increases fluid secretion to pathological levels. There are other toxins such as those produced by *Escherichia coli* which activate adenylate cyclase and cause diarrhea. Ordinarily, the action of cholera toxin is limited to the intestinal cells. However, cholera toxin will activate adenylate cyclase in other vertebrate cells after injection in vivo or addition to incubated cells.

The sequence of events in sensitive cells appears to involve an interaction of cholera toxin with the monosialo ganglioside GM_1 (galactosyl-*N*-acetylgalactosaminyl-(sialyl)-galactosyl-glucosylceramide) (130–132). The importance of specific gangliosides as receptors for cholera toxin was first recognized by Van Heyningen et al. (133). Van Heyningen (130) found that tetanus toxin also bound to gangliosides, but only to those with sialidase-sensitive bonds. In contrast, the ganglioside GM_1 which binds cholera toxin does not have sialidase-sensitive bonds.

Cuatrecasas (134) found that the sensitivity of fat cells to cholera toxin could be increased simply by incubating fat cells with gangliosides prior to addition of the toxin. Holmgren et al. (132) subsequently found that the amount of the ganglioside GM_1 present in mucosal cells from various species correlated with their ability to bind toxin. These data suggest that the cellular receptor which binds cholera toxin is probably ganglioside GM_1.

The cholera toxin molecule consists of two major proteins of 54,000 molecular weight (protein I) and 32,000 molecular weight (protein II). The larger molecular weight protein binds to the ganglioside and is composed of five subunits linked by noncovalent bonds (135).

There is little toxicity of either protein I or II alone in animals, but full toxicity can be obtained by recombination of the two proteins. However, Van Heyningen and King (136) and Gill and King (137) found that in pigeon erythrocyte lysates the protein II (small component) of cholera toxin was able to activate adenylate cyclase. This supports the hypothesis that the protein I component of cholera toxin is required for binding of the toxin to the cell surface receptors and for penetration of protein II, but is not required for activation of adenylate cyclase. The toxin binds rapidly, but there is a lag period at 37°C of about 15–60 min before adenylate cyclase is activated. The lag period varies with the cell type and apparently represents the time required for toxin to cross the cell membrane. The lag period is not seen when intact toxin or protein II is added to lysed cells (136–138).

The protein II component activated the adenylate cyclase of lysed cells only in the presence of a small molecular weight component in the cytosol (138, 139). Sattler and Wiegandt (135) found that mercaptoethanol could split the protein II to yield a 25,000 and a 7,000 molecular weight component. When intact cholera toxin was incubated with mercaptoethanol, only a 25,000 molecular weight component was released, which indicates that the smaller component links the 25,000 molecular weight component of protein II to protein I.

The sequence of events in cholera toxin action may involve a rapid binding of intact toxin to the ganglioside, slow transit of this complex through the plasma membrane, followed by dissociation of the 32,000 component from the ganglioside-55,000 molecular weight complex. The next step may be a reduction of the S-S bridges connecting the 7,000 to the 25,000 subunits of the 32,000 complex. The dissociation of the 32,000 component from the ganglioside-cholera toxin complex and/or reductive cleavage to release the 25,000 component may require the presence of unknown enzymes. Activation of adenylate cyclase appears to result from a tight binding of the 25,000 component of cholera toxin to the cyclase. Sahyoun and Cuatrecasas (141) found that there was substantial precipitation of solubilized adenylate cyclase from fat cell membrane particles by antisera against the "active" subunit after prior exposure of fat cells to toxin. Interestingly, there was substantial adenylate cyclase activity in the membrane particles precipitated by the double antibody procedure (138).

Bitensky et al. (139) have described a macromolecular cyclase-activating factor (MCAF) which is probably the reduced 25,000 component of cholera toxin. Activation of adenylate cyclase by the 25,000 component of cholera toxin has been demonstrated only in ascites cancer cell membrane fragments (139). Why membrane preparations from various mouse tissues which respond to the cholera toxin in vivo fail to respond to the 25,000 component is not known.

A mobile receptor hypothesis has been postulated to explain cholera toxin action (140). This hypothesis is based on assumptions which are plausible but unproven. The theory postulates that the toxin-ganglioside diffuses laterally within the plane of the membrane until it reacts with adenylate cyclase. Whether lateral diffusion of toxin-receptor complexes occurs or is even necessary remains to be established. The best evidence against this hypothesis comes from the work of Craig and Cuatrecasas (142). They found that inhibitors of lymphocyte capping, a phenomenon supposedly involving lateral mobility, were rather ineffective as inhibitors of adenylate cyclase activation due to cholera toxin (142).

Flores and Sharp (143) have suggested that cholera toxin activates adenylate cyclase at the same site as GTP or its nonhydrolyzable analog guanylylimido-phosphate (Gpp(NH)p). Rodbell et al. (144) demonstrated that under appropriate conditions GTP enhanced the stimulation of adenylate cyclase by hormones as well as basal activity. Subsequently, the Gpp(NH)p analog, which mimics the effects of GTP, activated adenylate cyclase by an irreversible process (145). Flores and Sharp (143) pointed out that cholera toxin and Gpp(NH)p are irreversible activators and the activated adenylate cyclase can be solubilized with retention of activity. They found that in liver homogenates the addition of cholera toxin blocked activation by Gpp(NH)p and vice versa (143). Pfeuffer and Helmreich (146) found a guanyl nucleotide-binding protein which they suggested might regulate adenylate cyclase. Possibly the interaction of cholera toxin with the guanyl nucleotide-binding protein is involved in its activation of adenylate cyclase.

Super- and Subsensitivity It has been recognized for some time that repetitive stimulation of a nerve decreased the sensitivity of the end organ to the relevant neurotransmitter. On the other hand, denervation leads to an increased sensitivity to neurotransmitters. Trendelenburg (147) has reviewed some of the pre- and postganglionic changes in sensitivity, which have been termed sub- and supersensitivity.

The phenomena of super- and subsensitivity have also been used to describe alterations in the response of cyclic nucleotides to hormones. Subsensitivity is defined under these conditions as a condition in which the normal rise in cyclic nucleotide due to a hormone is markedly reduced. Supersensitivity is defined as a condition in which the elevation of tissue cyclic nucleotide by hormones is greatly exaggerated. The mechanisms underlying these alterations could be at the level of phosphodiesterase, adenylate cyclase, hormone receptor, or at the level of coupling between hormone receptor and adenylate cyclase. In several tissues, cyclic AMP levels increase and then decline even in the continued presence of agonist (148–157). The level of cyclic AMP was unresponsive to the second addition of agonist. In some cases, there is evidence that a soluble inhibitory factor is formed during the first increase in cyclic AMP level (150). The inhibitory factor is released into the incubation medium and inhibits cyclic AMP accumulation when added to fresh tissue preparations.

Soluble feedback regulators of adenylate cyclase are discussed in later sections. This phenomenon is mentioned here to indicate that it could be an explanation for altered tissue sensitivity to hormones. Increased levels of the soluble inhibitor would be associated with subsensitivity, and, conversely, decreased levels of the inhibitor would be associated with supersensitivity. It should be apparent that this type of inhibitor would not be agonist-specific since it appears to be linked to increased cyclic AMP (150).

Another type of altered sensitivity has been demonstrated in a number of cell types and is agonist-specific. Clark et al. (158) reported that treatment of a subclone of a human astrocytoma cell line with catecholamines led to a decreased sensitivity to restimulation by catecholamines but not prostaglandins. Agonist-specific desensitization also has been reported for macrophages (159), lung fibroblasts (157, 160), thymocytes (161), and frog erythrocytes (162). Although the decreased sensitivity reported by Clark et al. (158) was agonist-specific, it was not associated with a change in the adenylate cyclase or phosphodiesterase activity detectable in whole homogenates. On the other hand, specific desensitization to agonists in macrophages, thymocytes, and frog erythrocytes is detectable in broken cell preparations at the level of adenylate cyclase. Agonist-specific subsensitivity of adenylate cyclase is probably not due to alterations in intracellular guanine nucleotides (163). Changes in receptor number, receptor accessibility, or coupling mechanism between hormone receptor and adenylate cyclase are more likely as sites of modification.

Recently, Mickey et al. (162) and Mukherjee et al. (164) reported that agonist-specific desensitization of frog erythrocyte adenylate cyclase to isoproterenol was associated with a decrease in the number of specific β-adrenergic receptors as determined from [^{3}H] alprenolol binding. The decrease in catecholamine receptors is analogous to the decrease seen in the number of cholinergic receptors in muscle tissue after chronic administration of acetylcholine (165). Similarly, hyperinsulinemia is associated with a decrease in the number of insulin receptors (166). Modulation of receptor number by a given agonist may be a general phenomenon. How this modulation is achieved is not known. It is known that it is very rapid and probably not linked to the level of cyclic AMP. Agonist-specific desensitization to agents which all elevate cyclic AMP cannot be mediated through a cyclic AMP-dependent mechanism.

DeVellis and Brooker (167) reported that in the Sb subclone of RGC6 rat glioma cells a second addition of catecholamine did not increase cyclic AMP. This was associated with a decreased sensitivity to catecholamines of adenylate cyclase in broken cell preparations. DeVellis and Brooker (167) also reported that the loss of catecholamine sensitivity was prevented by inhibitors of protein and RNA synthesis. This finding suggests that a protein which turns over rapidly is essential for development of catecholamine insensitivity in cultured glioma cells. The protein could be an inhibitor of adenylate cyclase.

The foregoing examples of decreased sensitivity to agonists were discussed only in terms of altered receptors, adenylate cyclase or cyclic AMP. Obviously, these are only the initial steps in the continuum between hormone action at the cell surface and the physiological response elicited by the hormone.

Axelrod's laboratory (168, 169) has reported both super- and subsensitivity in the rat pineal. Under conditions of increased catecholamine concentration (i.e., constant darkness, injection or addition of catecholamines), there was a decrease in the sensitivity of the pineals to catecholamine both in terms of cyclic AMP and N-acetyltransferase activities. Conditions of lowered catecholamine concentration (i.e., constant light, denervation, or reserpine treatment) potentiated the elevation of both cyclic AMP and N-acetyltransferase levels seen after the addition of low concentrations of catecholamines. These alterations in sensitivity were observed in both in vitro and in vivo experiments. Treatment with catecholamines also modified the inducibility of N-acetyltransferase by exogenous dibutyryl cyclic AMP.

It is apparent that super- and subsensitivity are seen in a wide variety of tissues, and explanations may be as diverse as the tissues involved. Efforts to explain these phenomena will clearly be one of the more important areas for investigation in the future.

Regulation of Adenylate Cyclase by Free Fatty Acids   Long chain fatty acids inhibit rat fat cell adenylate cyclase activity (170,171) but not rat liver adenylate cyclase (172). Marked inhibition of rat fat cell adenylate cyclase occurred as the ratio of fatty acid to albumin was increased from 2 to 6 (170,171). Inhibition of fat cell adenylate cyclase by sodium lauryl sulfate was not seen until the molar ratio of detergent to albumin exceeded 10 (172).

The inhibition of fat cell adenylate cyclase by fatty acid to albumin molar ratios above 2–3 can account for most of the feedback regulation of cyclic AMP accumulation seen when fat cells are incubated with lipolytic agents. Burns et al. (173) first pointed out that the addition of oleate to human fat cells mimicked the inhibition of adenylate cyclase seen with the use of medium which had previously been incubated with fat cells in the presence of lipolytic agents. Fain and Shepherd (170) found similar results with rat fat cells. Triglyceride lipase is also inhibited by fatty acid to albumin molar ratios above 2–3 (171). Since lipolysis virtually ceases after the primary sites on medium albumin are saturated with fatty acids, it is not surprising that adenylate cyclase is also inhibited.

Ho et al. (150, 174, 175) have described a feedback regulator of adenylate cyclase which is released to the medium during incubation of fat cells with lipolytic agents. Like fatty acids, the feedback regulator is bound to albumin and is both heat-stable and nondialyzable. The regulator was extracted from albumin with lipid solvents and purified by chromatography on Sephadex LH-20. Ho et al. (174) claimed, without presenting data, that the feedback regulator could be separated on Sephadex LH-20 columns from fatty acids, prostaglandins, phospholipids, and triglycerides. We prefer to think that their feedback regulator is either free fatty acids or products derived from free fatty acids during the procedures used to prepare the feedback regulator. Fain and Shepherd (170) found that extensive dialysis of albumin containing fatty acids against distilled water followed by lyophilization resulted in appearance of a potent inhibitor of adenylate cyclase. It was not necessary to incubate the buffer containing albumin with fat cells in order to obtain this inhibitor. Ho et al. (174) used albumin for incubation from which all fatty acids had been extracted. Under these conditions, the inhibitory effect on adenylate cyclase only appeared if fat cells had been incubated with lipolytic agents such as hormones or dibutyryl 3':5'-AMP. The possibility that the feedback regulator of Ho et al. (174) is a derivative of fatty acids rather than fatty acids themselves is supported by their report that the inhibitor was destroyed by incubation for 10 s at pH 1 (175).

Free fatty acids do not affect the activity of rat liver adenylate cyclase. The addition of 4 mM oleate to lysed rat liver cells (4 mg of protein/ml) did not affect basal adenylate cyclase activity or the increases due to norepinephrine, glucagon, or fluoride (172). Under identical conditions, 1 mM sodium lauryl sulfate (SDS) did inhibit adenylate cyclase (172).

Orly and Schramm (176) have shown that certain unsaturated fatty acids markedly enhanced the activation of turkey erythrocyte membrane adenylate cyclase by isoproterenol. Saturated long chain fatty acids such as palmitate or stearate were without effect if added as the free acids dissolved in ethanol. Linoleic acid was less active in potentiating adenylate cyclase activation by isoproterenol, whereas palmitoleic, oleic, and cis-vaccenic were the most active fatty acids. There was no correlation between the melting point and activation of adenylate cyclase by the various fatty acids. The effects of all fatty acids were more pronounced at 20° than at 37°.

These results indicate that fatty acids have marked effects on adenylate cyclase activity of various tissues. Adenylate cyclase activity is either enhanced or inhibited by long chain fatty acids depending upon the tissue.

Solubilization of Adenylate Cyclase and Role of Lipids in Hormone Action Sutherland et al. (177) first reported in 1962 that adenylate cyclase from bovine brain could be partially solubilized with detergents. The solubilized adenylate cyclase was activated by fluoride but not by hormones. It was postulated that adenylate cyclase was a membrane-bound enzyme dependent upon membrane lipids for activity.

Levey (178,179) used Lubrol detergents to solubilize adenylate cyclase from heart muscle. The solubilized adenylate cyclase had a molecular weight of about 160,000. After removal of the Lubrol, the enzyme was responsive to hormones in the presence of specific phospholipids. Although the addition of phosphatidylinositol restored the catecholamine-responsive activity, other phospholipids such as phosphatidylethanolamine, sphingomyelin, phosphatidylcholine, and cardiolipin were ineffective. The solubilized heart preparation bound glucagon. However, the hormone was not bound to adenylate cyclase but to a smaller protein in the solubilizing preparation since electrophoresis in the presence of sodium lauryl sulfate showed that glucagon was bound to a protein fraction with a molecular weight of 24,000–28,000.

Queener et al. (180) solubilized calcitonin-responsive adenylate cyclase activity from pork renal cortex membranes by the use of Lubrol-PX detergent. The calcitonin-responsive cyclase activity was still present in a high molecular weight complex which was excluded from Sephadex G-200 columns. Sensitivity to calcitonin was dependent upon the presence of fluoride and dithiothreitol, which acted in part by preventing dissociation or degradation of adenylate cyclase activity into inactive species with molecular weights between 100,000 and 200,000. The small molecular weight adenylate cyclase responded to fluoride but not to hormones and also failed to bind calcitonin. The findings can best be explained by the hypothesis that the native adenylate cyclase complex consists of a hormone receptor, enzyme catalytic subunit, and lipid which acts as a coupler between the hormone receptor and the adenylate cyclase. However, thus far only Levey has been successful in reconstituting hormonally responsive adenylate cyclase activity from a binding fraction and a catalytic fraction by the use of lipids or lipoproteins.

If specific phospholipids are required for the stimulation of adenylate cyclase by a given hormone, the sensitivity of a tissue to that hormone might be modulated by changing the concentration of the phospholipid. A variety of hormones alter the turnover of phospholipids in their target tissues (181–183). For example, cholinergic agonists elevate phosphatidylinositol turnover in a number of tissues (181,184). In some of these tissues, cholinergic agonists inhibit the increased accumulation of cyclic AMP caused by β-adrenergic agonists (53,185). If phosphatidylinositol is required for β-adrenergic activation of adenylate cyclase as suggested by Levey (178) for cardiac muscle, then cholinergic agonists might inhibit β-adrenergic stimulation of adenylate cyclase by altering phosphatidylinositol levels.

This type of model could be extended to include any agent which alters the sensitivity of adenylate cyclase to hormones. For example, α-adrenergic agonists

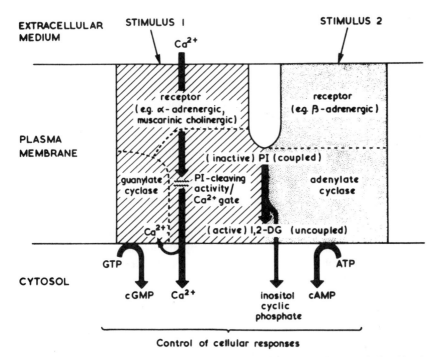

Control of cellular responses

Figure 2. A speculative model which attempts to indicate possible interrelationships between phosphatidylinositol breakdown and agonist-receptor interaction at the plasma membrane. Reprinted from Michell (189) with permission of Elsevier-North Holland Biomedical Press. Abbreviations: PI, phosphatidylinositol; 1,2-DG, 1,2-diacyglycerol. *Stimulus 1* and *stimulus 2* refer to a number of stimuli which might alter the rates of the reactions listed under each stimulus. Examples for each stimulus are given beneath the receptor.

block increases in the levels of cyclic AMP caused by β-adrenergic agonists in a variety of tissues (67,185,186). In many of these tissues, α-adrenergic agonists also affect phospholipid turnover (187,188).

Michell (189) proposed a role for phosphatidylinositol in regulating hormone action at the membrane receptor level and some of the breakdown products of phosphatidylinositol at an intracellular site. Figure 2 is Michell's speculative model which indicates some possible points of interaction between phosphatidylinositol or its metabolites and hormones. According to this model, increased turnover of phosphatidylinositol caused by *stimulus 1* inhibits the action of *stimulus 2* on adenylate cyclase. In addition, breakdown of phosphatidylinositol might increase the concentration of free calcium by freeing the calcium bound to membrane phosphatidylinositol. The increased concentration of free calcium could elevate guanylate cyclase or modify the activity of other calcium-sensitive steps. Another consequence of phosphatidylinositol breakdown could be an increased level of inositol 1,2-cyclic phosphate, inositol 1-phosphate, or inositol 2-phosphate.

These inositol phosphates might serve a role analogous to cyclic AMP in mediating the intracellular action of hormones. Exogenous inositol phosphate might be ineffective unless a critical level of cyclic GMP or cyclic AMP was also attained. This would make it very difficult to detect effects of any of the exogenously added inositol phosphates.

Regulation by Adenosine Sattin and Rall (190) reported that adenosine increased both basal cyclic AMP accumulation by slices of guinea pig brain and accumulation due to catecholamines and histamine. They suggested that the rise in cyclic AMP seen during electrical stimulation of brain slices was due to adenosine release. A striking difference between adenosine and other activators of cyclic AMP accumulation was that theophylline blocked the elevation in cyclic AMP due to adenosine (190). This suggested that theophylline might inhibit the uptake of adenosine by brain slices. However, 1 mM theophylline only blocked adenosine uptake by 25% under conditions in which cyclic AMP accumulation was markedly decreased (191). Future studies should be performed under conditions in which adenosine binding to receptors not involved in adenylate cyclase activation is minimized. Dipyridamole blocked the incorporation of adenosine into ATP but potentiated the stimulatory effect of adenosine on brain cyclic AMP (191).

The antagonism of adenosine-induced cyclic AMP accumulation in brain slices by theophylline or other methylxanthines may be unrelated to their inhibitory effects on cyclic AMP-phosphodiesterase. Dipyridamole and papaverine are potent inhibitors of cyclic AMP-phosphodiesterase, but they enhanced rather than inhibited adenosine action on brain slices (191). Similar results were seen in cultured mouse neuroblastoma cells in which adenosine-stimulated cyclic AMP accumulation and theophylline antagonized this rise (192). However, Blume et al. (192) found that the adenosine-induced increase in cyclic AMP was potentiated by the cyclic AMP-phosphodiesterase inhibitor 4-(3-butoxy-4-methoxybenzyl)-2-imidazolidinone.

Brain slices differ from many other tissues in that cyclic AMP accumulation can be increased by either an α- or a β-adrenergic mechanism (193). However, only α-adrenergic stimulation in brain slices is potentiated by adenosine (193).

Apparently, the increase in cyclic AMP produced by depolarizing agents such as veratridine, ouabain, high K^+, or electrical stimulation is secondary to adenosine release (194). This is supported by the finding that the addition of adenosine deaminase to the medium blocked the increase in cyclic AMP due to all of the agents except ouabain (194). The ouabain effect was blocked by theophylline, as was that of veratridine. It is not clear why adenosine deaminase failed to reverse the effects of ouabain.

In blood platelets, adenosine has also been shown to elevate cyclic AMP accumulation and to inhibit platelet aggregation (195). In platelets, as in brain slices, inhibition of adenosine uptake by papaverine or dipyridamole potentiated the stimulation of cyclic AMP accumulation by adenosine.

Adenosine stimulates adenylate cyclase in preparations from mouse neuroblastoma (196). The activation of adenylate cyclase by adenosine or 2-chloroadenosine, but not that due to prostaglandin E_1, was inhibited by theophylline

(196). The rise in cyclic AMP due to adenosine probably results from direct stimulation of adenylate cyclase via a process which is blocked by methyl-xanthines.

Fain et al. (197) reported that adenosine was a potent inhibitor of cyclic AMP accumulation and lipolysis by rat fat cells. Adenosine inhibited cate-cholamine-activated adenylate cyclase of fat cell ghosts by about 22% at a concentration of 73 μM (197). In contrast, 2',5'-dideoxyadenosine inhibited adenylate cyclase by 50% at a concentration of only 5 μM, whereas N^6-(phenyl-isopropyl)adenosine was inactive in inhibiting adenylate cyclase even at a con-centration of 73 μM (198). However, as little as 0.05 μM N^6-(phenyliso-propyl)adenosine inhibited cyclic AMP accumulation by 50% in intact cells, whereas 2 μM 2':5'-dideoxyadenosine gave only a 30% inhibition of cyclic AMP accumulation (198). These data suggest that the mechanism by which adenosine inhibits cyclic AMP accumulation in intact cells is different from that for adenylate cyclase inhibition in fat cell ghosts. This conclusion was based on the differences between the effects of N^6-(phenylisopropyl)adenosine and 2':5'-dideoxyadenosine and the finding that the amount of adenosine required to inhibit adenylate cyclase activity of fat cell ghosts by 50% was about 500–1,000 times greater than that required to reduce cyclic AMP accumulation in intact cells. The mechanism by which adenosine inhibits cyclic AMP ac-cumulation in intact fat cells is not known but is similar to that for nicotinic acid and prostaglandins of the E series in that none of these agents work in the available cell-free systems (33).

Relationship of Intracellular Cyclic AMP Concentration and Activation of Protein Kinase

Several investigators have reported that intracellular concentrations of cyclic AMP would approach 10^{-6} M. On the basis of these observations, it appeared that the basal intracellular level of cyclic AMP was sufficient to maintain protein kinase in a fully activated state. However, basal protein kinase activity in vivo was low, and there was a good correlation between increases in intracellular cyclic AMP concentrations and protein kinase activity (199,200). One possible explanation for this apparent paradox is that the protein kinase and cyclic AMP are sequestered in separate pools. The work from Steiner's laboratory with the use of immunocytochemical localization techniques to demonstrate unique and discrete cellular binding sites for both cyclic AMP and cyclic GMP reinforced the concept of cyclic nucleotide pools (201,202). The relationship between the cyclic nucleotide pools, demonstrable by immunocytochemical techniques, and the localization of protein kinase is not yet known.

Recently, three independent reports suggested that the concentration of cyclic AMP required to produce half-maximal activation of the protein kinase is not a constant (18, 203, 204). Actually, the concentration of cyclic AMP required for half-maximal activation of protein kinase is a function of protein kinase concentration. For example, Beavo et al. (204) showed that the amount of cyclic AMP required for half-maximal activation of 9 nM protein kinase was 300 nM cyclic AMP, whereas if the kinase concentration was increased to 150 nM the amount of cyclic AMP required was 1,500 nM. Since muscle tissue levels of protein kinase approach 150 nM and basal cyclic AMP levels are about 250 nM, there would be only about 20% activation of the kinase (204). The presence of the heat-stable protein kinase inhibitor would act to reduce the effect of basal cyclic AMP levels on protein kinase activation.

Since the concentrations of cyclic AMP (under basal conditions) and protein kinase are nearly equal, a large portion of cyclic AMP would be bound to the protein kinase (204). Cyclic AMP bound to protein kinase is not hydrolyzed by cyclic AMP-phosphodiesterase, at least in muscle (205). Therefore, agents which alter the equilibrium between free cyclic AMP and cyclic AMP bound to protein kinase might alter the concentration of cyclic AMP by making it more or less available to the phosphodiesterase. Several hormones elicit maximal or near maximal responses from their respective target cells without detectable increases in cyclic AMP. It is possible that these hormones act to alter the equilibrium between cyclic AMP, protein kinase, and the heat-stable inhibitor of protein kinase such that there is an elevated kinase activity without a detectable change in the total cyclic AMP concentration. Haddox et al. (206) and Beavo et al. (204) found that 4 mM Mg-ATP increased the K_d for cyclic AMP binding to skeletal muscle protein kinase. Apparently, the kinetic constants for cyclic AMP binding or activation of protein kinase activity can be altered in several ways. These observations might explain the apparent discrepancy between the amounts of cyclic AMP required for in vitro versus in vivo activation of protein kinase.

Relationship of Total Cyclic AMP Levels to Hormone Action

Sutherland and his associates (4) originally suggested four criteria which should be satisfied before it is concluded that a particular effect of a hormone is mediated through cyclic AMP.

1. The hormone should stimulate adenylate cyclase in broken cell preparations. Hormones which are inactive should not stimulate adenylate cyclase.
2. Physiological levels of the hormone should produce an elevation of cyclic AMP which occurs before or concurrently with the physiological response. There should be a correlation between the ability of various hormones or hormone analogs to increase cyclic AMP and the particular response.
3. Methylxanthines should potentiate the hormone response.
4. Exogenous cyclic AMP or its analogs should mimic the effect of the hormone. We would add a fifth criterion as follows:
5. Cholera toxin should mimic the hormone effect after a lag period of 1–2 hr.

Recently there has been considerable discussion about the role of cyclic AMP in hormone action because of difficulties with criterion 2. For example, in heart, adrenal cortex, and fat cells, all the other criteria listed above are easily fulfilled. However, in all of these tissues a significant hormone effect can be seen on the particular metabolic parameter being measured under circumstances in which there is no rise in total cyclic AMP. Robison et al. (4) originally pointed out that the levels of cyclic AMP which are physiologically important are small in relationship to the changes which can occur under certain experimental conditions. In fact, there is now evidence that a hormone response which appears to involve cyclic AMP can occur without any detectable rise in total cyclic AMP. Namm et al. (207) and Shanfeld et al. (208) pointed out a lack of correlation between cyclic AMP and the inotropic response to catecholamines in the heart. Øye and Langslet (209) suggested that only a small part of total cyclic AMP in the heart is involved in the regulation of contraction by catecholamines. The results of Venter et al. (210) support this hypothesis since immobilized isoproterenol caused a significant positive inotropic response without any change in total cyclic AMP in isolated cat papillary muscles. This is hardly surprising since the immobilized isoproterenol interacted with less than 0.01% of the cell population (210). Cyclic AMP may increase in those few cells which are directly in contact with isoproterenol but not in the other cells to which the inotropic response is transmitted. Alternatively, the inotropic response to catecholamines could result from shifts in intracellular Ca^{2+} with cyclic AMP serving to amplify the action of Ca^{2+}.

There is an inotropic effect of catecholamines which is mediated through α receptors and does not involve cyclic AMP (211–213). Phenylephrine, which is predominantly a stimulator of α receptors, weakly stimulated cyclic AMP accumulation. However, in the presence of propranolol, the rise in cyclic AMP was blocked without any depression in the inotropic response (211).

Hepatic glycogenolysis is also stimulated by an α effect of phenylephrine which is not abolished by propranolol (Figure 3). Our conclusion is that there is an α effect of catecholamines on both hepatic glycogenolysis and cardiac contractility which may involved Ca^{2+}, and a β effect which is associated with cyclic AMP.

Beall and Sayers (214) found that in isolated adrenal cells low concentrations of ACTH stimulated steroidogenesis without affecting total cyclic AMP accumulation. More impressive were the data of Moyle et al. (215) who used an o-nitrophenylsulfenyl derivative of ACTH prepared by chemical modification of the single tryptophan residue. The derivative stimulated steroidogenesis, but was virtually ineffective in increasing cyclic AMP accumulation. Moyle et al. (215) postulated that either only very small increases in cyclic AMP are required for stimulation of steroidogenesis or there is some other factor beside cyclic AMP involved in ACTH action. Richardson and Schulster (216) found that low concentrations of ACTH gave a submaximal stimulation of steroidogenesis but did not increase protein kinase activity in isolated adrenal cells. Their results rule out the hypothesis that very small changes in cyclic AMP could lead to a magnified signal in terms of total protein kinase activity. However, it is difficult to be sure that changes in protein kinase activity of broken cell preparations reflected what was going on in the intact cell.

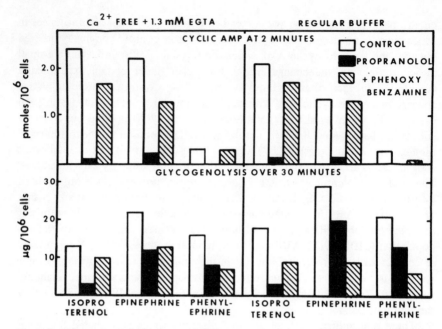

Figure 3. Effect of catecholamines and their antagonists on glycogenolysis and cyclic AMP accumulation. Liver cells (7×10^6 cells per tube) from normally fed rats were isolated as described by Pointer et al. (56) and incubated in regular Krebs-Ringer bicarbonate buffer (*right part* of figure) or in calcium-free buffer containing 1.3 mM EGTA (*left part* of figure). The cells were incubated with 1.5 μM epinephrine, 1.5 μM isoproterenol, or 20 μM phenylephrine either without (*open bars*) or with 10 μM 1-propranolol (*solid bars*) or with 10 μM phenoxybenzamine (*striped bars*). The values shown are the increments due to added catecholamines over basal values in the absence or presence of blocking drugs and are the means of seven paired experiments. (Pointer and Fain, unpublished experiments.)

Cholera toxin addition to isolated rat adrenal cells increased cyclic AMP accumulation at 40 min and steroidogenesis at 60 min (217,218). The ability of cholera toxin to mimic the action of ACTH after 60 min is impressive evidence that an increase in cyclic AMP can stimulate steroidogenesis. Calcium-free buffer abolished the stimulation of steroidogenesis by ACTH but inhibited cholera toxin action by only 66% (218).

Rubin et al. (219) suggested that ACTH acts by displacing Ca^{2+} bound to adenylate cyclase. This hypothesis is illustrated in Figure 4 and postulates that adenylate cyclase is linked to Ca^{2+} translocation. Possibly adenylate cyclase is present in an inhibited state due to bound Ca^{2+}, and activation of cyclase occurs by release from Ca^{2+} inhibition (Figure 4). Jaanus and Rubin (220) suggested that ACTH action on the adrenal was associated with a shift of Ca^{2+} from a rapidly exchanging to a more slowly exchanging cellular pool. Carchman et al. (221) showed that perfusion of cat adrenal glands with calcium-free buffer increased cyclic AMP by 3–6 fold but did not augment steroid release. In the absence of calcium, ACTH produced only a very small rise in cyclic AMP but

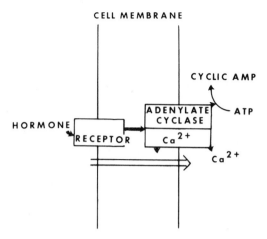

Figure 4. Model for coordinate activation of adenylate cyclase and Ca²⁺ influx based in part on the work of Rubin et al. (219).

markedly increased steroid release. The respiration-supported uptake of calcium stimulated pregnenalone formation by mitochondria isolated from rat adrenal glands (222). Further support for an elevation of cytosol Ca^{2+} by ACTH is the report that cyclic GMP is elevated by ACTH (73). These data are compatible with the hypothesis shown in Figure 4 that ACTH action on the adrenal involves both a rise in cytosol calcium and a rise in cyclic AMP.

The third system in which levels of cyclic AMP can be dissociated from hormone action is fat cells incubated with adenosine in the presence of lipolytic agents (198, 223, 224). Adenosine inhibits the lipolytic action of low concentrations of catecholamines. If the concentration of catecholamine is increased enough to detect a rise in cyclic AMP, addition of adenosine is not antilipolytic, but cyclic AMP accumulation is markedly inhibited (198, 223, 224). Ca^{2+} is probably not linked to adenylate cyclase activity in adipose tissue since extensive incubation of fat cells in calcium-free buffer containing 0.25 mM EGTA did not inhibit stimulation of lipolysis or cyclic AMP accumulation caused by norepinephrine (198). Similarly the inhibitory effect of adenosine on cyclic AMP accumulation in fat cells was not altered by the presence or absence of calcium (198).

There are still problems involved in understanding the details of the steps between cyclic AMP generation and the physiological responses caused by the hormones. In systems such as heart, adrenal cells, and fat cells, the bulk of the evidence indicates that cyclic AMP can mediate hormone action. Whether it is the sole factor remains to be established. Possibly, cyclic AMP is not the only signal generated by hormones. Activation of adenylate cyclase in the intact cell by hormone could result from or be linked to ion redistribution, as shown in Figure 4.

SELECTED ASPECTS OF HORMONE
ACTION INVOLVING CYCLIC NUCLEOTIDES

Hepatic Glucose Release

In fasting animals (including man), the main source of blood glucose is the liver (225). The glucose released by the liver comes primarily from breakdown of hepatic glycogen until stores are exhausted; then glucose is formed from amino acids and lactate by gluconeogenesis. The rate of glucose release by the liver appears to be regulated both by the level of blood glucose and the hormonal milieu (225). Insulin inhibits, whereas glucagon and catecholamines stimulate, glucose release. At the present time, there is a great emphasis on glucagon as the major stimulator of hepatic glucose release. However, there is evidence in man that norepinephrine released from sympathetic nerve endings is important under certain conditions (226).

The simple view that cyclic AMP alone mediates the regulation of hepatic glucose release by glucagon and catecholamines appears more untenable with the passage of time. Since there are marked species differences, the elucidation of the cyclic AMP story relied heavily on Sutherland and associates' choice of dog liver for most of their early work (227, 228). In dog liver preparations both glucagon and catecholamines increased adenylate cyclase activity, resulting in cyclic AMP activation of glycogen phosphorylase. However, in man and the rat there appear to be mechanisms which involve factors other than cyclic AMP by which hormones accelerate hepatic glucose release. This is particularly true with respect to catecholamine action.

On the basis of studies with perfused rat livers (154, 229, 230) and isolated liver cells (154, 231–234), it does not appear that cylic AMP mediates the stimulation of gluconeogenesis by catecholamines. In perfused rat livers epinephrine was able to stimulate gluconeogenesis, whereas isoproterenol was inactive (154). Furthermore, propranolol did not inhibit catecholamine-induced gluconeogenesis in perfused rat livers. Glucagon does elevate cyclic AMP and stimulate gluconeogenesis in rat liver cells (233). Dibutyryl cyclic AMP addition to liver cells at micromolar concentrations mimicked the effects of glucagon on gluconeogenesis (231, 233, 234). However, it remains unexplained why the rise in cyclic AMP due to isoproterenol does not stimulate gluconeogenesis (233,234).

There is substantial evidence that catecholamine-induced hepatic glycogenolysis in man (235–237) and rats (238, 239) is predominantly an α response which does not involve cyclic AMP. Isoproterenol (a predominantly β-adrenergic agonist) was relatively ineffective in activating hepatic glycogenolysis (238, 240) and glycogen phosphorylase in vivo (240) or in perfused rat livers (241). Isoproterenol was a much more potent activator of adenylate cyclase and cyclic AMP accumulation in rat liver (242) than epinephrine. The effects of isoproterenol on rat hepatic adenylate cyclase in vitro and on phosphorylase were effectively blocked by the β blocker propranolol (240). However, propranolol blocked the epinephrine-stimulated increases in rat adenylate cyclase and cyclic AMP release by perfused rat liver (241) but not the increase in hepatic phosphorylase in vivo (240) or in perfused liver (241). Phenylephrine, a predominantly α agonist, increased glycogen phosphorylase in perfused liver but did not stimulate cyclic AMP release or accumulation (241). Furthermore, the α-adrenergic antagonist phentolamine reduced the increase in phosphorylase activity, but not cyclic AMP accumulation (241), by epinephrine.

Shimazu and Amakawa (243) have shown that electrical stimulation of the splanchnic nerve (sympathetic innervation) of rabbits activated hepatic glycogenolysis. Intraportal injection of epinephrine or glucagon increased hepatic glycogenolysis and elevated cyclic AMP, glycogen phosphorylase, and liver dephosphophosphorylase kinase. In contrast, electrical stimulation also increased hepatic phosphorylase without affecting cyclic AMP or dephosphophosphorylase kinase (243). The increase in phosphorylase due to electrical stimulation was accompanied by a marked decrease in the activity of hepatic phosphorylase phosphatase (243). Epinephrine or glucagon did not affect the activity of hepatic phosphorylase phosphatase (243). Previously, it had been observed that cyclic AMP did not affect the activity of this enzyme in liver (244). The activation of glycogen phosphorylase due to splanchnic nerve stimulation was not inhibited by a β-adrenergic antagonist (243); under the same conditions, the activation due to catecholamine injection was blocked (245).

Edwards (246) has shown that the glycogenolytic effect of splanchnic nerve stimulation in dogs and cats depended upon the integrity of the hepatic innervation. Interestingly, the response to nerve stimulation was little affected by adrenalectomy of dogs or cats (246).

Studies on the catecholamine activation of glycogenolysis in isolated rat liver cells indicated that glycogenolysis is predominantly an α effect (229 and Figure 3). Exton and Harper (229) reported that isoproterenol was completely ineffective in stimulating glycogenolysis but was a good activator of cyclic AMP accumulation. Our results were more comparable to those seen in perfused rat livers (241) or in vivo (238, 239) since isoproterenol did activate glycogenolysis but epinephrine was considerably more effective (Figure 3).

The rise in cyclic AMP due to epinephrine was not required for its glycogenolytic action because it could be blocked by propranolol (a β blocker) without a sizeable inhibition of glycogenolysis. Phenoxybenzamine is an α blocker which markedly reduced glycogenolysis due to epinephrine without affecting cyclic AMP accumulation. These data (Figure 3) suggest that there are both α- and β-adrenergic mechanisms for the acceleration of glycogenolysis in rat liver.

Phenylephrine and epinephrine could increase glycogenolysis in the presence of propranolol if there were other factors besides cyclic AMP which were capable of increasing glycogen breakdown (Figure 3). An increase in intracellular Ca^{2+} possibly could activate glycogenolysis and potentiate the effects of cyclic

Table 5. Summary of effects of various agents on isolated rat liver cells[a]

Agent	Gluconeogenesis over 2 hr Starved rats	Glycogenolysis over 30 min[b]	Cyclic AMP[c] at 2 min	Cyclic GMP[d] at 2 min
A23187	Inhibited	Increased	No change	Increased
Insulin	No change	Inhibited	No change	Increased
Carbachol	No change	Decreased	Decreased	Increased
Epinephrine	Increased via alpha effect	Increased via alpha and beta effects	Increased	Greatly increased
Isoproterenol	No change	Increased via beta effect	Increased	Increased
Glucagon	Increased	Increased	Greatly increased	Increased

[a]The table is based on studies with isolated rat liver cells (56, 232–235).
[b]Only the increase in glycogenolysis due to A23187 was abolished in calcium-free buffer.
[c]The increases in cyclic AMP were unaffected in calcium-free buffer.
[d]Basal cyclic GMP was reduced by only 15% in calcium-free buffer while the increases due to A23187 and glucagon were inhibited by about 65% and those due to epinephrine and insulin by 85%.

AMP. Thus, a very large elevation of either cyclic AMP or Ca^{2+} alone could activate glycogenolysis. In the presence of epinephrine, both might be elevated.

Since it has been suggested that α effects of catecholamines are secondary to an elevation of cyclic GMP (14), we investigated the role of this nucleotide in glycogenolysis by rat liver cells (56). Our initial findings were in agreement with this hypothesis as epinephrine was a potent stimulator of cyclic GMP accumulation (56). However, as summarized in Table 5, a variety of other agents stimulated cyclic GMP accumulation in liver cells. Furthermore, insulin inhibited glycogenolysis, whereas carbachol had no effect, despite the finding that both elevated cyclic GMP. The conclusion from these studies was that alterations in cyclic GMP accumulation did not mediate the glycogenolytic effect of hormones.

Both isoproterenol and phenylephrine elevated cyclic GMP, but the rise due to these catecholamines was about half that due to epinephrine (56). The rise in cyclic GMP conformed to the criteria for an α effect in that the increase due to all catecholamines was blocked by phentolamine but not by propranolol (56).

A prominent role for extracellular calcium in mediating α stimulation of glycogenolysis appears unlikely. Extracellular Ca^{2+} is required for the rise in cyclic GMP in liver cells incubated with catecholamines (56). In contrast, in our hands the effects of omission of extracellular calcium (achieved by incubating cells in calcium-free buffer containing 1 mM concentration of the calcium chelator EGTA) on hepatic glycogenolysis or cyclic AMP accumulation have been unimpressive (Figure 3). The only agent which required calcium in the medium in order to stimulate glycogenolysis was the divalent cation ionophore A-23187 (56). Apparently the ionophore activated glycogenolysis by increasing calcium influx. The free cytosol concentration of calcium is less than 1 μM, whereas the extracellular calcium is usually above 1 mM. If glucagon or epinephrine acted by increasing cytosol calcium, they apparently caused the release of bound or sequestered calcium rather than increasing flux of calcium through the plasma membrane since both hormones were effective in calcium-free buffer.

Secretion by Parotid

The rat parotid gland secretes macromolecules (mostly α-amylase), water, and ions. The composition of the fluid released by the acinar cells is regulated by both the sympathetic and parasympathetic branches of the autonomic nervous system. Sympathetic stimulation increases the release of protein, fluid, and ions from the parotid, whereas parasympathetic stimulation produces primarily fluid and ion release. Sympathetic nerve stimulation increased both cyclic AMP and cyclic GMP in the rat parotid (J. P. Durham and F. R. Butcher, unpublished observations). Similarly, in vivo administration of adrenergic or cholinergic agonists increased the cyclic AMP or cyclic GMP (247) in the mouse parotid gland. Although it is possible to measure in vivo changes of cyclic nucleotides and a variety of physiological responses in the parotid gland after either neural stimulation or injection of test compounds, it is much easier to employ a slice or isolated cell preparation to investigate control by neurotransmitters in the parotid.

Bdolah and Schramm (248) first demonstrated that dibutyryl cyclic AMP increased α-amylase release. They suggested that the elevations of intracellular cyclic AMP mediated the increased α-amylase release due to adrenergic agonists. It has since been shown that adrenergic agonists increase the levels of cyclic AMP (247, 249–252) in the parotid. The elevations of cyclic AMP and α-amylase release have been classified as β_1-adrenergic responses (249). Although cyclic AMP most likely mediates the effects of β-adrenergic agents on α-amylase release, Butcher et al. (249) have shown that near maximal increases in α-amylase release can be attained even though cyclic AMP levels increased only 20% above basal values. This suggests that small increases in cyclic AMP are sufficient to cause maximal changes in α-amylase release. In vivo experiments by Durham et al. (247) suggested a similar relationship between alterations in parotid cyclic AMP levels and increased DNA synthesis. However, alterations in cyclic GMP levels may be more important than cyclic AMP in the control of DNA synthesis in the parotid (247).

It is possible that cyclic AMP is only one of the intracellular signals for increased α-amylase release caused by β-adrenergic agents. Selinger and Naim (253) have reported that intracellular calcium was required for α-amylase release caused by either β-adrenergic agonists or dibutyryl cyclic AMP. This suggests that both cyclic AMP and intracellular calcium are required for control of α-amylase release.

Calcium alone does not appear sufficient to provoke α-amylase release to the same degree as β-adrenergic agonists. Selinger et al. (254) and Butcher (81) have reported that the divalent cation ionophore A-23187 does not mimic the action of β-adrenergic agonists on α-amylase release. If alterations in intracellular calcium alone were sufficient to cause large increases in α-amylase release, then the ionophore should have mimicked the β-adrenergic agonists. The ionophore did not have deleterious effects on the parotid since isoproterenol was just as effective on α-amylase release in the presence, as in the absence, of the ionophore (254 and F. R. Butcher, unpublished observations).

Cyclic AMP does not seem to be required for increased α-amylase release from the exocrine pancreas (255–257). Acetylcholine and pancreozymin both cause α-amylase release, but neither agent increased cyclic AMP (255, 256). Furthermore, exogenous dibutyryl cyclic AMP did not cause α-amylase release from the exocrine pancreas (257). Calcium plays a key role in the control of enzyme release from the exocrine pancreas. The divalent cation ionophore A-23187 increased α-amylase release from exocrine pancreas to the same extent as acetylcholine or pancreozymin (258, 259).

In addition to its role in the release of α-amylase from the parotid, calcium is also required for maximal stimulation by β-adrenergic agents of adenylate cyclase in broken cell preparations (260) and for maximal increases in the level of cyclic AMP (261) in the parotid. The optimal concentration of calcium for stimulation of adenylate cyclase is low (10 μM), and high concentrations are actually inhibitory (260). Similar results have been observed with intact cells. Harfield and Tenenhouse (261) reported that removal of calcium from the incubation buffer and inclusion of EGTA blocked the increase of cyclic AMP in the parotid due to epinephrine. When EGTA was omitted from the calcium-free incubation buffer, there was a large rise in cyclic AMP due to epinephrine which was greater than that seen if slices were incubated in buffer containing 1.2 mM calcium. Modification of the buffer calcium concentrations did not affect α-amylase release due to β-adrenergic agonists (F. R. Butcher, unpublished observations).

The parotid also contains α-adrenergic (67, 250, 262, 263) and cholinergic receptors (181, 263, 264). Although the α-adrenergic and cholinergic receptors are distinct physical entities, the effects of both types of agonists on the parotid gland are very similar. As depicted in Figure 5, the predominant effect of cholinergic (carbachol) and α-adrenergic (phenylephrine) agonists is increased K^+ efflux (262–264). These two types of agonists also cause massive fluid release (265), but it is not possible to measure fluid release with the slice system. Neither phenylephrine nor carbachol increases the parotid levels of cyclic AMP. Both agonists inhibit the rise in parotid cyclic AMP caused by isoproterenol (67, 185) and increase cyclic GMP levels (see ref. 81 for summary table). It is not

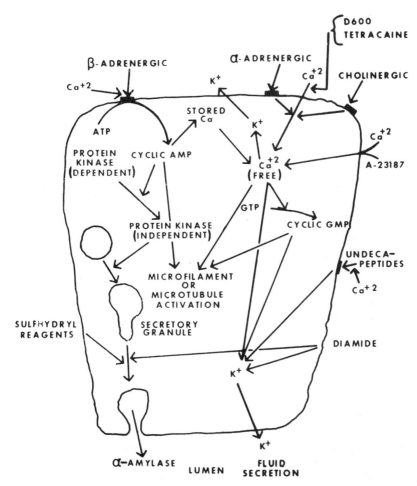

Figure 5. Diagrammatic representation of the effects of agonists on cyclic nucleotide levels, α-amylase release, and K^+ efflux with rat parotid acinar cells. Particularly important are the proposed roles of calcium. These effects should be studied with reference to Figure 1.

clear at this point whether or not the increases in cyclic GMP are responsible for increased K^+ efflux caused by cholinergic and α-adrenergic agonists. High concentrations (0.5–2.0 mM) of 8-bromocylic GMP cause increased K^+ efflux, but the amount of K^+ released was about one-third that observed with phenylephrine or carbachol (67).

The action of cholinergic and α-adrenergic agonists on K^+ efflux (263) and cyclic GMP (F. R. Butcher, unpublished observations) levels requires calcium in the incubation buffer. Consequently, it is possible, as suggested by Schramm and Selinger (263), that α-adrenergic and cholinergic agonists affect the parotid by increasing calcium influx. This argument is not only supported by the requirement for buffer calcium for agonist action, but also by the fact that the ionophore A-23187 effectively mimicked the effect of α-adrenergic and cholinergic agonists of K^+ efflux (254) and cyclic GMP levels in the parotid (81). The effect of the ionophore in both instances was calcium-dependent. The importance of calcium influx for the action of α-adrenergic and cholinergic agonists is also suggested by the observation that tetracaine and D-600 are competitive antagonists of cholinergic and α-adrenergic agonists on K^+ efflux (F. R. Butcher, unpublished observations). The relationship of cyclic GMP levels to increased K^+ efflux is not clear. It is possible that increased free intracellular calcium causes both increased K^+ efflux and cyclic GMP levels. Alternatively, it is possible to envision a sequential mechanism in which increases in free intracellular calcium cause a high level of cyclic GMP which in turn stimulates K^+ efflux.

The undecapeptides substance P and eledoisin mimic the effects of α-adrenergic and cholinergic agonists (266). Injection of either of the undecapeptides into intact animals caused copious saliva release (267, 268). In vitro the undecapeptides cause a calcium-dependent K^+ efflux which resembles the action of α-adrenergic and cholinergic agonists with respect to magnitude and time course (266). Since effects of the undecapeptides were not blocked by β-adrenergic, α-adrenergic, or cholinergic antagonists, their action appears pharmacologically distinct from the β-adrenergic, α-adrenergic, and cholinergic agonists. Unlike carbachol and phenylephrine, the undecapeptides do not increase parotid levels of cyclic GMP (266). This suggests that increased cyclic GMP levels might not be necessary for increased K^+ efflux.

Not all effects of α-adrenergic and cholinergic agonists on the parotid gland are calcium-dependent. Both α-adrenergic and cholinergic, but not β-adrenergic, agonists increase the rate of phosphoinositol turnover in the parotid (184, 187). The increases in phosphoinositol turnover were calcium-independent by the same criteria which established that the action of phenylephrine and carbachol on K^+ efflux and cyclic GMP levels was calcium-dependent.

As noted in Figure 5, diamide caused both α-amylase release and K^+ efflux whereas sulfhydryl reagents altered only α-amylase release (F. R. Butcher, unpublished observations). Since these reagents react fairly selectively with sulfhydryl groups, they have the potential of serving as fruitful probes into the mechanism of α-amylase release and K^+ efflux. The precise role of Ca^{2+} and cyclic nucleotides in regulation of parotid gland secretion remains to be established.

Opiates and Cyclic Nucleotides

The discovery of a link between cyclic nucleotides and morphine addiction has provided exciting clues to the biochemical basis of opiate action. The studies on opiate action have even led to isolation of the natural opiate receptor agonist in brain which may regulate pain and emotion.

There had been hints for several years that cyclic AMP metabolism was altered by morphine, but the data were unconvincing until Collier and Roy (269) reported in March, 1974, that morphine inhibited the prostaglandin E_1 - or

E_2-induced rise in cyclic AMP in rat brain homogenates. Furthermore, they demonstrated that heroin was more and methadone less active than morphine. Dextrophan was inactive. The effect of morphine was antagonized by naloxone (269). Collier and Roy (270) suggested that morphine analgesia was due to inhibition of adenylate cyclase activation by endogenous prostaglandins.

Morphine and other opiates act at the same receptors as a natural pentapeptide to inhibit adenylate cyclase. At least three laboratories have reported the existence of such a factor in brain extracts (271–274). Hughes et al. (272) have called this substance enkephalin and have shown that it is composed of the two pentapeptides H-Tyr-Gly-Gly-Phe-Met-OH and H-Tyr-Gly-Gly-Phe-Leu-OH (275).

The neuroblastoma X glioma hybrid cell line is a useful model system to study morphine action (78, 276–278). In cells cultured for 4 days in the presence of morphine, the basal level of cyclic AMP was the same as in the control cells. However, the rise in cyclic AMP due to prostaglandins of the E type or adenosine, although still appreciable in addicted cells, was about half that seen in control cells (277). In contrast, naloxone, a potent morphine antagonist, had little effect on control cells but increased by 300–500% of normal the rise in cyclic AMP due to concurrent addition of prostaglandins or adenosine to addicted cells (277). This suggests that opiates bind tightly to some factor which regulates adenylate cyclase activity, and when they are displaced from this factor by opiate antagonists there is a massive overproduction of cyclic AMP.

Several groups have sought unsuccessfully to find changes in opiate binding to receptors in addicted animals (277, 279). In the addicted state, the biochemical alterations are apparently not at the receptor level but at some subsequent step.

What is the mechanism by which opiates inhibit the stimulation by prostaglandins or other activators of adenylate cyclase of cyclic AMP accumulation? Most workers have suggested that cylic AMP is involved (269, 270, 276, 277), but Gullis et al. (78) have implicated cyclic GMP. Gullis et al. (78) claimed that the addition of low concentrations of morphine to a neuroblastoma X glioma hybrid cell line elevated cyclic GMP and lowered cyclic AMP. Acetylcholine and norepinephrine also elevated cyclic GMP in the hybrid cells and antagonized the stimulation of cyclic AMP accumulation due to prostaglandins (78) (see footnote 1).

The elevation of cyclic GMP due to many agents appears to be secondary to an elevation of intracellular Ca^{2+} (23). Possibly carbamylcholine, catecholamines, and morphine increase cytosol Ca^{2+}-dependent factors which regu-

---

[1] The increases in cyclic GMP reported by Gullis et al. (ref. 78) in neuroblastoma and neuroblastoma X glioma hybrid cells now turn out to have been invented by Gullis. In an unusual statement which appeared in *Nature*, vol. 265, p. 764 (1977) Gullis admits that he invented the results of all his experiments on cyclic GMP in neuroblastoma cells.

late both adenylate cyclase and cyclic AMP-phosphodiesterase activities of brain (280, 281). However, another group of investigators (M. Nirenberg, personal communication) was unable to confirm the report that cyclic GMP was elevated in neuroblastoma X glioma hybrid cell lines and also observed no effect of Ca^{2+} on the inhibition of adenylate cyclase by opiates.

Cardenas and Ross (282) were able to show a marked decrease in total brain calcium after a single dose of morphine. The effect of morphine was blocked by naloxone and was stereospecific (282). Pretreatment of rats with morphine 1 or 3 days earlier inhibited the calcium-depleting effects of morphine (283). These results are more in line with the hypothesis that inhibition of adenylate cyclase and the subsequent reduction in tissue cyclic AMP by morphine might result in increased release of calcium from intracellular organelles. This might temporarily elevate cytosol calcium and result in net efflux of calcium from the cells in the presence of morphine.

Morphine directly inhibits adenylate cyclase activity of cell-free homogenates (276). This weak inhibitory effect of morphine on adenylate cyclase activity in a purified membrane fraction might be due to the loss of opiate-binding proteins (276). Interestingly, Gpp(NH)p, which is a stable analog of GTP, could reverse the inhibition of adenylate cyclase activity due to morphine (276).

Some of the confusion about the effects of opiates on cyclic nucleotide metabolism comes from their apparent activity as weak agonists. This is particularly true at high concentrations since Gullis et al. (78) found that 0.1 or 1 mM morphine elevated cyclic AMP and lowered cyclic GMP in a neuroblastoma X glioma hybrid cell line.

In addicted animals, the administration of a morphine antagonist should result in hyperactivity of adenylate cyclase, leading to excess accumulation of cyclic AMP. If this is the case, inhibitors of cyclic AMP-phosphodiesterase activity might potentiate the withdrawal symptoms seen after the administration of opiate antagonists. Theophylline administration has been shown to do this (284–286). Naloxone precipitated a quasi-morphine abstinence syndrome in rats which had never been given opiates if the potent phosphodiesterase inhibitor 1-methyl-3-isobutylxanthine was administered subcutaneously 1 hr prior to naloxone (284). Naloxone presumably antagonized enkephalin action in naive rats which resulted in an increased adenylate cyclase activity.

The intracerebroventricular injection of cyclic AMP also produced withdrawal symptoms in animals. Dibutyryl cyclic 3′:5′-AMP was less effective than cyclic AMP (285). Even intravenous injection of 10 mg/kg of cyclic 3′:5′-AMP into mice enhanced tolerance and dependence development (285). Administration of cyclic 2′:3′-AMP or cyclic 3′:5′-GMP was ineffective, but no controls with the use of 5′-AMP or adenosine were run (285). The possibility that the effect of cyclic AMP was due to the latter must be considered since adenosine could raise cyclic AMP by activation of adenylate cyclase.

Morphine effects on cyclic nucleotide metabolism are not restricted to the central nervous system. Low concentrations of morphine (3–30 μM) antagonized the ability of prostaglandin E_1 to inhibit epinephrine-induced aggregation of human platelets (287). However, morphine at a concentration of 133 μM actually enhanced the effect of prostaglandin E_1 on platelet aggregation (287). Thomas et al. (288) reported that the basal cyclic AMP concentration in mouse prostate glands was markedly elevated by prior treatment with morphine or the addition of 20 μM morphine in vitro. The acute administration of morphine to rats lowered the plasma free fatty acids (FFA) values in normal rats, had no effect in rats treated chronically with morphine, but elevated plasma FFA in addicted rats from which morphine had been withheld for 4 days (abstinent rats) (289). Interestingly, injection of the morphine antagonist nalorphine doubled the plasma FFA 1 hr following its administration (289). In isolated rat liver cells, the rise in cyclic AMP seen 1 or 2 min after the addition of glucagon was reduced about 23% by the concomitant presence of 0.1 μM morphine and 42% by 0. 33μM morphine (J N. Fain, unpublished results). The basal level of cyclic AMP was unaffected by 0.1 or 0.33 μM morphine but was reduced 45% by 1 μM morphine. These results indicate that opiates, like methylxanthines, affect cyclic nucleotide metabolism in a variety of cells outside the central nervous sytem at concentrations higher than those which affect the central nervous system. However, except at toxic levels of these drugs, the major effects of opiates and of methylxanthines are on the central nervous system in man.

Opiates and opiate antagonists clearly affect adenylate cyclase activity in morphine-sensitive neurons. Whether the endogenous stimulator of adenylate cyclase is adenosine, prostaglandin E_1, or some other substance in these neurons is not clear (290). Opiates appear to act as tight-binding but reversible inhibitors which react with the enkephalin receptors to inactivate adenylate cyclase. Opiate dependency appears to arise through a "biochemical hypertrophy" of proteins which regulate adenylate cyclase activity. Marked elevations in cyclic AMP occur when the balance between association and dissociation of opiates with this regulatory protein is altered by opiate antagonists or discontinuation of opiate administration.

REFERENCES

1. Drummond, G. I., Greengard, P., and Robison, G. A. (eds.) (1975). Adv. Cyclic Nucleotide Res. 5:1–872.
2. Weiss, B. (ed.) (1975). Cyclic Nucleotides in Disease. University Park Press, Baltimore.
3. Fain, J. N. (ed.) (1975). Metabolism 24:1–221.
4. Robison, G. A., Butcher, R. W., and Sutherland, E. W. (1971). Cyclic AMP. Academic Press, New York.
5. Perkins, J. P. (1973). Adenyl cyclase. Adv. Cyclic Nucleotide Res. 3:1.
6. Birnbaumer, L., Pohl, S. L., and Kaumann, A. J. (1974). Receptors and acceptors: a necessary distinction in hormone binding studies. Adv. Cyclic Nucleotide Res. 4:239.
7. Helmreich, E. J. M., Zenner, H. P., Pfeuffer, T., and Cori, C. F. (1976).

Signal transfer from hormone receptor to adenylate cyclase. Curr. Top. Cell. Reg. 10:41.

8. Appleman, M. M., Thompson, W. J., and Russell, T. R. (1973). Cyclic nucleotide phosphodiesterase. Adv. Cyclic Nucleotide Res. 3:65.

9. Langan, T. A. (1973). Protein kinases and protein kinase substrates. Adv. Cyclic Nucleotide Res. 3:99.

10. Rubin, C. S., and Rosen, O. M. (1975). Protein phosphorylation. Annu. Rev. Biochem. 44:831.

11. Cohen, P., Antoniw, J. F., Nimmo, H. G., and Yeaman, S. J. (1976). Protein phosphorylation and hormone action. Ciba Found. Symp. on Peptide Hormones 41:281.

12. Krebs, E. G., and Stull, J. T. (1975). Protein phosphorylation and metabolic control. Ciba Found. Symp. 321:355.

13. Corbin, J. D., Soderling, T. R., Sugden, P. H., Keely, S. L., and Park, C. R. (1976). Control of metabolic processes by cAMP-dependent protein phosphorylation. In J. E. Dumont, B. Brown, and N. Marshall (eds.), Eukaryotic Cell Functions and Growth, pp. 231–247. Plenum Press, New York.

14. Goldberg, N. D., O'Dea, R. F., and Haddox, M. K. (1973). Cyclic GMP. Adv. Cyclic Nucleotide Res. 3:155.

15. Goldberg, N. D., Haddox, M. K., Nicol, S. E., Ascott, T. S., Zeilig, C. E., and Glass, D. B. (1975). Cyclic GMP and cyclic AMP in biological regulation. In F. Fox and D. McMahon (eds.), Proceedings ICN-UCLA Symposia on Molecular and Cellular Biology, vol. 2, pp. 440–472. W. A. Benjamin Inc., Menlo Park, Calif.

16. Goldberg, N. D. (1974). Cyclic nucleotides and cell function. Hosp. Practice. May, 1974, p. 127.

17. Pastan, I. H., Johnson, G. S., and Anderson, W. B. (1975). Role of cyclic nucleotides in growth control. Annu. Rev. Biochem. 44:491.

18. Soderling, T. R., and Park, C. R. (1974). Recent advances in glycogen metabolism. Adv. Cyclic Nucleotide Res. 4:283.

19. Wicks, W. D. (1974). Regulation of protein synthesis by cyclic AMP. Adv. Cyclic Nucleotide Res. 4:335.

20. Simon, L. N., Shuman, D. A., and Robins, R. K. (1973). The chemistry and biological properties of nucleotides related to nucleoside 3',5'-cyclic phosphates. Adv. Cyclic Nucleotide Res. 3:225.

21. Rasmussen, H., Goodman, D. B. P., and Tenenhouse, A. (1972). The role of cyclic AMP and calcium in cell activation. CRC Crit. Rev. Biochem. 1:95.

22. Rasmussen, H. (1974). Ions as second messengers. Hosp. Practice. June, 1974, p. 99.

23. Berridge, M. M. (1975). The interaction of cyclic nucleotides and calcium in the control of cellular activity. Adv. Cyclic Nucleotide Res. 6:1.

24. Parker, C. W., Sullivan, T. J., and Wedner, H. J. (1974). Cyclic AMP and the immune response. Adv. Cyclic Nucleotide Res. 4:1.

25. Bär, H. P. (1974). Cyclic nucleotides and smooth muscle. Adv. Cyclic Nucleotide Res. 4:195.

26. Halkerston, I. D. K. (1975). Cyclic AMP and adrenocortical functions. Adv. Cyclic Nucleotide Res. 6:99.

27. Marsh, J. M. (1975). The role of cyclic AMP in gonadal function. Adv. Cyclic Nucleotide Res. 6:137.

28. Entman, M. L. (1974). The role of cyclic AMP in the modulation of cardiac contractility. Adv. Cyclic Nucleotide Res. 4:163.

29. Montague, W., and Howell, S. J. (1975). Cyclic AMP and the physiology of the islets of Langerhans. Adv. Cyclic Nucleotide Res. 6:201.

30. Voorhees, J. J., Duell, E. A., Stawiski, M., and Harrell, E. R. (1974). Cyclic nucleotide metabolism in normal and proliferating epidermis. Adv. Cyclic Nucleotide Res. 4:117.

31. Chlapowski, F. J., Kelly, L. A., and Butcher, R. W. (1975). Cyclic nucleotides in cultured cells. Adv. Cyclic Nucleotide Res. 6:245.

32. Daly, J. (1975). Role of cyclic nucleotides in the nervous system. Handbook of Psychopharmacology, Vol. 5, p. 47. Plenum Press, New York.

33. Fain, J. Cyclic nucleotides and the regulation of adipose tissue metabolism. *In* H. Cramer and J. Schultz (eds.), Cyclic Nucleotides: Mechanisms of Action. Wiley and Sons, London, in press.

35. Sutherland, E. W., and Rall, T. W. (1958). Fractionation and characterization of a cyclic adenine ribonucleotide formed by tissue particles. J. Biol. epinephrine or glucagon. J. Am. Chem. Soc. 79:3608.

35. Sutherland, E. W., and Rall, T. W. (1958). Fractionation and characterization of a cyclic adenine ribonucleotide formed by tissue particles. J. Biol. Chem. 232:1077.

36. Ashman, D. F., Lipton, R., Melicow, M. M., and Price, T. D. (1963). Isolation of adenosine $3',5'$-monophosphate and guanosine $3',5'$-monophosphate from rat urine. Biochem. Biophys. Res. Commun. 11:330.

37. Hardman, J. G., and O'Malley, B. W. (eds.) (1974). Hormone action, Part C, Cyclic nucleotides. Methods Enzymol., Vol. 38. Academic Press, New York.

38. Greengard, P., Robison, G. A., and Paoletti, R. (eds.) (1972). New assay methods for cyclic nucleotides. Adv. Cyclic Nucleotide Res., Vol. 2. Raven Press, New York.

39. Chasin, M. (ed.) (1972). Methods in Cyclic Nucleotide Research. Dekker, New York.

40. Gilman, A. G. (1970). A protein binding assay for adenosine $3':5'$-cyclic monophosphate. Proc. Natl. Acad. Sci. U. S. A. 67:305.

41. Brown, B. L., Albano, J. D. M., Ekins, R. P., and Sgherzi, A. M. (1971). A simple and sensitive saturation assay method for the measurement of adenosine $3':5'$-cyclic monophosphate. Biochem. J. 121:561.

42. Steiner, A. L., Parker, C. W., and Kipnis, D. M. (1972). Radioimmunoassay for cyclic nucleotides. I. Preparation of antibodies and iodinated cyclic nucleotides. J. Biol. Chem. 247:1106.

43. Cailla, H. L., Racine-Weisbuch, M. S., and Delaage, M. A. (1973). Adenosine $3',5'$-cyclic monophosphate assay at 10^{-15} mole level. Anal. Biochem. 56:394.

44. Harper, J. F., and Brooker, G. (1975). Femtomole sensitive radioimmunoassay for cyclic AMP and cyclic GMP after $2'0$ acetylation by acetic anhydride in aqueous solution. J. Cyclic Nucleotide Res. 1:207.

45. White, A. A., and Zenser, T. V. (1971). Separation of cyclic $3',5'$-nucleotide monophosphates from other nucleotides on aluminum oxide columns: application to the assay of adenyl cyclase and guanyl cyclase. Anal. Biochem. 41:372.

46. Murad, F., Manganiello, V., and Vaughan, M. (1971). A simple, sensitive protein-binding assay for guanosine $3':5'$-monophosphate. Proc. Nat. Acad. Sci. U. S. A. 68:736.

47. Jakobs, K. H., Böhme, E., and Schultz, G. (1976). Determination of cyclic GMP in biological material. *In* J. E. Dumont, B. Brown, and N. Marshall

(eds.), Eukaryotic Cell Functions and Growth, pp. 295–311. Plenum Press, New York.

48. Albano, J. D. M., Barnes, G. D., Maudsley, D. V., Brown, B. L., and Etkins, R. P. (1974). Factors affecting the saturation assay of cyclic AMP in biological systems. Anal. Biochem. 60:130.

49. Kuo, J. F., and Kuo, W.-N. (1973). Regulation by β-adrenergic receptor and muscarinic cholinergic receptor activation of intracellular cyclic AMP and cyclic GMP levels in rat lung slices. Biochem. Biophys. Res. Commun. 55:660.

50. Stoner, J., Manganiello, V. C., and Vaughan, M. (1974). Guanosine cyclic 3',5'-monophosphate and guanylate cyclase activity in guinea pig lung: effects of acetylcholine and cholinesterase inhibitors. Mol. Pharmacol. 10:155.

51. George, W. J., Polson, J. B., O'Toole, A. G., and Goldberg, N. D. (1970). Elevation of guanosine 3',5'-cyclic phosphate in rat heart after perfusion with acetylcholine. Proc. Natl. Acad. Sci. 66:398.

52. George, W. J., Wilkerson, R. D., and Kadowitz, P. J. (1973). Influence of acetylcholine on contractile force and cyclic nucleotide levels in the isolated perfused rat heart. J. Pharma. Exp. Ther. 184:228.

53. Lee, T.-P., Kuo, J. F., and Greengard, P. (1972). Role of muscarinic cholinergic receptors in regulation of guanosine 3':5'-cyclic monophosphate content in mammalian brain, heart muscle, and intestinal smooth muscle. Proc. Natl. Acad. Sci. U. S. A. 69:3287.

54. Schultz, G., Hardman, J. G., Schultz, K., Baird, C. E., and Sutherland, E. W. (1973). The importance of calcium ions for the regulation of guanosine 3':5'-cyclic monophosphate and the action of insulin and acetylcholine. Proc. Natl. Acad. Sci. U. S. A. 70:3889.

55. Illiano, G., Tell, G. P. E., Siegel, M. I., and Cuatrecasas, P. (1973). Guanosine 3':5'-cyclic monophosphate and the action of insulin and acetylcholine. Proc. Natl. Acad. Sci. U. S. A. 70:2443.

56. Pointer, R. H., Butcher, F. R., and Fain, J. N. (1976). Studies on the role of cyclic GMP and extracellular Ca^{2+} in the regulation of glycogenolysis in rat liver cells. J. Biol. Chem. 251:2987.

57. Yamashita, K., and Field, J. B. (1972). Elevation of cyclic guanosine 3',5'-monophosphate levels in dog thyroid slices caused by acetylcholine and sodium fluoride. J. Biol. Chem. 247:7062.

58. Fain, J. N., and Butcher, F. R. (1976). Cyclic guanosine 3',5'-monophosphate and the regulation of lipolysis in rat fat cells. J. Cyclic Nucleotide Res. 2:71.

59. Goldberg, N. D., Haddox, M. K., Dunham, E., Lopez, C., and Hadden, J. W. (1974). The Ying Yang hypothesis of biological control: opposing influences of cyclic GMP and cyclic AMP in the regulation of cell proliferation and other biological processes. In R. Baserga and R. Paoletti (eds.), p. 490. Cold Spring Harbor Press, Cold Spring Harbor, New York.

60. Ignarro, L. J., and George, W. J. (1974). Hormonal control of lysosomal enzyme release from human neutrophils: elevation of cyclic nucleotide levels by autonomic neurohormones. Proc. Natl. Acad. Sci. U. S. A. 71:2027.

61. Murad, F., and Kimura, H. (1974). Cyclic nucleotide levels in incubations of guinea pig trachea. Biochim. Biophys. Acta 343:275.

62. Lochmann, S. M., Miech, R. P., and Butcher, F. R. (1977). Regulation of

cyclic nucleotide levels and contractibility in bovine tracheal muscle, in press.

63. Kuo, J. F., and Kuo, W. N. (1975). Regulation of cyclic nucleotide systems in pancreatic islets of langerhans: implication of insulin secretion. *In* B. Weiss (ed.), Cyclic Nucleotides in Disease, p. 211. University Park Press, Baltimore.

64. Robberecht, P., Deschodt-Lanckman, M., DeNeef, P., Borgeat, P., and Christophe, J. (1974). In vivo effects of pancreozymin, secretin, vasoactive intestinal polypeptide and pilocarpine on the levels of cyclic AMP and cyclic GMP in the rat pancreas. FEBS Lett. 43:139.

65. Schultz, G., Schultz, K., and Hardman, J. G. (1975). Effects of norepinephrine on cyclic nucleotide levels in ductus deferens of the rat. Metabolism 24:429.

66. Ball, J. H., Kaminsky, N. I., Hardman, J. G., Broadus, A. E., Sutherland, E. W., and Liddle, G. W. (1972). Effects of catecholamines and adrenergic blocking agents on plasma and urinary cyclic nucleotides in man. J. Clin. Invest. 51:2124.

67. Butcher, F. R., Rudich, L. K., Emler, C., and Nemerovski, M. Effects of adrenergic agents on cyclic nucleotide levels, K^+ release and α-amylase release from rat parotid tissue slices. Molec. Pharmacol. 12:862.

68. Kaneko, T., Oka, H., Munemura, M., Suzuki, S., Yasuda, H., and Oda, T. (1974). Stimulation of guanosine 3',5'-cyclic monophosphate accumulation in rat anterior pituitary gland in vitro by synthetic somatostatin. Biochem. Biophys. Res. Commun. 61:53.

69. Seifert, W. F., and Rudland, P. S. (1974). Possible involvement of cyclic GMP in growth control of cultured mouse cells. Nature (Lond.) 248:138.

70. Seifert, W., and Rudland, P. S. (1974). Cyclic nucleotides and growth control in cultured mouse cells: correlation of changes in intracellular 3':5'-cGMP concentration with a specific phase of the cell cycle. Proc. Natl. Acad. Sci. U. S. A. 71:4920.

71. Hadden, J. W., Hadden, E. M., Haddox, M. K., and Goldberg, N. D. (1972). Guanosine 3':5'-cyclic monophosphate: a possible intracellular mediator of mitogenic influences in lymphocytes. Proc. Natl. Acad. Sci. U. S. A. 69:3024.

72. Ferrendelli, J. A., Kinscherf, D. A., and Chang, M. M. (1973). Regulation of levels of guanosine cyclic 3',5'-monophosphate in the central nervous system: effects of depolarizing agents. Mol. Pharmacol. 9:445.

73. Sharma, R. K., Ahmed, N. K., Sutliff, L. S., and Brush, J. S. (1974). Metabolic regulation of steroidogenesis in isolated adrenal cells of the rat: ACTH regulation of cGMP and cAMP levels and steroidogenesis. FEBS Lett. 45:107.

74. Honn, K. V., and Chavin, W. (1975). ACTH control of adrenocortical c-GMP. Gen. Comp. Endocrinol. 26:374.

75. Kuehl, F. A., Jr., Ham, E. A., Zanetti, M. E., Sanford, C. H., Nicol, S. E., and Goldberg, N. D. (1974). Estrogen-related increases in uterine guanosine 3':5'-cyclic monophosphate levels. Proc. Natl. Acad. Sci. U. S. A. 71:1866.

76. Sandler, J. A., Gallin, J. I., and Vaughan, M. (1975). Effects of serotonin, carbamylcholine, and ascorbic acid on leukocyte cyclic GMP and chemotaxis. J. Cell Biol. 67:480.

77. Clyman, R. I., Blacksin, A. D., Sandler, J. A., Manganiello, V. C., and

Vaughan, M. (1975). The role of calcium in regulation of cyclic nucleotide content in human umbilical artery. J. Biol. Chem. 250:4718.
78. Gullis, R., Traber, J., and Hamprecht, B. (1975). Morphine elevates levels
of cyclic GMP in a neuroblastoma X glioma hybrid cell line. Nature
(Lond.) 256:57.
79. Sandler, J. A., Clyman, R. I., Manganiello, V. C., and Vaughan, M. (1975).
The effect of serotonin (5-hydroxytryptamine) and derivatives on
guanosine 3',5'-monophosphate in human monocytes. J. Clin. Invest.
55:431.
80. Stoner, J., Manganiello, V. C., and Vaughan, M. (1973). Effects of bradykinin and indomethacin on cyclic GMP and cyclic AMP in lung slices.
Proc. Natl. Acad. Sci. U. S. A. 70:3830.
81. Butcher, F. R. (1975). The role of calcium and cyclic nucleotides in
α-amylase release from slices of rat parotid: studies with the divalent
cation ionophore A-23187. Metabolism 24:409.
82. Sande, J. V., Decoster, C., and Dumont, J. E. (1975). Control and role of
cyclic 3',5'-guanosine monophosphate in the thyroid. Biochem. Biophys.
Res. Commun. 62:168.
83. Smith, R. J., and Ignarro, L. J. (1975). Bioregulation of lysosomal enzyme
secretion from human neutrophils: role of guanosine 3':5'-mono-
phosphate and calcium in stimulus-secretion coupling. Proc. Natl. Acad.
Sci. U. S. A. 72:108.
84. Hardman, J. G., Davis, J. W., and Sutherland, E. W. (1969). Effects of
some hormonal and other factors on the excretion of guanosine
3',5'-monophosphate and adenosine 3',5'-monophosphate in rat urine.
J. Biol. Chem. 244:6354.
85. Goldberg, N. D., Dietz, S. B., and O'Toole, A. G. (1969). Cyclic guanosine
3',5'-monophosphate in mammalian tissues and urine. J. Biol. Chem.
244:4458.
86. Pinkett, M. O., and Perlman, R. L. (1975). Stimulation of sugar transport
in rat diaphragm by 8-bromoguanosine 3',5'-monophosphate. Biochim.
Biophys. Acta 399:473.
87. Estensen, R. D., Hill, H. R., Quie, P. G., Hogan, N., and Goldberg, N. D.
(1973). Cyclic GMP and cell movement. Nature (Lond.) 245:458.
88. Hill, R. H., Estensen, R. D., Quie, P. G., Hogan, N. A., and Goldberg, N. D.
(1975). Modulation of human neutrophil chemotactic responses by
cyclic 3',5' guanosine monophosphate and cyclic 3',5'-monophosphate.
Metabolism 24:447.
89. Gamow, E., and Barnes, F. S. (1974). Chemotactic responses of human
polymorphonuclear leukocytes to cyclic GMP and other compounds.
Exp. Cell Res. 87:1.
90. Ignarro, L. J., and Colombo, C. (1973). Enzyme release from polymorphonuclear leukocyte lysosomes: regulation by autonomic drugs and cyclic
nucleotides. Science 180:1181.
91. Zurier, R. B., Wiessmann, G., Hoffstein, S., Kammerman, S., and Tai, H. H.
(1974). Mechanism of lysosomal enzyme release from human leukocytes.
II. Effects of cAMP and cGMP, autonomic agonists, and agents which
affect microtubule function. J. Clin. Invest. 53:297.
92. Kaliner, M., Orange, R. P., and Austen, K. F. (1972). Immunological
release of histamine and slow reacting substance of anaphylaxis from
human lung. IV. Enhancement by cholinergic and alpha adrenergic
stimulation. J. Exp. Med. 136:556.

93. Kram, R., and Tomkins, G. (1973). Pleiotypic control of cyclic AMP interaction with cyclic GMP and possible role of microtubules. Proc. Natl. Acad. Sci. U. S. A. 70:1659.
94. McAfee, D. A., and Greengard, P. (1972). Adenosine 3',5'-monophosphate: electrophysiological evidence for a role in synaptic transmission. Science 178:310.
95. Stone, T. W., Taylor, D. A., and Bloom, F. E. (1975). Cyclic AMP and cyclic GMP may mediate opposite neuronal responses in the rat cerebral cortex. Science 187:845.
96. Weinstein, Y., Chambers, D. A., Bourne, H. R., and Melmon, K. L. (1974). Cyclic GMP stimulates lymphocyte nucleic acid synthesis. Nature (Lond.) 251:352.
97. Diamantstein, T., and Ulmer, A. (1975). The antagonistic action of cyclic GMP and cyclic AMP on proliferation of B and T lymphocytes. Immunology 28:113.
98. Johnson, E. M., and Hadden, J. W. (1975). Phosphorylation of lymphocyte nuclear acidic proteins: regulation by cyclic nucleotides. Science 18:1198.
99. Kimura, H., and Murad, F. (1975). Subcellular localization of guanylate cyclase. Life Sci. 17:837.
100. Kimura, H., and Murad, F. (1974). Evidence for two different forms of guanylate cyclase in rat heart. J. Biol. Chem. 249:6910.
101. Kimura, H., and Murad, F. (1975). Increased particulate and decreased soluble guanylate cyclase activity in regenerating liver, fetal liver, and hepatoma. Proc. Natl. Acad. Sci. U. S. A. 72:1965.
102. Kimura, H., and Murad, F. (1975). Localization of particulate guanylate cyclase in plasma membranes and microsomes of rat liver. J. Biol. Chem. 250:4810.
103. Chrisman, T. D., Garbers, D. L., Parks, M. A., and Hardman, J. G. (1975). Characterization of particulate and soluble guanylate cyclases from rat lung. J. Biol. Chem. 250:374.
104. Durham, J. P. (1976). Guanylate cyclase: assay and properties of the particulate and supernatant enzymes in mouse parotid. Eur. J. Biochem. 61:535.
105. Thompson, W. J., Williams, R. H., and Little, S. A. (1973). Activation of guanyl cyclase and adenyl cyclase by secretin. Biochim. Biophys. Acta 302:329.
106. Howell, S. L., and Montague, W. (1974). Regulation of guanylate cyclase in guinea-pig islets of langerhans. Biochem. J. 142:379.
107. Böhme, E., Jung, R., and Mechler, I. (1974). Guanylate cyclase in human platelets. Methods Enzymol. 38:199.
108. White, A. A., and Lad, P. J. (1975). Activation of the soluble guanylate cyclase from rat lung by preincubation. Fed. Proc. 34:232 (Abstr.).
109. Czech, M. P., Lawrence, J. C., Jr., and Lynn, W. S. (1974). Evidence for the involvement of sulfhydryl oxidation in the regulation of fat cell hexose transport by insulin. Proc. Natl. Acad. Sci. U. S. A. 71:4173.
110. Kimura, H., Mittal, C. K., and Murad, F. (1975). Activation of guanylate cyclase from rat liver and other tissues by sodium azide. J. Biol. Chem. 250:8016.
111. Kuo, J. F., and Greengard, P. (1970). Cyclic nucleotide-dependent protein kinases. J. Biol. Chem. 245:2493.

112. Kuo, J. F. (1974). Guanosine $3':5'$-monophosphate-dependent protein kinases in mammalian tissues. Proc. Natl. Acad. Sci. U. S. A. 71:4037.

113. Walsh, D. A., Ashby, C. D., Gonzalez, C., Calkins, D., Fisher, E. H., and Krebs, E. G. (1971). Purification and characterization of a protein inhibitor of adenosine $3',5'$-monophosphate-dependent protein kinases. J. Biol. Chem. 246:1977.

114. Hofmann, F., and Sold, G. (1972). A protein kinase activity from rat cerebellum stimulated by guanosine $3',5'$ monophosphate. Biochem. Biophys. Res. Commun. 49:1100.

115. Kuo, J. F. (1975). Changes in activities of modulators of cyclic AMP-dependent and cyclic GMP-dependent protein kinases in pancreas and adipose tissue from alloxan-induced diabetic rats. Biochem. Biophys. Res. Commun. 65:1214.

116. Takai, Y., Nishiyama, K., Yamahura, H., and Nishizuka, Y. (1975). Guanosine $3':5'$-monophosphate-dependent protein kinase from bovine cerebellum. J. Biol. Chem. 250:4690.

117. Casnellie, J. E., and Greengard, P. (1974). Guanosine $3':5'$-cyclic monophosphate-dependent phosphorylation of endogenous substrate proteins in membranes of mammalian smooth muscle. Proc. Natl. Acad. Sci. U. S. A. 71:1891.

118. Johnson, E. M., and Hadden, J. W. (1975). Phosphorylation of lymphocyte nuclear acidic proteins: regulation by cyclic nucleotides. Science 187:1198.

119. Gill, G. N., and Kanstein, C. B. (1975). Guanosine $3',5'$-monophosphate receptor protein: separation from adenosine $3',5'$-monophosphate receptor protein. Biochem. Biophys. Res. Commun. 63:1113.

120. Thomas, E. W., Murad, F., Looney, W. B., and Morris, H. P. (1973). Adenosine $3',5'$-monophosphate and guanosine $3',5'$-monophosphate: concentrations in Morris hepatomas of different growth rates. Biochim. Biophys. Acta 297:564.

121. Goldberg, M. L., Burke, G. C., and Morris, H. P. (1975). Cyclic AMP and cyclic GMP content and binding in malignancy. Biochem. Biophys. Res. Commun. 62:320.

122. Voorhees, J. J., Stawiski, M., and Duell, E. A. (1973). Increased cyclic GMP and decreased cyclic AMP levels in the hyperplastic, abnormally differentiated epidermis of psoriasis. Life Sci. 13:639.

123. Murad, F., Kimura, H., Hopkins, H. A., Looney, W. B., and Kovacs, C. J. (1975). Increased urinary excretion of cyclic guanosine monophosphate in rats bearing Morris hepatoma 3924A. Science 190:58.

124. Moens, W., Vokaer, A., and Kram, R. (1975). Cyclic AMP and cyclic GMP concentrations in serum and density restricted fibroblast cultures. Proc. Natl. Acad. Sci. U. S. A. 72:1063.

125. Balk, S. D., Whitefield, J. F., Youdale, T., and Braun, A. C. (1973). Roles of calcium, serum, plasma, and folic acid in the control of proliferation of normal and rous sarcoma virus-infected chicken fibroblasts. Proc. Natl. Acad. Sci. U. S. A. 70:675.

126. Parker, C. W. (1974). Correlation between mitogenicity and stimulation of calcium uptake in human lymphocytes. Biochem. Biophys. Res. Commun. 61:1180.

127. Dulbecco, R., and Elkington, J. (1975). Induction of growth in resting fibroblastic cell cultures by Ca^{++}. Proc. Natl. Acad. Sci. U. S. A. 72:1584.

128. Freedman, M. H., Raff, M. C., and Gomperts, B. (1975). Induction of

increased calcium uptake in mouse T lymphocytes by concanavalin A and its modulation by cyclic nucleotides. Nature (Lond.) 255:378.

129. Pierce, N. F., Greenough, W. B., III, and Carpenter, C. C. J., Jr. (1971). Vibrio cholerae enterotoxin and its mode of action. Bacteriol. Rev. 35:1.

130. Van Heyningen, W. E. (1973). On the similarity of tetanus and cholera toxins. Nauyn Schmiedebergs Arch. Pharmacol. 276:289.

131. Cuatrecasas, P. (1973). Interaction of vibrio cholerae enterotoxin with cell membranes. Biochemistry 12:3547.

132. Holmgren, J., Lonnroth, I., Mansson, J.-E., and Svennerholm, L. (1975). Interaction of cholera toxin and membrane G_{M1} ganglioside of small intestine. Proc. Natl. Acad. Sci. U. S. A. 72:2520.

133. Van Heyningen, W. E., Carpenter, C. C. J., Pierce, N. F., and Greenough, W. B., III. (1971). Deactivation of cholera toxin by ganglioside. J. Infect. Dis. 124:415.

134. Cuatrecasas, P. (1973). Gangliosides and membrane receptors for cholera toxin. Biochemistry 12:3558.

135. Sattler, J., and Wiegandt, H. (1975). Studies of the subunit structure of choleragen. Eur. J. Biochem. 57:309.

136. Van Heyningen, S., and King, A. C. (1975). Subunit A from cholera toxin is an activator of adenylate cyclase in pigeon erythrocytes. Biochem. J. 146:269.

137. Gill, D. M., and King, C. A. (1975). The mechanism of action of cholera toxin in pigeon erythrocyte lysates. J. Biol. Chem. 250:6424.

138. Gill, D. M. (1975). Involvement of nicotinamide adenine dinucleotide in the action of cholera toxin in vitro. Proc. Natl. Acad. Sci. U. S. A. 72:2064.

139. Bitensky, M. W., Wheeler, M. A., Mehta, H., and Miki, N. (1975). Cholera toxin activation of adenylate cyclase in cancer cell membrane fragments. Proc. Natl. Acad. Sci. U. S. A. 72:2572.

140. Bennett, V., O'Keefe, E., and Cuatrecasas, P. (1975). Mechanism of action of cholera toxin and the mobile receptor theory of hormone receptor-adenylate cyclase interactions. Proc. Natl. Acad. Sci. U. S. A. 72:33.

141. Sahyoun, N., and Cuatrecasas, P. (1975). Mechanism of activation of adenylate cyclase by cholera toxin. Proc. Natl. Acad. Sci. U. S. A. 72:3438.

142. Craig, S. W., and Cuatrecasas, P. (1975). Mobility of cholera toxin receptors on rat lymphocyte membrane. Proc. Natl. Acad. Sci. U. S. A. 72:3844.

143. Flores, J., and Sharp, G. W. G. (1975). Effects of cholera toxin on adenylate cyclase. J. Clin. Invest. 56:1345.

144. Rodbell, M., Lin, M. C., Salomon, Y., Londos, C., Harwood, J. P., Martin, B. R., Rendell, M., and Berman, M. (1975). Role of adenine and guanine nucleotides in the activity and response of adenylate cyclase systems to hormones: evidence for multisite transition states. Adv. Cyclic Nucleotide Res. 5:3.

145. Londos, C., Salomon, Y., Lin, M. C., Harwood, J. P., Schramm, M., Wolff, J., and Rodbell, M. (1974). 5'-Guanylylimidodiphosphate, a potent activator of adenylate cyclase systems in eukaryotic cells. Proc. Natl. Acad. Sci. U. S. A. 71:3087.

146. Pfeuffer, T., and Helmreich, E. J. M. (1975). Activation of pigeon erythrocyte membrane adenylate cyclase by guanylnucleotide analogues and separation of a nucleotide binding protein. J. Biol. Chem. 250:867.

147. Trendelenburg, U. (1966). I. Mechanisms of supersensitivity and subsensitivity to sympathomimetic amines. Pharmacol. Rev. 18:629.
148. Kakiuchi, S., and Rall, T. W. (1968). The influence of chemical agents on the accumulation of adenosine $3',5'$ phosphate in slices of rabbit cerebellum. Mol. Pharmacol. 4:367.
149. Manganiello, V. C., Murad, F., and Vaughan, M. (1971). Effects of lipolytic and antilipolytic agents on cyclic $3',5'$-monophosphate in fat cells. J. Biol. Chem. 246:2195.
150. Ho, R. J., and Sutherland, E. W. (1971). Formation and release of a hormone antagonist by rat adipocytes. J. Biol. Chem. 246:6822.
151. Schultz, J., and Daly, J. W. (1973). Cyclic adenosine $3',5'$-monophosphate in guinea pig cerebral cortical slices. III. Formation, degradation, and reformation of cyclic adenosine $3',5'$-monophosphate during sequential stimulations by biogenic amines and adenosine. J. Biol. Chem. 248:860.
152. Peytremann, A., Nicholson, W. E., Brown, R. D., Liddle, G. W., and Hardman, J. G. (1973). Comparative effects of angiotensin and ACTH on cyclic AMP and steroidogenesis in isolated bovine adrenal cells. J. Clin. Invest. 52:835.
153. Espiner, E. A., Livesey, J. H., Ross, J., and Donald, R. A. (1974). Dynamics of cyclic adenosine $3',5'$-monophosphate release during adrenocortical stimulation in vivo. Endocrinology 95:838.
154. Exton, J. H., Robison, G. A., Sutherland, E. W., and Park, C. R. (1971). Studies on the role of adenosine $3',5'$-monophosphate in hepatic actions of glucagon and catecholamines. J. Biol. Chem. 246:6166.
155. Siddle, K., Kane-Maguire, B., and Campbell, A. K. (1973). The effects of glucagon and insulin on adenosine $3',5'$-cyclic monophosphate concentrations in an organ culture of mature rat liver. Biochem. J. 132:765.
156. Manganiello, V., and Vaughan, M. (1972). Prostaglandin E_1 effects on adenosine $3',5'$-cyclic monophosphate concentration and phosphodiesterase activity in fibroblasts. Proc. Natl. Acad. Sci. U. S. A. 69:269.
157. Franklin, T. J., and Foster, S. J. (1973). Hormone induced desensitization of the hormonal control of cyclic AMP levels in human diploid fibroblasts. Nature (New Biol.) 246:146.
158. Clark, R. B., Su, Y.-F., Ortman, R., Cubeddu, L., Johnson, G. L., and Perkins, J. P. (1975). Factors influencing the effect of hormones on the accumulation of cyclic AMP in cultured human astrocytoma cells. Metabolism 24:343.
159. Remold-O'Donnell, E. (1974). Stimulation and desensitization of macrophage adenylate cyclase by prostaglandins and catecholamines. J. Biol. Chem. 249:3615.
160. Franklin, T. J., Morris, W. P., and Twose, P. A. (1975). Desensitization of beta adrenergic receptors in human fibroblasts in tissue culture. Mol. Pharmacol. 11:485.
161. Makman, M. H. (1971). Properties of adenylate cyclase of lymphoid cells. Proc. Natl. Acad. Sci. U. S. A. 68:885.
162. Mickey, J., Tate, R., and Lefkowitz, R. J. (1975). Subsensitivity of adenylate cyclase and decreased β-adrenergic receptor binding after chronic exposure to (−)-isoproterenol in vitro. J. Biol. Chem. 250:5727.
163. Rendell, M., Saloman, Y., Lin, M. C., Rodbell, M., and Berman, M. (1975). The hepatic adenylate cyclase system. III. A mathematical model for the steady state kinetics of catalysis and nucleotide regulation. J. Biol. Chem. 250:4235.

164. Mukherjee, C., Caron, M. G., and Lefkowitz, R. J. (1975). Catecholamine-induced subsensitivity of adenylate cyclase associated with loss of β-adrenergic receptor binding sites. Proc. Natl. Acad. Sci. U. S. A. 72:1945.

165. Berg, D. K., and Hall, Z. W. (1974). Fate of α-bungarotoxin bound to acetylcholine receptors of normal and denervated muscle. Science 184:473.

166. Kahn, C. R., Neville, D. M., and Roth, J. (1973). Insulin-receptor interaction in the obese-hyperglycemic mouse: a model of insulin resistance. J. Biol. Chem. 248:244.

167. DeVellis, J., and Brooker, G. (1974). Reversal of catecholamine refractoriness by inhibitors of RNA and protein synthesis. Science 186:1221.

168. Deguchi, T., and Axelrod, J. (1973). Supersensitivity and subsensitivity of the β-adrenergic receptor in pineal gland regulated by catecholamine transmitter. Proc. Natl. Acad. Sci. U. S. A. 70:2411.

169. Romero, J. A., and Axelrod, J. (1975). Regulation of sensitivity to beta-adrenergic stimulation in induction of pineal N-acetyltransferase. Proc. Natl. Acad. Sci. U. S. A. 72:1661.

170. Fain, J. N., and Shepherd, R. E. (1975). Free fatty acids as feedback regulators of adenylate cyclase and cyclic 3':5'-AMP accumulation in rat fat cells. J. Biol. Chem. 250:6586.

171. Malgieri, J. A., Shepherd, R. E., and Fain, J. N. (1975). Lack of feedback regulation of cyclic 3':5'-AMP accumulation by free fatty acids in chicken fat cells. J. Biol. Chem. 250:6593.

172. Shepherd, R. E., Sauer, V. A., and Fain, J. N., unpublished observations.

173. Burns, T. W., Langley, P. E., and Robison, G. A. (1975). Site of free-fatty-acid inhibition of lipolysis by human adipocytes. Metabolism 24:265.

174. Ho, R. J., Bomboy, J. D., Wasner, H. K., and Sutherland, E. W. (1975). Preparation and characterization of a hormone antagonist from adipocytes. Methods Enzymol. 39:431.

175. Ho, R. J., Russell, T. R., Asakawa, T., and Hucks, M. W. (1975). Inhibition of cyclic nucleotide phosphodiesterase activity by an endogenous factor. J. Cyclic Nucleotide Res. 1:81.

176. Orly, J., and Schramm, M. (1975). Fatty acids as modulators of membrane functions: catecholamine-activated adenylate cyclase of the turkey erythrocyte. Proc. Natl. Acad. Sci. U. S. A. 72:3433.

177. Sutherland, E. W., Rall, T. W., and Menon, T. (1962). Adenyl cyclase. I. Distribution, preparation, and properties. J. Biol. Chem. 237:1220.

178. Levey, G. S. (1975). The glucagon receptor and adenylate cyclase. Metabolism 24:301.

179. Levey, G. S., Fletcher, M. A., Klein, I., Ruiz, E., and Schenk, A. (1974). Characterization of [125] I-glucagon binding in a solubilized preparation of cat myocardial adenylate cyclase. J. Biol. Chem. 249:2665.

180. Queener, S. F., Fleming, J. W., and Bell, N. H. (1975). Solubilization of calcitonin-responsive renal cortical adenylate cyclase. J. Biol. Chem. 250:7586.

181. Hokin, L. E. (1966). Effects of calcium omission on acetylcholine-stimulated secretion and phospholipid synthesis in pigeon pancreas slices. Biochim. Biophys. Acta 115:219.

182. DeTorrentegui, G., and Berthet, J. (1966). The action of insulin on the incorporation of (^{32} P) phosphate in the phospholipids of rat adipose tissue. Biochem. Biophys. Acta 116:477.

183. Gaut, Z. N., and Huggins, C. G. (1966). Effect of epinephrine on the metabolism of the inositol phosphatides in rat heart in vivo. Nature (Lond.) 212:612.

184. Jones, L. M., and Michell, R. H. (1974). Breakdown of phosphatidylinositol provoked by muscarinic cholinergic stimulation of rat parotid-gland fragments. Biochem. J. 142:583.

185. Butcher, F. R., Rudich, L. K., and McBride, A. (1976). Effect of cholinergic agonists on cyclic nucleotide levels, α-amylase release and K^+ efflux from rat parotid slices. Molec. Cell. Endo. 5:243.

186. Haslam, R. J., and Taylor, A. (1971). Effects of catecholamines on the formation of adenosine $3',5'$-cyclic monophosphate in human blood platelets. Biochem. J. 125:377.

187. Oron, Y., Lowe, M., and Selinger, Z. (1973). Involvement of the α-adrenergic receptor in the phospholipid effect in rat parotid. FEBS Lett. 34:198.

188. Deykin, D., and Snyder, D. (1973). Effect of epinephrine on platelet lipid metabolism. J. Lab. Clin. Med. 82:554.

189. Michell, R. H. (1975). Inositol phospholipids and cell surface receptor function. Biochim. Biophys. Acta 415:81.

190. Sattin, A., and Rall, T. W. (1970). The effect of adenosine and adenine nucleotides on the cyclic adenosine $3',5'$-phosphate content of guinea pig cerebral cortex slices. Mol. Pharmacol. 6:13.

191. Huang, M., and Daly, J. W. (1974). Adenosine-elicited accumulation of cyclic AMP in brain slices: potentiation by agents which inhibit uptake of adenosine. Life Sci. 14:489.

192. Blume, A. J., Dalton, C., and Sheppard, H. (1973). Adenosine-mediated elevation of cyclic $3',5'$-adenosine monophosphate concentrations in cultured mouse neuroblastoma cells. Proc. Natl. Acad. Sci. U. S. A. 70:3099.

193. Skolnick, P., and Daly, J. W. (1975). Stimulation of adenosine $3',5'$-monophosphate formation in rat cerebral cortical slices by methoxamine: interaction with an alpha adrenergic receptor. J. Pharmacol. Exp. Ther. 193:549.

194. Huang, M., Gruenstein, E., and Daly, J. W. (1973). Depolarization-evoked accumulation of cyclic AMP in brain slices: inhibition by exogenous adenosine deaminase. Biochem. Biophys. Acta 329:147.

195. Mills, D. C. B., and Smith, J. B. (1971). The influence on platelet aggregation of drugs that affect the accumulation of adenosine $3':5'$-cyclic monophosphate in platelets. Biochem. J. 121:185.

196. Blume, A. J., and Foster, C. J. (1975). Mouse neuroblastoma adenylate cyclase. J. Biol. Chem. 250:5003.

197. Fain, J. N., Pointer, R. H., and Ward, W. F. (1972). Effects of adenosine nucleosides on adenylate cyclase, phosphodiesterase, cyclic adenosine monophosphate accumulation, and lipolysis in fat cells. J. Biol. Chem. 247:6866.

198. Fain, J. N. (1973). Inhibition of adenosine cyclic $3',5'$-monophosphate accumulation in fat cells by adenosine, N^6-(phenylisopropyl) adenosine, and related compounds. Mol. Pharmacol. 9:595.

199. DoKhac, L., Harbon, S., and Clauser, H. J. (1973). Intracellular titration of cyclic AMP bound to receptor proteins and correlation with cyclic AMP levels in the surviving rat diaphragm. Eur. J. Biochem. 40:177.

200. Soderling, T. R., Corbin, J. D., and Park, C. R. (1973). Regulation of

adenosine $3',5'$ monophosphate-dependent protein kinase. J. Biol. Chem. 248:1822.

201. Steiner, A. L., Whitley, T. A., Ong, S. H., and Stowe, N. W. (1975). Cyclic AMP and cyclic GMP: studies utilizing immunohistochemical teachings for the localization of the nucleotides in tissue. Metabolism 24:419.

202. Fallon, E. F., Agarawal, R., Furth, E., Steiner, A. L., and Cowden, R. (1974). Cyclic guanosine and adenosine $3',5'$-monophosphates in canine thyroid: localization by immunofluorescence. Science 184:1089.

203. Swillens, S., Van Cauter, E., and Dumont, J. E. (1974). Significance of binding and activation constants. Biochim. Biophys. Acta 364:250.

204. Beavo, J. A., Bechtel, P. J., and Krebs, E. G. (1974). Activation of protein kinase by physiological concentrations of cyclic AMP. Proc. Natl. Acad. Sci. U. S. A. 71:3580.

205. O'Dea, R. F., Haddox, M. K., and Goldberg, N. D. (1971). Interaction with phosphodiesterase of free and kinase-complexed cyclic adenosine $3',5'$-monophosphate. J. Biol. Chem. 246:6183.

206. Haddox, M. K., Newton, N. E., Hartle, D. K., and Goldberg, N. D. (1972). ATP (Mg^{2+}) induced inhibition of cyclic AMP reactivity with a skeletal muscle protein kinase. Biochem. Biophys. Res. Commun. 47:653.

207. Namm, D. H., Mayer, S. E., and Maltbie, M. (1968). The role of potassium and calcium ions in the effect of epinephrine on cardiac cyclic adenosine $3',5'$-monophosphate, phosphorylase kinase, and phosphorylase. Mol. Pharmacol. 4:522.

208. Shanfeld, J., Frazer, A., and Hess, M. E. (1969). Dissociation of the increased formation of cardiac adenosine $3',5'$-monophosphate from the positive inotropic effect of norepinephrine. J. Pharmacol. Exp. Ther. 169:315.

209. Øye, I., and Langslet, A. (1972). The role of cyclic AMP in the inotropic response to isoprenaline and glucagon. Adv. Cyclic Nucleotide Res. 1:291.

210. Venter, J. C., Ross, J., Jr., and Kaplan, N. O. (1975). Lack of detectable change in cyclic AMP during the cardiac inotropic response to isoproterenol immobilized on glass beads. Proc. Natl. Acad. Sci. U. S. A. 72:824.

211. Osnes, J.-B., and Øye, I. (1975). Relationship between cyclic AMP metabolism and inotropic response of perfused rat hearts to phenylephrine and other adrenergic amines. Adv. Cyclic Nucleotide Res. 5:415.

212. Rabinowitz, B., Chuck, L., Kligerman, M., and Parmley, W. W. (1975). Positive inotropic effects of methoxamine: evidence for alpha-adrenergic receptors in ventricular myocardium. Am. J. Physiol. 229:582.

213. Benfey, B. G. (1973). Characterization of α-adrenoceptors in the myocardium. Br. J. Pharmacol. 48:132.

214. Beall, R. J., and Sayers, G. (1972). Isolated adrenal cells: steroidogenesis and cyclic AMP accumulation in response to ACTH. Arch. Biochem. Biophys. 148:70.

215. Moyle, W. R., Kong, Y. C., and Ramachandran, J. (1973). Steroidogenesis and cyclic adenosine $3',5'$-monophosphate accumulation in rat adrenal cells. J. Biol. Chem. 248:2409.

216. Richardson, M. C., and Schulster, D. (1973). The role of protein kinase activation in the control of steroidogenesis by adrenocorticotrophic hormone in the adrenal cortex. Biochem. J. 136:993.

217. Palfreyman, J. W., and Schulster, D. (1975). On the mechanism of action

of cholera toxin on isolated rat adrenocortical cells: comparison with the effects of ACTH. Biochim. Biophys. Acta 404:221.

218. Haksar, A., Maudsley, D. V., and Person, F. G. (1975). Stimulation of cyclic adenosine 3′:5′-monophosphate and corticosterone formation in isolated rat adrenal cells by cholera enterotoxin: comparison with the effects of ACTH. Biochim. Biophys. Acta 381:308.

219. Rubin, R. P., Carchman, R. A., and Jaanus, S. D. (1972). Role of calcium and adenosine cyclic 3′-5′phosphate in action of adrenocorticotropin. Nature (New Biol.) 240:150.

220. Jaanus, S. D., and Rubin, R. P. (1971). The effect of ACTH on calcium distribution in the perfused cat adrenal gland. J. Physiol. 213:581.

221. Carchman, R. A., Jaanus, S. D., and Rubin, R. P. (1971). The role of adrenocorticotropin and calcium in adenosine cyclic 3′,5′-phosphate production and steroid release from the isolated, perfused cat adrenal gland. Mol. Pharmacol. 7:491.

222. Simpson, E. R., and Williams-Smith, D. L. (1975). Effect of calcium (ion) uptake by rat adrenal mitochondria on pregnenolone formation and spectral properties of cytochrome P-450. Biochim. Biophys. Acta 404:309.

223. Stock, K., and Prilop, M. (1974). Dissociation of catecholamine-induced formation of adenosine 3′,5′-monophosphate and release of glycerol in fat cells by prostaglandin E_1, E_2 and N^6-phenylisopropyladenosine. Nauyn Schmiedebergs Arch. Pharmacol. 282:15.

224. Fain, J. N., and Wieser, P. B. (1975). Effects of adenosine deaminase on cyclic adenosine monophosphate accumulation, lipolysis, and glucose metabolism of fat cells. J. Biol. Chem. 250:1027.

225. Cahill, G. F., Jr. (1971). Physiology of insulin in man. Diabetes 20:785.

226. Brodows, R. G., Pi-Sunyer, F. X., and Campbell, R. B. (1975). Sympathetic control of hepatic glycogenolysis during glucopenia in man. Metabolism 24:617.

227. Rall, T. W., Sutherland, E. W., and Wosilait, W. D. (1956). The relationship of epinephrine and glucagon to liver phosphorylase. III. Reactivation of liver phosphorylase in slices and in extracts. J. Biol. Chem. 218:483.

228. Rall, T. W., Sutherland, E. W., and Berthet, J. (1957). The relationship of epinephrine and glucagon to liver phosphorylase. IV. Effect of epinephrine and glucagon on the reactivation of phosphorylase in liver homogenates. J. Biol. Chem. 224:463.

229. Exton, J. H., and Harper, S. C. (1975). Role of cyclic AMP in the actions of catecholamines on hepatic carbohydrate metabolism. Adv. Cyclic Nucleotide Res. 5:519.

230. Hagino, Y., and Nakashima, M. (1973). Adrenergic receptors in rat liver. I. Effects of epinephrine and adrenergic blocking agents on gluconeogenesis in perfused liver. Jap. J. Pharmacol. 23:543.

231. Fain, J. N., Tolbert, M. E. M., Pointer, R. H., Butcher, F. R., and Arnold, A. (1975). Cyclic nucleotides and gluconeogenesis by rat liver cells. Metabolism 24:395.

232. Johnson, M. E. M., Das, N. M., Butcher, F. R., and Fain, J. N. (1972). The regulation of gluconeogenesis in isolated rat liver cells by glucagon, insulin, dibutyryl cyclic adenosine monophosphate, and fatty acids. J. Biol. Chem. 247:3229.

233. Tolbert, M. E. M., Butcher, F. R., and Fain, J. N. (1973). Lack of correlation between catecholamine effects on cyclic adenosine

3′,5′-monophosphate and gluconeogenesis in isolated rat liver cells. J. Biol. Chem. 248:5686.

234. Tolbert, M. E. M., and Fain, J. N. (1974). Studies on the regulation of gluconeogenesis in isolated rat liver cells by epinephrine and glucagon. J. Biol. Chem. 249:1162.

235. Pilkington, T. R. E., Lowe, R. D., Robison, B. F., and Titterington, E. (1962). Effect of adrenergic blockage on glucose and fatty-acid mobilization in man. Lancet 2:316.

236. Day, J. L. (1975). The metabolic consequences of adrenergic blockade: a review. Metabolism 24:987.

237. Gothelf, B., and Ellis, S. (1974). Effects of propranolol and sotalol on epinephrine-induced hyperglycemia and glycogen depletion of liver and muscle in the rat. Proc. Soc. Exp. Biol. Med. 147:259.

238. Arnold, A., and McAuliff, J. P. (1968). Positive correlation of responsiveness to catecholamines of the rat liver glycogenolytic receptor with other α-receptor responses. Experientia 24:674.

239. Kennedy, B. L., and Ellis, S. (1969). Interactions of catecholamines and adrenergic blocking agents at receptor sites mediating glycogenolysis in the rat. Arch. Int. Pharmacodyn. Ther. 177:390.

240. Newton, N. E., and Hornbrook, K. R. (1972). Effects of adrenergic agents on carbohydrate metabolism of rat liver: activities of adenyl cyclase and glycogen phosphorylase. J. Pharmacol. Exp. Ther. 181:479.

241. Sherline, P., Lynch, A., and Glinsmann, W. H. (1972). Cyclic AMP and adrenergic receptor control of rat liver glycogen metabolism. Endocrinology 91:680.

242. Murad, F., Chi, Y.-M., Rall, T. W., and Sutherland, E. W. (1962). Adenyl cyclase. III. The effect of catecholamines and choline esters on the formation of adenosine 3′,5′-phosphate by preparations from cardiac muscle and liver. J. Biol. Chem. 237:1233.

243. Shimazu, T., and Amakawa, A. (1975). Regulation of glycogen metabolism in liver by the autonomic nervous system. VI. Possible mechanism of phosphorylase activation by the splanchnic nerve. Biochim. Biophys. Acta 385:242.

244. Merlevede, W., Goris, J., and DeBrandt, C. (1969). Interconversion in vitro of two forms of liver phosphorylase phosphatase. Eur. J. Biochem. 11:499.

245. Shimazu, T., and Amakawa, A. (1968). Regulation of glycogen metabolism in liver by the autonomic nervous system. III. Differential effects of sympathetic-nerve stimulation of catecholamines on liver phosphorylase. Biochim. Biophys. Acta 165:349.

246. Edwards, A. V. (1972). The hyperglycaemic response to stimulation of the hepatic sympathetic innervation in adrenalectomized cats and dogs. J. Physiol. 220:697.

247. Durham, J. P., Baserga, R., and Butcher, F. R. (1974). The effect of isoproterenol and its analogs upon adenosine 3′,5′-monophosphate and guanosine 3′,5′-monophosphate levels in mouse parotid gland in vivo: relationship to the stimulation of DNA synthesis. Biochim. Biophys. Acta 372:196.

248. Bdolah, A., and Schramm, M. (1965). The function of 3′,5′ cyclic AMP in enzyme secretion. Biochem. Biophys. Res. Commun. 18:452.

249. Butcher, F. R., Goldman, J. A., and Nemerovski, M. (1975). Effect of adrenergic agents on α-amylase release and adenosine 3′,5′-monophos-

phate accumulation in rat parotid tissue slices. Biochim. Biophys. Acta 392:82.

250. Batzri, S., Selinger, Z., Schramm, M., and Robinovitch, M. R. (1973). Potassium release mediated by the epinephrine α-receptor in rat parotid slices. J. Biol. Chem. 248:361.

251. Monnard, P., and Schorderet, M. (1973). Cyclic adenosine $3',5'$-monophosphate concentration in rabbit parotid slices following stimulation by secretagogues. Eur. J. Pharmacol. 23:306.

252. Malamud, D. (1972). Amylase secretion from mouse parotid and pancreas: role of cyclic AMP and isoproterenol. Biochim. Biophys. Acta 279:373.

253. Selinger, Z., and Naim, E. (1970). The effect of calcium on amylase secretion by rat parotid slices. Biochim. Biophys. Acta 203:335.

254. Selinger, Z., Eimerl, S., and Schramm, M. (1974). A calcium ionophore simulating the action of epinephrine on the α-adrenergic receptor. Proc. Natl. Acad. Sci. U. S. A. 71:128.

255. Benz, L., Eckstein, B., Matthews, E. K., and Williams, J. A. (1972). Control of pancreatic anylase release in vitro: effects of ions, cyclic AMP and colchicine. Br. J. Pharmacol. 46:66.

256. Deschodt-Lanckman, M., Robberecht, P., DeNeff, P., Labrie, F., and Christophe, J. (1975). In vitro interactions of gastrointestinal hormones on cyclic adenosine $3':5'$-monophosphate levels and anylase output in the rat pancreas. Gastroenterology 68:318.

257. Case, R. M., and Schratcherd, T. (1972). The actions of dibutyryl cyclic adenosine $3',5'$-monophosphate and methyl xanthines on pancreatic exocrine secretion. J. Physiol. 223:649.

258. Eimerl, S., Savion, N., Heichal, O., and Selinger, Z. (1974). Induction of enzyme secretion in rat pancreatic slices using the ionophore A-23187 and calcium. J. Biol. Chem. 249:3991.

259. Williams, J. A., and Lee, M. (1974). Pancreatic acinar cells: use of a Ca^{++} ionophore to separate enzyme release from the earlier steps in stimulus-secretion coupling. Biochem. Biophys. Res. Commun. 60:542.

260. Franks, D. J., Perrin, L. S., and Malamuc, D. (1974). Calcium ion: a modulator of parotid adenylate cyclase activity. FEBS Lett. 42:267.

261. Harfield, B., and Tenenhouse, A. (1973). Effect of EGTA on protein release and cyclic AMP accumulation in rat parotid gland. Can. J. Physiol. Pharamcol. 51:997.

262. Mangos, J. A., McSherry, N. R., Barber, T., Arvanitakis, S. N., and Wagner, V. (1975). Dispersed rat parotid acinar cells. II. Characterization of adrenergic receptors. Am. J. Physiol. 229:560.

263. Schramm, R., and Selinger, Z. (1975). The functions of cyclic AMP and calcium as alternative second messengers in parotid and pancreas. J. Cyclic Nucleotide Res. 1:181.

264. Mangos, J. A., McSherry, N. R., and Barber, T. (1975). Dispersed rat parotid acinar cells. III. Characterization of cholinergic receptors. Am. J. Physiol. 229:566.

265. Burgen, A. S. V. Secretory processes in salivary glands. In C. Code (ed.), Handbook of Physiology, Section B, Vol. II, p. 561. American Physiological Society, Washington, D.C.

266. Rudich, L. K., and Butcher, F. R. (1976). Effect of substance P and eledoisin on cyclic nucleotide levels, α-amylase release and K^+ efflux from rat parotid tissue slices. Biochim. Biophys. Acta 444:704.

267. Bertaccini, G., and DeCaro, G. (1965). The effect of physalaemin and related polypeptides on salivary secretion. J. Physiol. 181:68.

268. Emmelin, N., and Lenninger, S. (1967). The "direct" effect of physalaemin on salivary gland cells. Br. J. Pharmacol. Chemother. 30:676.
269. Collier, H. O. J., and Roy, A. C., (1974). Morphine-like drugs inhibit the
stimulation by E prostaglandins of cyclic AMP formation by rat brain
homogenate. Nature (Lond.) 248:24.
270. Collier, H. O. J., and Roy, A. C. (1974). Hypothesis inhibition of E
prostaglandin-sensitive adenyl cyclase as the mechanism of morphine
analgesia. Prostaglandins 7:361.
271. Pasternak, G. W., Goodman, R., and Snyder, S. H. (1975). An endogenous
morphine-like factor in mammalian brain. Life Sci. 16:1965.
272. Hughes, J., Smith, T., Morgan, B., and Fothergill, L. (1975). Purification
and properties of enkephalin: the possible endogenous ligand for the
morphine receptor. Life Sci. 16:1753.
273. Hughes, J. (1975). Isolation of an endogenous compound from the brain
with pharmacological properties similar to morphine. Brain Res. 88:295.
274. Terenius, L., and Wahlstrom, A. (1975). Search for an endogenous ligand
for the opiate receptor. Acta Physiol. Scand. 94:74.
275. Hughes, J., Smith, T. W., Kosterlitz, H. W., Fothergill, L. A., Morgan, B.
A., and Morris, H. R. (1975). Identification of two related pentapeptides
from the brain with potent opiate agonist activity. Nature (Lond.)
258:577.
276. Sharma, S. K., Nirenberg, M., and Klee, W. A. (1975). Morphine receptors
as regulators of adenylate cyclase activity. Proc. Natl. Acad. Sci. U. S. A.
72:590.
277. Klee, W. A., Sharma, S. K., and Nirenberg, M. (1975). Opiate receptors as
regulators of adenylate cyclase. Life Sci. 16:1869.
278. Traber, J., Gullis, R., and Hamprecht, B. (1975). Influence of opiates on
the levels of adenosine $3':5'$-cyclic monophosphate in neuroblastoma X
glioma hybrid cells. Life Sci. 16:1863.
279. Snyder, S. H. (1975). Opiate receptor in normal and drug alteree brain
function. Nature (Lond.) 257:185.
280. Wickson, R. D., Boudreau, R. J., and Drummond, G. I. (1975). Activation
of $3':5'$-cyclic adenosine monophosphate phosphodiesterase by calcium
ion and a protein activator. Biochemistry 14:669.
281. Brostrom, C. O., Huang, Y.-C., Breckenridge, B. M., and Wolff, D. J.
(1975). Identification of a calcium-binding protein as a calcium-dependent regulator of brain adenylate cyclase. Proc. Natl. Acad. Sci. U. S. A.
72:64.
282. Cardenas, H. L., and Ross, D. H. (1975). Morphine induced calcium
depletion in discrete regions of rat brain. J. Neurochem. 24:487.
283. Ross, D. H. (1975). Tolerance to morphine-induced calcium depletion in
regional brain areas: characterization with reserpine and protein synthesis inhibitors. Br. J. Pharmacol. 55:28.
284. Francis, D. L., Roy, A. C., and Collier, H. O. J. (1975). Morphine
abstinence and quasi-abstinence effects after phosphodiesterase inhibitors and naloxone. Life Sci. 16:1901.
285. Ho, I. K., Loh, H. H., Bhargava, H. N., and Way, E. L. (1975). Effect of
cyclic nucleotides and phosphodiesterase inhibition on morphine tolerance and physical dependence. Life. Sci. 16:1895.
286. Collier, H. O. J., and Francis, D. L. (1975). Morphine abstinence is
associated with increased brain cyclic AMP. Nature (Lond.) 255:159.
287. Gryglewski, R. J., Szczeklik, A., and Bieron, K. (1975). Morphine antago-

nizes prostaglandin E_1-mediated inhibition of human platelet aggregation. Nature (Lond.) 256:56.

288. Thomas, J. A., Dombrosky, J. T., Mawhinney, M. G., and Hossaini
     (Shahid-Salles), K. S. (1975). Effects of morphine on cyclic AMP levels
     in the prostate glands of the mouse. Life Sci. 16:1157.

289. Sable-Amplis, R., Agid, R., and Abadie, D. (1975). Some effects of
     morphine on lipid metabolism in normal, tolerant and abstinent rats.
     Life Sci. 16:1477.

290. Roy, A. C., and Collier, H. O. J. (1975). Prostaglandins, cyclic AMP and
     the biochemical mechanism of opiate agonist action. Life Sci. 16:1857.

Index

Catecholamines
  as possible PIF, 60
  and sodium excretion, 185–186
α-Cell hypersecretion, 153, 155
Cell proliferation, regulation, and
  cyclic nucleotides, 253–254
Cells, isolation of, 117–120
Central nervous system
  effects of HHH on, 58–59
  role of, in release of CRF, 95–97
p-Chlorophenylalanine, 55
Cholera, and adenylate cyclase
  activation, 254–256
Circadian rhythm, and neurotransmitter content, 96
Circhoral rhythm, 46
CNS, see Central nervous system
Coitus, oxytocin release during, 14
Cold, and TRH secretion, 49–50
Collecting duct, sodium reabsorption
  in, 179–180
Copper, possible role of, in hormone
  release, 99–100
Corticotropin-releasing factor
  activation of pituitary gland,
    100–103
  assays for, 120–123
  biochemical characterization of, 60
  distribution, 98
  hypothalamic, nature of, 98–100
  modulation of effects of, 50–51
  nature of, 97–100
Cortisol, concentration, as possible
  CNS control mechanism, 109–111
Cow, lactation in, 10
CRF-ACTH, secretion, and
  neurotransmitters, 57
Cyclic AMP
  and ACTH, tropic action of,
    129–130
  and adenylate cyclase regulation,
    254–263
  intracellular concentration of, and
    protein kinase, 263–264
  regulation, and adenosine, 262–263
  and regulation of cell proliferation,
    253–254
  relationship of total levels of to
    hormone action, 264–267
  and steroidogenesis, 126–129
  see also Cyclic nucleotides
Cyclic GMP
  accumulation in liver, 270

agents that elevate, 249
analogs, tissues responding to, 250
control of tissue levels, 248–250
exogenous, tissues responding to,
  249–250
and regulation of cell proliferation,
  253–254
Cyclic nucleotides
  and Ca^{2+}, 244–246
  methodology for, 246–248
  and opiates, 274–277

Dehydration, and vasopressin level,
  15
Diabetes, glucagon-insulin interactions
  in, 160–164
Diabetes insipidus, 7, 15, 16
  and hormone levels, 4
16α-18-Dihydroxydeoxycortico-
  sterone, 182
Distal convoluted tubule, and sodium
  reabsorption, 178–179
Dog
  lactation in, 10
  osmoregulation in, 15
  serum vasopressin level in, 15
  vasopressin response in, 19
Drug administration
  effects of site of, 96
  effect of time of, 96

Enkephalin, 275
Epinephrine, action in liver, 268, 269
Episodic secretion, defined, 109
Escherichia coli, 255
Estrogen
  and LRH effect, 46, 47
  and mineral metabolism, 221
  and oxytocin release, 13–14
  and regulation of sodium excretion,
    182–183
Exocytosis, 6

Fasting, glucagon levels during,
  154–155
Free fatty acids, regulation of
  adenylate cyclase by, 258–259

Gastrointestinal tract, calcitonin
  action in, 212
Glucagon
  big plasma, 152